D1565685

Progress in Pain Research and Management
Volume 11

Sickle Cell Pain

Mission Statement of IASP Press

The International Association for the Study of Pain (IASP) is a non-profit, interdisciplinary organization devoted to understanding the mechanisms of pain and improving the care of patients with pain through research, education, and communication. The organization includes scientists and health care professionals dedicated to these goals. The IASP sponsors scientific meetings and publishes newsletters, technical bulletins, the journal *Pain*, and books.

The goal of IASP Press is to provide the IASP membership with timely, high-quality, low-cost publications relevant to the problem of pain. These publications are also intended to appeal to a wider audience of scientists and clinicians interested in the problem of pain.

Previous volumes in the series
Progress in Pain Research and Management

Progress in Pain Research and Management
Volume 11

Sickle Cell Pain

Samir K. Ballas, MD

Department of Medicine
Cardeza Foundation for Hematologic Research
Jefferson Medical College
Thomas Jefferson University
Philadelphia, Pennsylvania, USA

IASP PRESS • SEATTLE

Library of Congress Cataloging-in-Publication Data

Ballas, Samir K., 1938–
    Sickle cell pain / Samir K. Ballas.
      p. cm. — (Progress in pain research and management ; v. 11)
    Includes bibliographical references and index.
    ISBN 0-931092-22-1 (cloth)
    1. Sickle cell anemia—Complications. 2. Pain. I. Title. II. Series.
    [DNLM: 1. Anemia, Sickle Cell—therapy. 2. Pain—therapy.   WH170 B189s 1998]
    RC641.7.S5B35 1998
    616.1'527—dc21
    DNLM/DLC
    for Library of Congress   98-2595

Published by:

IASP Press
International Association for the Study of Pain
909 NE 43rd St., Suite 306
Seattle, WA 98105 USA
Fax: 206-547-1703

Printed in the United States of America

To my patients with sickle cell disease,
whose pain and suffering prompted me to write this book.

CHWECHWECHE II

(language of Ghana for relentless, perpetual chewing;
also sickle cell disease)

Just an ache,
Maybe it'll break;
Only a pang,
Perhaps if I sang . . .
Now it's a stitch;
You damn witch.

Just a twinge,
But I wanna cringe;
Oooh, it's aching,
Backbreaking;
Oooh, it's stabbing,
Bedpost I'm grabbing;
Oooh, it's sharp,
Think I'm gonna barf.

Shooting pains in my head,
Wish I were dead;
Elbow swelling,
No wonder I'm yelling;
Rib pain racking,
Might be cracking;
Now it's my belly,
Legs feel like jelly;
Excruciating, feel like fainting . . .
Now I'm cryin'
Maybe I'm dyin'

Chwechweche!
Unchain me, unshackle me,
Unbind me, discharge me,
Disenthrall me, disimprison me,
Detach me, disencumber me,
Liberate me—
Chwechweche, set me free!

—Adapted from Elliott Perlin, MD
   Howard University

Contents

Preface

Pain and suffering are the hallmarks of sickle cell disease. For most patients who are afflicted with this illness, pain is their nemesis, their unpredictable master, and ruthless dictator. For many patients and their families, pain is a chore and a major component of routine activities of daily living. It has to be factored into every plan, project, activity, dream, ambition, and relationship. In adults, sickle cell pain becomes the major driving force of life. Persistent, severe sickle cell pain is a poor prognostic sign and a predictor of death.

This book will describe sickle cell disease from the perspective of its major symptom. To that end, the word *pain* is included in the title of most chapters to emphasize its role in this disease and its magnitude in the life of affected persons. The history of sickle cell pain, its hematology, pathophysiology, classification, types, complications, management, and associated issues will be reviewed in detail. I wish Pauling had referred to sickle cell disease as the first *painful* molecular disease and not simply the first molecular disease. This descriptor might have emphasized the morbid clinical picture and stimulated more research on pain. I hope this book will impress upon the reader the significant role of pain in the life of patients with sickle cell disease and will stimulate investigators to conduct more basic and clinical research on sickle cell pain.

Acknowledgments

For secretarial assistance
Carole Ayling
Kim Berger
Barbara Scott

For artistic and photographic input
Andrew Likens

For assistance in collecting data for the illustrative cases
Nadia S. Ballas

For assistance in production
Louisa E. Jones
Leslie N. Bond
Sandra Marvinney
Dale A. Schmidt

For editorial comments and suggestions
Howard L. Fields, MD, PhD

For reviewing selected chapters
Oswaldo Castro, MD
Roy N. Gay, MD
Ahmed A. Mallouh, MD
Narla Mohandas, PhD

For contribution of pain descriptions and related issues
Many patients and their families
Walter Brandon, DCSW, MDiv
Zemoria Brandon
Timothy M. Carlos, MD
Oswaldo Castro, MD
Carlton Dampier, MD
Roy N. Gay, MD
Ahmed A. Mallouh, MD
Elliot Perlin, MD

For valuable personal support
My wife, Nida, and daughter, Nadia, whose tolerance and support
made this book a reality.

Part I

Basic Considerations

1

Sickle Cell Pain in Historical Perspective

Pain has an element of blank;
It cannot recollect
When it began, or if there were
A day when it was not.

It has no future but itself,
Its infinite realms contain
Its past, enlightened to perceive
New periods of pain.
— Emily Dickinson, 1830–1886

After great pain, a formal feeling comes —
The Nerves sit ceremonious, like Tombs —
— Emily Dickinson, 1830–1886

HISTORY

Sickle cell disease has an interesting history that spans the twentieth century. Our understanding of the disease evolved through four periods: the tribal medicine period in Africa, clinical recognition by Western medicine, an era of biochemical/molecular research and characterization, and now an era of molecular therapy (Table I). As highlighted below, progress has thus proceeded from the bedside to the bench and, recently, has returned to the bedside with possible curative therapy. Unfortunately, the laudatory progress in basic research in sickle cell disease is marred by the lack of research on sickle pain, the hallmark of the disease and the major concern of patients and their families. This book reviews what is known about sickle pain with the hope of stimulating others to investigate this area.

Sickle cell disease was known in Africa before the twentieth century. Inhabitants of West Africa realized that the disease was hereditary and gave it specific names listed in Table II (Konotey-Ahulu 1969, 1974). These tribal names are characterized by alliteration of letters that apparently signifies the recurrent clinical manifestations of the disease; the most probable English meaning of these names include "body biting," "body chewing,"

3

Table I

Major clinical milestones in the history of sickle cell disease

Initial Observations, before 1910

African tribes' terminology, e.g., onomatopoetic names of sickle cell disease in Ghana
Medicine man
    Iatrogenic tattoos as diagnostic markers of sickle cell disease
    Anecdotes related to belief in reincarnation

Clinical Period, 1910–1949

First case report by Herrick, 1910
Introduction of the term "sickle cell anemia" by Mason, 1922
Introduction of the term "crisis" by Sydenstricker, 1924a
Characterization of the clinical picture by Diggs (1932–1956) and others

Biochemical/Molecular Period, 1949–1990

Identification of Hb S by electrophoresis (Pauling et al. 1949)
Introduction of the concept that sickle cell anemia is a molecular disease
Inheritance of sickle cell anemia follows Mendelian principles (Neel 1951)
Deoxy Hb S has decreased solubility (Perutz and Mitchison 1950)
Hb S differs from normal Hb by incorporating valine instead of glutamic acid
    (Ingram 1956)
Description of the subunit composition of Hb and its primary, secondary, tertiary, and
    quaternary structure, 1950s–1970s
Localization of the sickle mutation at the sixth residue of the β-globin chain
Description of other hemoglobinopathies and thalassemias, 1960s–1980s
Prenatal and neonatal diagnosis by globin chain synthesis, 1970s
Prenatal and neonatal diagnosis by restriction fragment length polymorphism (RFLP),
    1970s (Kan and Dozy 1978).
Introduction of molecular technology: analysis by restriction endonucleases, Southern
    blotting, polymerase chain reaction (PCR), and dot blots, 1980s
Prevention of infection: vaccination and antibiotic prophylaxsis, 1980s (Gaston et al.
    1986)
Description of the natural history of sickle cell disease, 1980s–1990
Description of the molecular basis of the variability among sickle cell syndromes:
    role of α genotype and β haplotypes, 1980s
Focus on pathophysiology and management of organ damage, 1980s–1990s

Molecular Therapy, 1990–Present

Induction of Hb F
    5-Azacytidine
    Hydroxyurea
    Erythropoietin
    Butyrate and derivatives
    Other compounds
Bone marrow transplantation
Transgenic mouse model
Gene therapy

Table II
African tribal names for sickle cell anemia

Name	Tribe	Probable Meaning
Chwechweechwe	Ga	"relentless, perpetual chewing"
Ahotutuo	Twi	"Aoo, I'm dying"
Nwiiwii	Fante	"I will die, eeh"
Nuidudui	Ewe	"body chewing"
Adep	Banyangi (Cameroon)	"beaten up"
HemKom	Adangme	"body biting"

and "beaten up" (Konotey-Ahulu 1974). Legend has it that native medicine men in some African tribes marked patients with limb girdle tattoos (Fig. 1) (Konotey-Ahulu 1969, 1991) to allow a spot diagnosis whenever they presented screaming and writhing in pain to the medicine man, who would treat them accordingly without undue delay. Horton (1874) described what seems to be the first report of sickle cell disease in Africa. His description included blood abnormality, fever, joint pains, and precipitation of painful episodes during the rainy season.

Isichei (1976) and Onwubalili (1983) suggested a connection between sickle cell anemia and reincarnation beliefs in Nigeria. The term "reincarnating child," known as *Ogbanje* in the Ibo tribe and *Abiku* in the Yoruba tribe, refers to children destined to die and be reborn repeatedly to the world as their own siblings (Isichei 1976; Edelstein and Stevenson 1983; Onwubalili 1983). The reincarnated child was normal at birth but soon developed signs and symptoms reminiscent of sickle cell anemia (growth retardation, convulsions, protuberant abdomen, yellow eyes, and recurrent episodes of fever and body aches and pain) and died before the age of 5 or 10 years. Disheartened parents often inflicted a physical mark on their dead child before burial to enable identification if reborn. Moreover, children preceded by two or three deceased siblings were ritualistically treated by amputating the distal phalanx of the left little finger and were referred to as *Ogbanje* children.

In North America the first two reports highly suggestive of sickle cell disease (Lebby 1846; Hodenpyl 1898) described two black males with anatomic asplenia (autosplenectomy) found at autopsy. In the nineteenth and early twentieth centuries, it is conceivable that patients with sickle cell disease who had frequent painful episodes were mistaken as cases of acute rheumatism. Dr. James Herrick of Chicago (1910) truly ushered in the clinical period with the first accepted report of sickle cell disease. He described a young Negro student from Grenada in the West Indies who presented with cough and fever. This case report is significant because it illustrated (Fig. 2) and described "peculiar elongated and sickle-shaped red blood corpuscles in

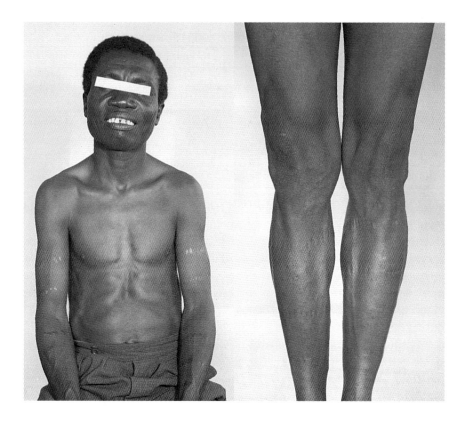

Fig. 1. Konotey-Ahulu's iatrogenic upper (left) and lower (right) limb-girdle tattoos of a patient in Ghana that afford a spot diagnosis of sickle cell disease (Konotey-Ahulu 1969 with permission).

a case of severe anaemia," and thus left no doubt that the patient described had a severe variety of sickle cell syndrome, probably sickle cell anemia.* Washburn (1911) and Cook and Meyer (1915) reported the second and third cases, respectively, and the fourth case was described by Mason (1922), who summarized the four case reports and coined the term sickle cell anemia. Interestingly, the clinical picture of these first four cases of sickle cell anemia was not dominated by recurrent attacks of painful episodes but was characterized by severe anemia, weakness, jaundice, leg ulcers, and numerous sickle-shaped, oat-shaped, and elliptical erythrocytes in the peripheral smears. Two of these patients had attacks of pain in the right upper quadrant

*Savitt and Goldberg (1989) identified Herrick's patient as Walter Clement Noel, who entered Chicago College of Dental Surgery in 1904. A respiratory infection later led to his admission to the Presbyterian Hospital, where the intern, Dr. Irons, noted the abnormal shape of the red cells in the peripheral smear. After graduating in 1907, Noel returned to Grenada and established private dental practice. He died of pneumonia ("acute chest syndrome") at age 32.

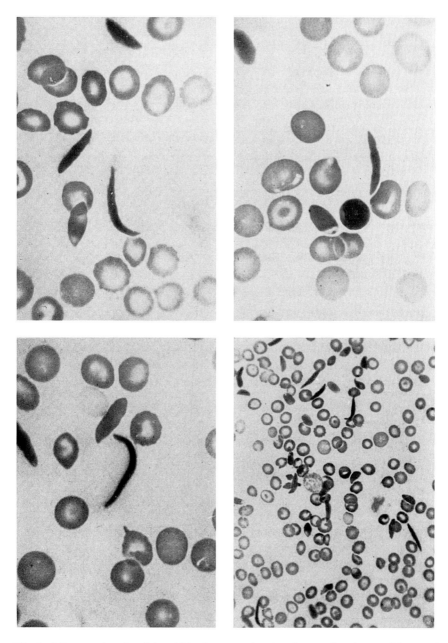

Fig. 2. Micrographs of peripheral blood smears showing the peculiar elongated forms of the red cell corpuscles originally reported by Herrick (1910) (reprinted with permission).

associated with jaundice and fever; these signs and symptoms were relieved in one instance by the removal of gall stones. Thus, Mason was the first to describe what is nowadays known as the right upper quadrant syndrome (described in Chapter 5).

Several cases of sickle cell anemia were described after 1922. It was Sydenstricker (1923, 1924a,b,c, 1929), however, who used the word *crisis* to describe the abdominal pains and jaundice in sickle cell anemia that resembled the crises in congenital hemolytic jaundice. He also noted that sickle cell anemia is characterized by two phases that he called "latent" and "active" depending on the severity of symptoms. Subsequently the words *hemolytic* and *crisis* were used frequently to describe the recurrent paroxysms of illness in sickle cell anemia, and the concept of hemolytic crisis— implying accelerated hemolysis and worsening anemia during painful episodes—became prevalent among students of sickle cell disease.

Based on his extensive clinical experience, Diggs made valuable contributions to the understanding of sickle cell disease (1932, 1934, 1937, 1954, 1956, 1965, 1967). He noted that the hallmark of sickle cell anemia is the recurrent and painful vascular occlusive crisis interspersed with periods of stable steady state with no symptoms or signs other than those due to chronic hemolytic anemia. Diggs also noted that hemolytic crises in sickle cell anemia are usually precipitated by infection and may occur with or independent of the painful crises. With one exception, all complications of sickle cell disease were described between 1910 and 1950 (Serjeant 1992) and included painful episodes, hyperhemolytic episodes, leg ulcers, priapism, bone infarction, avascular necrosis, lesions in the central nervous system, and multiple organ infarctions (lungs, kidneys, and spleen). The exception was severe retinopathy, first recognized in 1966 (Welch and Goldberg 1966).

The biochemical and molecular period in the history of sickle cell disease was ushered in by Pauling and his associates (1949), who introduced the concept of sickle cell anemia as a molecular disease. They demonstrated that hemoglobin isolated from red cells of patients with sickle cell disease differed electrophoretically from the hemoglobin of normal persons and that the hemoglobin of those with sickle cell trait was a mixture of normal and sickle hemoglobin. Neel (1951) showed that the inheritance of sickle cell anemia followed simple Mendelian genetics. Perutz and Mitchison (1950) reported that crystals of deoxy sickle hemoglobin were birefringent and had decreased solubility. Ingram (1956) reported that the only difference between normal and sickle hemoglobin was the replacement of glutamic acid by valine. The work of several groups (Bunn and Forget 1986) established the subunit structure and primary sequences of the subunits ($\alpha,\beta,\gamma,\delta$) of human hemoglobin and localized the sickle mutation to the sixth residue of the β-globin chain ($\beta^{6\ Glu \rightarrow Val}$). The interaction of the sickle mutation with other hemoglobin abnormalities clarified the spectrum of sickle cell syndromes. The advent of DNA technology in the 1970s and the 1980s paved the way for the molecular diagnosis of sickle cell disorders, prenatal diagnosis, and the identification of α-gene deletions and β^S haplotypes and their effect on the clinical picture of sickle cell disease. By the 1980s it had become clear that sickle cell disease is a highly heterogeneous disorder not only at the clinical level but also at the cellular and molecular levels.

The remarkable advances in our understanding of the biochemical and molecular aspects of sickle cell disease have lead to the inevitable question: Can sickle cell disease be cured? The attempt to answer this question launched the period of molecular therapy. Induction of fetal hemoglobin, bone marrow transplantation, and gene therapy are current approaches to achieve a cure of sickle cell disease and will be described in Chapter 12.

NOMENCLATURE

The English word sickle is derived from the Latin verb *secare*, which means to cut, and from *secula*, which means sickle. The word evolved from Old English (A.D. 450–1150) *sicol*, to Middle English (A.D. 1150–1475) *sikel*, and finally to *sickle* in Modern English (1475–present). Literally and classically, "sickle" refers to an agricultural implement with a short handle and a crescent-shaped blade that is used for reaping, lopping, or cutting down tall grasses and weeds. Before 1910, the word sickle was officially used as a noun, not as a verb nor an adjective. In his classic paper in 1910, Herrick referred to the abnormal elongated cells in his patient as "sickle-shaped" red blood cells or "crescent-shaped" red blood cells, and thus preserved the proper use of sickle (and crescent) as a noun. With the advent of the word sickle to the medical literature usage changed. Sickle now is not only a noun but also: (1) an adjective meaning having the form of a curved blade, as in a sickle cell instead of sickle-shaped cell; (2) a transitive verb that means to change into a sickle shape, as in saying a red blood cell sickles; or (3) an intransitive verb that means to change into a sickle cell, as in the ability of red blood cells to sickle.

Given use of the word sickle as a noun, verb, and an adjective, we would expect respective derivatives of these forms such as "sickling," "sickled," and "sickler." The word sickler, however, is controversial. Linguistically, sickler means a reaper or a person who uses a sickle. Some care providers and even prominent authorities in the field (Onwubalili 1983; Konotey-Ahulu 1991; Rees et al. 1995) used the term sickler to mean a patient with sickle cell disease. Some patients with sickle cell disease find no problem in referring to themselves as sicklers (see below). Other care providers and some patients abhor the term sickler and consider it an awkward and insulting adulteration of the word sickle. Recently a group of patients in Bronx, New York, USA, established their own commendable advocacy organization referred to as S.C.A.R.E. (Sickle Cell Advocates for Research and Empowerment) and produced literature and a home page on the internet. Their motto is "Turning Fear into Action." They refer to themselves as "sickle cell defiers" and reject all other terminologies, including sickler, sickle cell victim, sickle cell sufferer, and sickle cell patient (Pannell and Oster-Pannell, personal communication, 1997).

In Latin the word for sickle is *falx* and in Spanish it is *falce*. Sickle cell anemia in Spanish is referred to as *anemia falciforme* (sickle-shaped anemia). (Ironically, malaria and sickle cell anemia are related not only geographically, but also linguistically. The malaria-carrying parasite *Plasmodium falciparum* is so named because its gametes have the shape of a small sickle [*parum* means small]). If Herrick had been linguistically, rather than agriculturally, oriented he might have referred to the unusual scythe-shaped cells as falciforme and the new disease as falciparum anemia. The term *sicklemia,* meaning sickle cell trait, was used in the 1940s and 1950s but rarely after that (Bauer and Fisher 1943; Wasserman et al. 1952; Bauer 1974; Cresta 1974).

The word *crisis* is another controversial term that pertains to sickle cell disease. It originates from the Greek *krisis,* meaning a turning point in the course of a disease with the development of new signs and symptoms. Thus a painful crisis is defined as the sudden and striking onset of severe pain in a patient with sickle cell anemia or other sickle cell syndrome. Some prefer to replace "crisis" with "episode" because the former implies a sense of catastrophe (Shapiro 1997). In some patients, however, the combination of a severe acute painful episode with adverse financial, environmental, and medical factors may approach catastrophic proportions. From many patients' point of view, what matters is pain perception irrespective of the term used to describe it (Shapiro 1997). In this book "crisis" and "episode" will be used interchangeably.

DEFINITIONS

PAIN

In 1979 the International Association for the Study of Pain (IASP) defined pain as "an unpleasant sensory and emotional experience associated with actual or potential tissue damage or described in terms of such damage" (IASP 1979, 1982; Merskey 1983; de Jong 1980). This definition implies several important aspects of the pain experience: (1) unpleasantness is a major component; (2) sensation and emotion are two major aspects; (3) tissue damage may not be a visible factor of pain; and (4) patients may complain of pain in the absence of objective signs. This definition applies extremely well to patients with sickle cell disease as discussed below.

SICKLE PAIN

Sickle pain is unique (Ballas 1994b; Shapiro 1997). The above-mentioned definition applies well to sickle pain, which can be acute, chronic, intermittent, recurrent, or persistent (Benjamin 1989; Payne 1989b; Ballas 1993, 1994b, 1995a). Sensation and emotion in sickle pain are intertwined in an unusually complex manner that is specific to each person and affects behavior in every painful episode. Perhaps one way to appreciate the uniqueness of sickle pain is to consider how some patients have described it:

1. One patient with sickle cell anemia who had a hip fracture said: "Although the pain due to the fracture is severe, you have some control over it. You can assume a certain position and stay still and you feel no pain. Sickle pain, on the other hand, is uncontrollable. No matter what position you take, it hits you. It is as if you have one or more fractures and the involved part is uncontrollably set in constant motion" (Ballas 1994b).

2. Sickle pain is like a migraine headache, except that it affects all your body.

3. Sickle pain is enveloping. You can do nothing about it. It controls you, you have no control over it.

4. Sickle pain is like a toothache all over your body magnified hundred times.

5. To me sickle cell means pain and suffering.

6. To have sickle cell anemia means "living life in pain." When a sickle cell crisis attacks, "my body is submerged in intense pain. . . . There is relentless throbbing. . . . All I want to do is die. . . . The pain can be so severe that I feel like dying or cutting the painful part of the body off."

7. "My worst sickle cell crisis . . . was during my junior year of college . . . in winter . . . I felt a tremendous explosion in my body. . . . Pain was shooting out of my bones and muscles. . . . The pain was sharp and seemed to last forever. Every heart beat seemed to pump the pain machine and

squeeze my muscles tighter. Every muscle in my body, from the tip of my index finger to the bottom of my feet felt like they were in a vise, that kept being tightened every other second. . . . This painful episode had me scared to death, for I felt it would surely kill me. . . . This episode took seven days to run its course. . . . The first three days I got no sleep. . . . Being in this much pain . . . takes away all . . . your patience, calmness, and some of your sanity. . . . The seventh day took a month to arrive."

8.   An African American school teacher with sickle cell anemia died suddenly at the age of 35 years during hospitalization for a painful crisis. One year before his death he wrote an article titled "The Nature of the Beast," in which he described his sickle pain as follows: "During child-hood, (from age 4 years) I experienced sickle cell crises as bouts of curious discomfort involving the joints and extremities. The sensation was a continuous tingling numbness, identical to the sensation experienced when one awakens after having slept in an awkward position, inadvertently cutting off circulation to an arm or leg. . . . After the age of 6 the discomfort was characteristic of the typical sickle cell crisis. . . . The first warnings of a sickle cell crisis would be a burning behind the sternum, identical in nature to heartburn, but differing only in intensity. This warning lasts for only 15 minutes or so. After this it radiates downward into the abdomen and then spreads, like a belt, to . . . the back . . . and into the lower belly. . . . By this time the discomfort no longer resembles heartburn, but is a severe throb-bing . . . with each heart beat. This pain soon involves the entire torso, including the chest, sides, and back. . . . The internal organs also begin to ache, with a discomfort like severe stomach pain. . . . This is a separate and distinct visceral pain which continues simultaneously with the throbbing pain . . . (a severe cramping) . . . (which) results in a sympathetic tightening of muscles until . . . (I am) curled in the fetal position. The discomfort continues to radiate outward until the arms, legs, and head are involved. . . . (with) the characteristic throbbing pain and tightening of musculature. The pain concentrates itself in the joints: knees, elbows, shoulders, hips, ankles, and wrists. . . . While a sickle cell patient may be able to identify the joints or viscera as epicenters of severe pain, she/he may be unable to communicate that the pain is pervasive. Wherever . . . the system carries sickle hemoglobin there will be pain; from top to bottom . . . left to right, inside out."

9.   A 23-year-old Hispanic woman with sickle cell disease died suddenly at home within 24 hours after discharge from the hospital where she was treated for an acute painful episode. Her family found the following description of her disease in her diary:

SICKLE CELL ANEMIA PACKAGE DEAL

  1 Tiny Person
+ 1 Large Packet of Courage
  2 Understand a Sickler

In my life there are many questions, doubts and fears. Perhaps maybe just like you, but being disabled with Sickle Cell anemia has opened up new views.

As I am older now, and more capable of understanding, I often sit and question myself. However, no matter the quantity or quality of my questions, my train of thought will rarely give me an answer. My mind-boggling question is one that a person with Sickle Cell anemia will often ask themselves:

Why me?! Why do I deserve this torture of pain?

To this day, no one can answer this delicate question! Knowing there are so many goals in life just waiting to be accomplished by determination, this disease never seems to cooperate, or at least give your abilities and talents a chance to excel. This is when "Why me?" hits you again, but harder.

I have learned to become a fighter with a constant positive attitude, trying my hardest to obtain my desires in life. I struggle to do my finest job because what is mine is earned, not given. Don't get me wrong for there are many times I fail at what I'm trying to accomplish. There is also much fear which I try never to show; especially to loved ones. I don't fear death from the disease, but instead consider it a blessing. I fear what my tomorrow brings, however, and in what condition it will leave me.

Many tears are shed, but no matter how deep the pain or how hard the struggle, I thank God above for giving me the strength and determination He has. (He is a round-the-clock understanding entity.) If I could change one thing in life, it would be to delete pain for all. Especially the innocent babies being born with Sickle Cell. Just as I was born with it, I sympathize for I know what facing and accepting a life of unexpected painful hospitalizations is like.

I have a secret to this illness though. I try to live one day at a time, and plan ahead for the next. If my plans don't follow through, I over-look it and continue with my head up high. You learn to care and love about people: not for how they walk, talk, or act, but for who they are and not what they seem to be. I always manage to maintain a smile and often people ask how do I do this having been through so much at a young age. The reason I smile is so I don't cry. Yet, every night before I go to sleep I think of what my day has been like and thank God above for making me strong mentally and emotionally . . . and I let Him know I am grateful for one more day.

UNIQUE FEATURES OF SICKLE CELL PAIN

THE PATIENT POPULATION

The comprehensive management of sickle cell disease, especially in adults, presents certain difficulties because this patient population, in general, is faced with multiple disadvantages (Ballas 1994b, 1995a):

1. They suffer from an inherited, chronic, and incurable disease (except in children who received successful bone marrow transplantation described in Chapter 12).
2. Most patients are African Americans and are subject to the disadvantages associated with minorities.
3. Patients and their health care providers may have disparate sociocultural backgrounds. Most patients come from a poor psychosocial background and thus may not be able to negotiate the complex medical system to their advantage.
4. Some patients who use large doses of narcotic analgesics may find that some providers may misinterpret such consumption as maladaptive behavior.
5. Most patients lack good health insurance coverage.
6. Some institutions do not provide continuity of care.
7. Some providers fail to distinguish tolerance and physical dependence from addiction.
8. Although there is, to date, no curative therapy for sickle cell disease in adults, the sociocultural aspects of the disease, the poor continuity of care, and the negative attitude of some health care providers can be changed through education, support groups, advocates, counseling, and enhanced communication. It is with this goal and hope that this book is written.

SICKLE PAIN VS. CANCER PAIN

In contrast with their general empathy for patients with cancer pain, postoperative pain, and pain due to trauma, health care providers often have an inability to relate to sickle cell pain. This difference may result from a real or potential experience with the former syndromes in conjunction with

Table III
Comparative aspects of cancer pain and pain in sickle cell disease

	Cancer	Sickle Cell Disease
Type of pain	Mostly chronic	Acute crisis is a hallmark
	Somatic, visceral, or deafferentation	Somatic or visceral
Site	Usually localized	Varies with time, often generalized
Acute-phase reactants	Minor role	Play major role by decreasing efficacy of opioids
Life expectancy	Months to a few years	Decades
Psychosocial background	Variable	Usually poor
Attitude of care providers	Strongly positive	Negative

an abstract perception of an inherited disorder having remote or no personal relevance (Ballas 1994b; Payne 1997).

Although sickle cell pain and cancer pain share some similarities, their differences are significant (Table III). Most importantly, these two types of pain differ in pathophysiology. Chapters 3 and 4 will review the types of sickle cell pain and their pathophysiologies. Cancer pain can be divided into three major syndromes (Foley 1987). Deafferentation pain is associated with direct tumor involvement, commonly nerve compression or infiltration, hollow viscus involvement, or metastatic bone disease. Pain from cancer therapy includes postsurgical, postchemotherapy (e.g., peripheral neuropathy, steroid pseudorheumatism), and postradiation therapy pain (e.g., radiation fibrosis of the lumbosacral plexus). Pain may also result from incidental disease processes not related to cancer or its therapy.

Moreover, the prevalence of pain in patients with advanced or terminal cancer is about 74% (Bonica et al. 1990) compared to almost 100% in patients with sickle cell anemia (Table IV). Despite many clinical

Table IV
Prevalence of pain in various types of
malignant disease and in sickle cell anemia

Disease	Prevalance (%)
Bone cancer	85
Oral cavity cancer	80
Genitourinary cancer	75
Lymphomas	20
Leukemias	5
Sickle cell anemia	> 95

Table V
Similarities between patients with malignant disease and sickle cell disease

Complication/Parameter	Malignant Disease	Sickle Cell Anemia
CNS* complications	Yes (metastases)	Yes (stroke)
Pulmonary complications	Yes (metastases)	Yes (acute chest)
Hepatic complications	Yes (metastases)	Yes (hepatic crisis)
Infections	Yes	Yes
Bone marrow transplant	Yes	Yes
Severe pain	Yes	Yes
Opioid analgesics	Yes	Yes
Chemotherapy	Yes	Yes (hydroxyurea)
Transfusion	Yes	Yes
Potential gene therapy	Yes	Yes
Molecular diagnostics	Yes	Yes

Source: Ballas 1996a.
*Central nervous system.

similarities between patients with cancer and sickle cell disease (Table V), some providers refer patients with sickle cell disease to others but fight fiercely among themselves to retain patients with malignant disease. This state of affairs disrupts the continuity of care for patients with sickle cell syndromes and creates a barrier to the effective management of sickle pain.

Jacox et al. (1994) published comprehensive clinical practice guidelines for management of cancer pain. Despite its apparent specific focus, this publication is a meta-analysis of published reports and gives the impression that the guidelines are applicable to other types of incurable pain; Chapter 7 of that publication, for example, addressed pain in special populations, such as the elderly and patients with AIDS. Unfortunately, these guidelines never mentioned sickle pain and none of the 519 references pertain to the pain associated with sickle cell disease. This omission may, unwittingly, convince the average reader that sickle pain should be treated more like chronic nonmalignant pain syndrome than cancer pain.

SICKLE PAIN VS. POSTOPERATIVE PAIN

Postoperative pain is the result of local tissue damage with consequent release of mediators of inflammation that initiate the painful experience (Cousins 1994). The incidence, severity, and duration of postoperative pain vary with the type and site of surgery (Bonica 1990b). In major joint surgery, for example, up to 60% of patients may have severe steady pain, and up to 80% may have severe pain on movement and reflex spasm (Bonica

Table VI
Comparative aspects of sickle cell and postoperative pain

	Sickle Cell	Postoperative
Type	Nociceptive	Nociceptive
	Acute or chronic	Acute
	Acute crisis a hallmark	
	Somatic or visceral	Usually somatic
Site	Variable, often generalized	Localized to site of surgery
Frequency	Recurrent	Restricted to postsurgery period
Duration	Mean of acute crisis 9–11 days	Mean duration 0.5–8.0 days

1990b). The mean duration of postoperative pain varies between about 12 hours and eight days (Bonica 1990b). Although sickle pain varies greatly among patients and in the same patient over time, it is recurrent and the severe, acute painful crisis has a mean duration of nine to 11 days (Billet et al. 1988b; Davies 1990; Ballas 1995a,b). Table VI lists the major differences between postoperative and sickle pain. Moreover, analysis of a home-based diary system (Shapiro et al. 1995) revealed that children and adolescents experienced pain on a surprisingly high number of days (about 30% of completed diary days) and that nearly 90% of painful episodes were managed at home. Thus, unlike other types of pain, sickle cell pain is pervasive with acute, acute recurrent, and chronic components.

The difference between postoperative pain and the pain of the acute sickle cell episode is confirmed by patients who have experienced both. Patients with sickle cell disease have reported that pain associated with childbirth, Cesarean section, or cholecystectomy is milder than that of acute sickle cell episodes (Ballas 1994b; Shapiro et al. 1993). The efficacy of new opioid analgesics is often assessed by their effect on postoperative pain, so equivalent efficacy cannot be assumed for sickle cell pain.

SICKLE PAIN VS. CHRONIC NONMALIGNANT PAIN SYNDROME

Sickle pain is nonmalignant and thus is often confused with chronic benign pain syndrome (CBPS) by providers who have cursory experience with sickle cell disease. CBPS is an acquired condition typically seen (Vasudevan 1993) in middle-aged persons with the following characteristics: (1) persistent pain that lasts beyond the expected healing period of the condition that caused it; (2) no identifiable cause of the pain despite several investigative trials; (3) no identifiable curative approach; (4) typical lifestyle characterized by the so-called six Ds: deconditioning, disease, drug misuse, dependence, depression, and disability (Brena and Chapman 1985). More-

Table VII
Comparative aspects of sickle cell pain and chronic
benign pain syndrome (CBPS)

	Sickle Cell	CBPS
Identifiable etiology	Yes	No
Opioid analgesics	Required in acute episodes	Not recommended
Nonpharmacologic therapy	Desirable	Major role
Curative therapy	None in adults	None
	Bone marrow transplant in selected children	

over, CBPS has numerous associated psychosocial implications including workers' compensation and disability. Management of CBPS typically includes avoidance of opioids, implementation of progressive, graded physical activity, and the use of nonpharmocologic approaches such as relaxation training, diversionary techniques, biofeedback, and cognitive restructuring (Barton and Gallegos 1994; Turk and Meichenbaum 1994). Nevertheless, the role of opioids in the management of patients with CBPS is intensely controversial (Portenoy 1996). Limited clinical experience by few physicians suggests that some patients with CBPS can achieve partial analgesia from opioid therapy in the absence of major side effects or the development of maladaptive drug-seeking behavior (Portenoy 1996). Turk (1996) reviewed the subject of opioid therapy in CBPS and summarized reported proposed guidelines for chronic opioid therapy. Controlled studies for the assessment of chronic opioid therapy in nonmalignant pain are needed to clarify the issue.

Sickle cell pain is unique and should not be equated with CBPS. Although they share some characteristics, they have fundamental differences (Table VII). Major distinctions for sickle cell disease include an identifiable etiology, chronic anemia, recurrent acute episodes of severe pain, and progressive organ damage. Unfortunately, some care providers consider sickle cell pain as one type of CBPS and treat it accordingly. This is a tragic mistake because sickle cell crises are recurrent attacks of acute severe pain (of peripheral origin) for which relief (as for acute traumatic, postsurgical, or burn pain) is best achieved by short-term use of opioids (see Chapter 10).

2

The Hematology of Sickle Cell Pain: A Prototype of Bedside and Bench Interaction

For the person in pain, so incontestably and unnegotiably present is it that "having pain" comes to be thought of as the most vibrant example of what it is "to have certainty," while for the other person it is so elusive that "hearing about pain" may exist as the primary model of what it is "to have doubt." Thus pain comes unsharably into our midst as at once that which cannot be confirmed and that which cannot be denied.

— Elaine Scarry, *The Body in Pain*, 1985

CLASSIFICATION OF HEMOLYTIC ANEMIAS

Red cell destruction normally occurs after a life span of about 120 days when the senescent erythrocytes are removed extravascularly by the macrophages of the reticuloendothelial system (bone marrow, spleen, liver, lymph nodes). Hemolytic anemias are characterized by premature destruction of red blood cells, shortening their life span to a few days in severe cases. Table I represents a simplified classification of hemolytic anemias (Ballas 1978, 1990a) into two major classes of intrinsic and extrinsic membrane disorders (membranopathies). The former include primary disorders of the red cell membrane that may be hereditary or acquired. Extrinsic membrane disorders, i.e., those that arise from an abnormality not intrinsic to the membrane, could be cytoplasmic or extracellular in origin. The former include enzymopathies and hemoglobin disorders. Extracellular disorders are mostly acquired hemolytic anemias such as those caused by autoimmune abnormalities, liver disease, or induced by drugs. (Table I). Sickle cell syndromes are the prototype of hemoglobin disorders as will be explained below.

19

Table I
Classification of hemolytic anemias

Intrinsic Membrane Disorders
Hereditary
Hereditary spherocytosis
Hereditary elliptocytosis
Hereditary xerocytosis
Hereditary acanthocytosis
Rh null syndromes
Acquired
Paroxysmal nocturnal hemoglobinuria
Megaloblastic anemias
Extrinsic Membrane Disorders
Cytoplasmic abnormalities
Enzymopathies
Disorders of pentose phosphate shunt
Disorders of glycolytic pathways
Globin disorders
Defects in globin structure (hemoglobinopathies)
Sickle Cell syndromes
Defects in globin synthesis (thalassemias)
α-thalassemia
β-thalassemia
Heme disorders (porphyrias)
Extracellular abnormalities
Autoimmune hemolytic anemias
Drug-induced hemolytic anemias
Fragmentation syndromes
Anemia of liver disease
Infection
Physical agents
Other disorders

SIGNS AND SYMPTOMS OF HEMOLYTIC ANEMIA

CLINICAL FEATURES

The cardiovascular and respiratory symptoms of hemolytic anemia such as pallor, decreased exercise tolerance, easy fatigability, tiredness, palpitations, and dyspnea are similar to those seen in anemia in general and vary according to the severity, duration, and acuteness of disease and its specific cause. Acute hemolytic anemia, for instance, is accompanied by all these symptoms and their corresponding signs. Patients with moderate or mild chronic hemolysis, however, usually adapt well to the anemia and manifest few symptoms. Patients with compensated hemolysis and no anemia are symptom free unless they develop some of the complications of chronic hemolytic states described below.

Icterus and dark-colored urine are two signs that are characteristic of hemolysis. The presence of anemia in conjunction with jaundice and tea-colored urine should alert the physician to the possibility of hemolysis. Spleno-megaly with or without hepatomegaly may be present in certain congenital chronic hemolytic anemias such as hereditary spherocytosis, pyruvate kinase deficiency, or thalassemias, and in some patients with certain acquired forms such as autoimmune hemolytic anemia. Asplenia, whether functional or ana-tomic, is typical of the sickle cell syndromes. The sections below will men-tion the signs and symptoms characteristic of certain hemolytic disorders.

HEMATOLOGICAL FEATURES

LABORATORY SIGNS OF HEMOLYSIS

The red cell indices in hemolytic anemias show great heterogeneity. Acquired hemolytic anemias usually have normochromic, normocytic indi-ces but could have macrocytic red cells if the reticulocyte count is markedly increased. In thalassemias and in certain hemoglobinopathies, the red cells are microcytic hypochromic. In sickle cell anemia, the indices are normocytic despite a high reticulocyte count—a combination sometimes referred to as relative microcytosis (Glader et al. 1975). Hyperchromia (high MCHC) is unique to hereditary spherocytosis (Schafer et al. 1978) and xerocytosis (Ballas et al. 1982, 1987), whether primary or secondary to such disorders as sickle cell anemia (with no deletion of alpha globin genes) and hemoglobin C disorders (Hb SC, CC, AC, etc.).

Table II lists the important laboratory signs of hemolysis. The reticulo-cyte count is typically increased in hemolytic anemia. Examination of the

Table II
Laboratory signs of hemolysis

Reticulocytosis (polychromasia)
Unconjugated hyperbilirubinemia
Increased fecal and urine urobilinogen
Decreased serum haptoglobin
Decreased serum hemopexin
Increased serum methemalbumin
Elevated lactate dehydrogenase (LDH)
Mildly elevated serum aspartate aminotransferase (AST)
Hemoglobinemia
Hemoglobinuria
Hemosiderinuria
Increased production of endogenous carbon monoxide
Decreased survival of autologous RBC labeled with ^{51}Cr

peripheral smear shows polychromasia due to the presence of ribosomes in reticulocytes. The hyperbilirubinemia in hemolysis almost always consists of unconjugated bilirubin. The maximum serum bilirubin level caused by hemolysis is 5 to 6 mg/dL except during the neonatal period. Higher values suggest a coexisting hepatic dysfunction. Hemoglobinemia, hemoglobinuria, and hemosiderinuria indicate intravascular hemolysis. Increased production of endogenous carbon monoxide reflects an increased rate of heme catabolism and is a more sensitive and quantitative measure than the serum level of unconjugated bilirubin. This diagnostic method, however, is complex and is not available in the average clinical laboratory. The normal half-life (T½) of chromium 51 (^{51}Cr)-tagged red cells is 25 to 32 days, but decreases to less than 16 days in severe hemolysis.

In practice, evidence of reticulocytosis and unconjugated hyperbilirubinemia suggests hemolysis. Increased levels of urine urobilinogen, lactate dehydrogenase (LDH), serum aspartate aminotransferase (AST), methemalbumin, and decreased levels of haptoglobin and hemopexin support the diagnosis of hemolysis. Decreased T½ of ^{51}Cr-tagged red blood cells (RBC) offers definitive evidence of hemolysis. Hemoglobinemia, hemoglobinuria, and hemosiderinuria indicate intravascular hemolysis.

Signs of chronic hemolysis

Chronic hemolytic anemia is usually accompanied by a constellation of characteristic signs and symptoms including cholelithiasis, leg ulcers, aplastic crises, hyperhemolytic crises, megaloblastic crises, and skeletal abnormalities. Leg ulcers are particularly characteristic of sickle cell anemia (Chernoff et al. 1954) and hereditary spherocytosis (Beinhauer and Gruhn 1957). Aplastic crises are usually precipitated by an intercurrent infection, especially with human parvovirus B19 (Bertrand et al. 1985; Saarinen et al. 1986). Hyperhemolytic crises may also be precipitated by intercurrent infection or by increased splenic activity (Jandle et al. 1961). Megaloblastic crises are due to complicating folate deficiency resulting from increased use of folate by the active bone marrow, especially if the dietary habits of the affected patient exclude items rich in folic acid such as leafy vegetables and fruits. Skeletal abnormalities are particularly characteristic of severe thalassemia major and of sickle cell disorders. These abnormalities include hair-on-end appearance seen on radiographs of the skull, thickening and striation of parietal and frontal bones, gnathopthy, and maxillary and dental abnormalities.

HEMOGLOBIN STRUCTURE AND FUNCTION

BIOCHEMISTRY

Normal hemoglobin consists of globin polypeptides and heme moieties. The globin polypeptide chains are organized into a tetramer of two different pairs of globins: one pair of α chains in fetal and adult hemoglobins, and one pair of non-α chains ($\alpha_2 x_2$ where x could be β, γ, or δ). It is the non-α chain that determines the type of hemoglobin. Thus, if the non-α chain is β globin, then the hemoglobin in question is hemoglobin A. Each globin chain enfolds a single heme moiety that consists of a single molecule of protoporphyrin IX coordinately bound to a single ferrous (Fe^{2+}) ion. In methemoglobin the iron ion is oxidized to the ferric (Fe^{3+}) state. Table III lists the structure and levels of normal fetal and adult hemoglobins (Bunn and Forget 1986). Hb A ($\alpha_2\beta_2$) is the major adult hemoglobin whereas Hb F ($\alpha_2\gamma_2$) is the major fetal hemoglobin. Hb A2 ($\alpha_2\delta_2$) is a minor adult hemoglobin that may be elevated in certain types of thalassemia as will be discussed below.

Certain embryonic and nonfunctional hemoglobins have physiologic and diagnostic importance, respectively (Table IV). The embryonic hemoglobins Gower 1 ($\zeta_2\varepsilon_2$), Gower 2 ($\alpha_2\varepsilon_2$), and Portland ($\zeta_2\gamma_2$) are produced in early intrauterine life prior to the formation of the predominant Hb F. It is generally believed that embryonic hemoglobins are produced in the yolk sac, fetal hemoglobins in the liver and spleen, and adult hemoglobins in the bone marrow.

Hemoglobin Barts (γ_4) is a nonfunctional type occurring in neonates with α-thalassemia. Hb H (β_4) is another nonfunctional hemoglobin in adults with one type of α-thalassemia referred to as Hb H disease (see below).

Biochemical features of all globin polypeptide chains have been well characterized and their primary structure is known (Dayhoff 1975; Bunn and Forget 1986) (Table V). The γ chain occurs in two types, Gγ and Aγ, depending on whether glycine or alanine amino acid is at position 136 in the polypeptide chain. Gγ is predominant in fetal life, whereas Aγ is the major γ chain in adults. Sickle hemoglobin is characterized by the presence of valine

Table III
Normal hemoglobins

Hb Type	Structure	% at Birth	% in Adults
Hb A	$\alpha_2\beta_2$	10–40	95–97.5
Hb A2	$\alpha_2\delta_2$	<1	2.5–3.5
Hb F	$\alpha_2\gamma_2$	60–90	<1

Table IV
Structural features of human hemoglobins

Hb Type	Structure	Ontogenic Relevance
Gower 1	$\zeta_2\varepsilon_2$	Embryonic
Gower 2	$\alpha_2\varepsilon_2$	Embryonic
Portland	$\zeta_2\gamma_2$	Embryonic
Hb F	$\alpha_2\gamma_2$	Major fetal
Hb A	$\alpha_2\beta_2$	Major adult
Hb A2	$\alpha_2\delta_2$	Minor adult
Hb Barts	γ_4	Nonfunctional
Hb H	β_4	Nonfunctional

Table V
Primary structure and net charge of
normal globin polypeptide chains at alkaline pH

Globin	No. of AAs*	No. of Acidic AAs	No. of Basic AAs	Net Charge vs. α
α	141	12	24	0
β^A	146	15	23	−4
β^S	146	14	23	−3
β^C	146	14	24	−2
$G\gamma$	146	16	22	−6
$A\gamma$	146	16	22	−6
δ	146	14	22	−4

*AAs = amino acids.

Table VI
Effect of amino acid substitution on Hb net charge

Hb Type	Structure	β-Chain Sequence	Net Charge vs. Hb A
A	$\alpha_2\beta_2$	Val-His-Leu-Thr-Pro-Glu-Glu--	0
S	$\alpha_2\beta_2^S$	Val-His-Leu-Thr-Pro-**Val**-Glu	+1
C	$\alpha_2\beta_2^C$	Val-His-Leu-Thr-Pro-**Lys**-Glu	+2
J Baltimore	$\alpha_2\beta_2^{J\ Baltimore}$	β^{16} Gly→Asp	−1

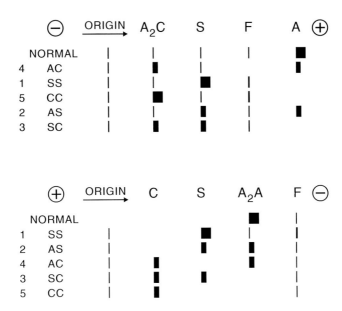

Fig. 1. Separation of hemoglobins by electrophoresis. **Top:** Cellulose acetate pH 9. **Bottom:** Citrate agar pH 6.2.

instead of glutamic acid at the sixth position of the β chain (Table VI). Another β-chain mutant, Hb C, has lysine instead of glutamic acid at the same position of the β chain. These two mutations result in changes in the net positive charge of the hemoglobin in question. In Hb J Baltimore the mutation ($\beta^{16\ Gly \to ASP}$) results in a net negative charge of the Hb molecule. Consequently, such hemoglobins can be separated easily by Hb electrophoresis (Fig. 1).

ONTOGENY

The composition of hemoglobin varies considerably between conception and postnatal development (Fig. 2) (Stamatoyannopoulos and Nienhuis 1993). Early in embryonic life ζ and ε globin polypeptides are synthesized in the yolk sac, which leads to the formation of Gower 1, Gower 2, and Portland (Table IV). The α and γ chains are the major chains synthesized in fetal life, primarily in the liver and to a lesser extent in the spleen. Around the time of birth a switch occurs such that the synthesis of the γ chain decreases and that of the β chain increases. About six months after birth the synthesis of these chains normally achieves adult values. Despite extensive research, the control mechanisms responsible for these switches are poorly understood.

Several clinical conclusions can be drawn by careful consideration of

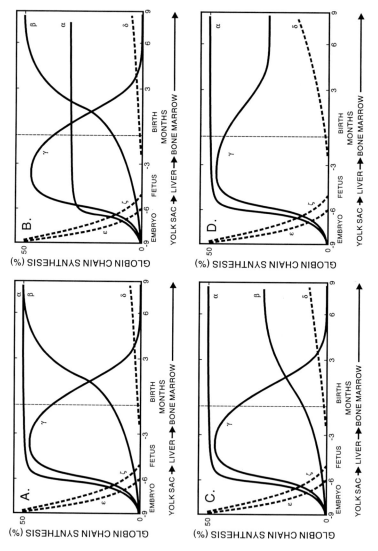

Fig. 2. Ontogeny of human globin chains in health and disease. **A:** Normal pattern of synthesis of globin chains in the fetus and the switching from γ and to β chain synthesis postnatally. **B:** Pattern of synthesis of globin chains in α-thalassemia trait: the excess γ chain in the fetus forms Hb Barts (γ₄) and the excess β chain in α-thalassemia with three α genes deleted forms Hb H (β₄). **C and D:** Patterns of globin chain synthesis in β thalassemia trait and thalassemia major (β°-thalassemia), respectively. Fig. 2A adapted from Steinberg (1994) with permission.

Fig. 2. Fetal survival depends heavily on the availability of α and γ globin polypeptide chains, which seems to be one explanation for the duplication of the α and γ globin genes (see below). Homozygous deficiency of either chain is incompatible with life and leads to hydrops fetalis. Abnormalities of the β chain do not pose serious problems to the fetus but assume importance postnatally, usually around the sixth month. Many parents of children with sickle cell anemia indicate that their problems began around the age of six months. Finally, reversal of the switch, i.e., turning off the synthesis of the β chain and activating the synthesis of the γ globin, is one approach to therapy of sickle cell disease as will be discussed in Chapter 12.

MOLECULAR BIOLOGY

The genes that control the synthesis of the globin chains occur in two clusters referred to as the β- and α-gene clusters (Fig. 3). The α-gene cluster (ζ and α genes) is located near the tip of the short arm of chromosome 16, whereas the β-gene cluster (ϵ, Gγ, Aγ, δ, and β) is located near the tip of the short arm of chromosome 11. The genes are arranged in the order they are expressed in prenatal life. Both the α genes (α_2 and α_1) and the γ genes (Gγ and Aγ) are duplicated, which seems to be an evolutionary trend to ensure fetal survival. Gγ activity is predominant in the fetus whereas Aγ activity is predominant postnatally. Alpha genes (α_2 and α_2) are both active in fetal and adult life and demonstrate high homology.

Each globin gene (Fig. 3) consists of three axons or coding regions and two introns (noncoding intervening sequences) referred to as IVS-1 and IVS-2. Initially, the entire gene is transcribed from both axons and introns into pre-mRNA. Subsequently the introns are removed from this transcript by a process known as splicing. Introns always begin with a G-T dinucleotide and end with an A-G dinucleotide, and the splicing process recognizes these sequences and the neighboring conserved axons. After splicing, the ends of the coding sequences are ligated together to yield the mature mRNA. Two structural modifications of mRNA, capping and polyadenylation, occur within the nucleus. Capping refers to the addition of a 7-methylguanosine group to the 5′ end of mRNA whereas polyadenylation refers to the addition of a poly (A) tail at the 3′ end of mRNA. Capping may be important for the attachment of mRNA to ribosomes whereas polyadenylation stabilizes it. Each gene has a promoter that is located 5′ to the gene, either close to or distal to the initiation site. Promoters are sites where RNA polymerases bind to catalyze gene transcription. Each gene also has an enhancer, a DNA sequence that increases the expression of the gene in cis-configuration. Enhancers may be located upstream or downstream from promoters.

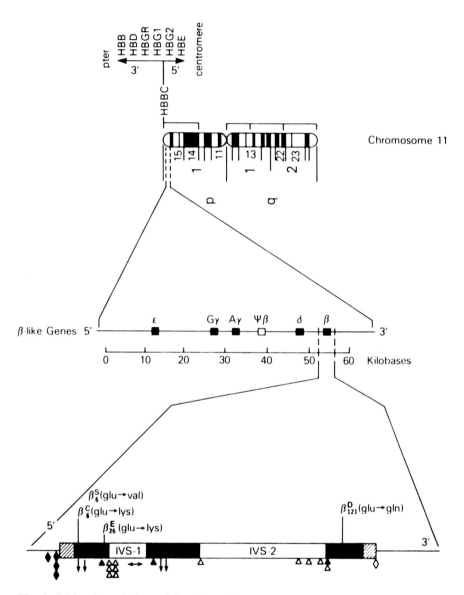

Fig. 3. Molecular pathology of disorders affecting the human β-globin gene. Location of lesions within the chromosome (upper diagram), the β-globin cluster (middle diagram), and the structural β-globin gene (lower diagram) account for the major hemoglobinopathies (above) and mutations resulting in β-thalassemias (below): (◆) transcription, (↓) frame-shift deletions, (Δ) splicing, (↔) deletion, (▲) nonsense. From McKusick (1987) with permission.

The mature, capped, and polyadenylated mRNA enters the cytoplasm and attaches to ribosomes where translation or the synthesis of globin chains occurs. This process is mediated by the attachment of transfer RNAs (tRNA), each with its individual amino acid, by codon/anticodon base pairing to an appropriate site on the mRNA template.

Mutations in the coding regions (axons) of the gene may yield structural hemoglobin variants or thalassemias. Alternatively, mutations within introns, at splice junctions, at the cap region, at the poly (A) tail, or at the promoter region usually affect the rate of transcription of mRNA and result in thalassemia. Deletion of an entire gene is another possible molecular mechanism.

PHYSIOLOGY

Hemoglobin is a respiratory pigment whose primary function is to transport oxygen from the lungs to all tissues where it is needed to maintain various metabolic processes. To achieve its mission as an oxygen transporter, Hb has five important properties (Table VII). Derangement in any of these properties impedes effective oxygen transport and usually leads to certain clinical disorders. As will be discussed below, mutations that alter any of these properties of Hb constitute certain classes of hemoglobinopathies.

Hb stability refers to its ability to maintain its quaternary structure due to stable and coordinated intramolecular bonds among its subunits ($\alpha_1\beta_2$ and $\alpha_1\beta_1$ contacts). Mutations at the $\alpha_1\beta_2$ interface are usually associated with changes in the oxygen affinity of hemoglobin, whereas mutations at the $\alpha_1\beta_1$ interface usually cause hemoglobin instability. Unstable hemoglobins break down into individual, poorly functioning globin polypeptide chains. These chains precipitate and attach themselves to the inner surface of the RBC as Heinz bodies that impair cell deformability and thus lead to premature destruction in the reticuloendothelial system.

The ability of Hb to bind oxygen reversibly seems to be the result of its capacity to carry different amounts of oxygen at different oxygen tensions that is best described by the oxygen dissociation curve (Fig. 4). The sigmoid

Table VII
Major properties of normal hemoglobin

Soluble in both the oxy and deoxy states
Stable
Binds oxygen reversibly with a P50 of about 27 torr
Maintains iron in the reduced ferrous state (Fe^{2+}) in the heme moiety
Contains balanced amounts of α- and non-α globin polypeptide chains

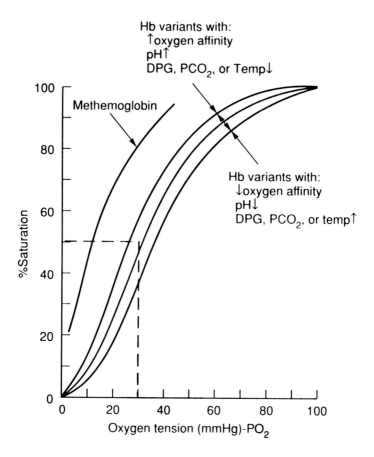

Fig. 4. Oxygen dissociation curve of hemoglobin. The P50 (the oxygen tension at which the hemoglobin molecule is half saturated) is about 27 torrs in normal RBC. Heterotopic modifiers of hemoglobin function can shift the curve leftward by increasing oxygen affinity or rightward by decreasing oxygen affinity. From Benz (1989) with permission.

shape of this curve is a result of heme-heme cooperativity or coordinated interaction among its subunits. Thus, the four heme groups do not undergo oxygenation or deoxygenation simultaneously, but sequentially depending on the state of each individual heme unit with regard to the presence or absence of bound oxygen on the other three globin chains. Normally, the P50 or the oxygen tension at which Hb is half saturated is about 27 torrs (mmHg). Increased P50 indicates decreased oxygen affinity and vice-versa.

Normally the ratio of a globin to non-α globin (α/non-α) is about 1. Significant changes in this ratio result in surplus intracellular globin chains that interfere with normal function and cellular survival. This aberration in the α/non-α ratio is the hallmark of thalassemias as will be discussed below.

CLASSIFICATION OF HEMOGLOBINOPATHIES

Traditionally, hemoglobin disorders have been broadly divided into two major categories: structural variants and thalassemias. Some structural variants, however, also demonstrate thalassemic features in their expression (Bunn and Forget 1986).

STRUCTURAL VARIANTS

Classification by extent of base mutations

Variants of hemoglobins result from a wide variety of mutations that are inherited as co-dominant traits in classic Mendelian fashion. About 199 α, 335 β, 68 γ, and 28 δ globin polypeptide variants have been described (Huisman et al. 1996). Some examples are illustrated in Table VIII.

Functional classification of Hb variants

A more relevant and clinically significant classification of structural hemoglobin variants pertains to derangement of the five major properties of

Table VIII
Classification of hemoglobinopathies
by extent of base mutation

Single Base Mutations
  One substitution
    Hb S ($\beta^{6\ Glu \rightarrow Val}$)
    Hb C ($\beta^{6\ Glu \rightarrow Lys}$)
    Hb M Boston ($\alpha^{58\ His \rightarrow Tyr}$)
  Two substitutions
    Hb C Harlem ($\beta^{6\ Glu \rightarrow Val}$ and $\beta^{73\ ASP \rightarrow ASn}$)
Elongated Subunits
  Base substitutions in termination codon
    Hb constant spring: 30 extra amino acids in α chain
  Frame shift mutations
    Hb Wayne: α 139–141 extended chain
    Hb Grady: α 115–118 extended chain
  Retention of initiation methionine
    Hb South Florida: $\beta^{1\ Val \rightarrow Met}$
Shortened Subunits
  Hb Gun Hill: β 91–95 deletion
Fusion Subunits
  Hb Lepore: $\delta\beta$ fusion
  Hb Miyada: $\beta\delta$ fusion

Table IX
Functional classification of hemoglobin variants

Hemoglobins with decreased solubility
  Hb S, Hb C
Unstable hemoglobins
  Hb Gun Hill
Hemoglobins with abnormal oxygen affinity
  Increased oxygen affinity: Hb Wayne
  Decreased oxygen affinity: Hb Kansas
M Hemoglobins
  Hb M Boston
Structural variants with thalassemic phenotype
  Hb E
  Hb Lepore
  Hb Constant Spring

normal Hb listed in Table VII. Consequently, clinically significant and common structural variants of hemoglobin are listed in Table IX and include those that are insoluble in the oxy or deoxy state, unstable, those with abnormal oxygen affinity, those that have oxidized heme (Fe^{3+}), and those that result in a thalassemic phenotype.

THALASSEMIAS

Thalassemias are characterized by decreased or absent synthesis of at least one globin polypeptide chain. They consist of a wide variety of genetic abnormalities that may involve axons, introns, splice junctions, promoter region, or flanking regions of the gene (cap site and poly-A tail). Thalassemia is a compound word derived from Greek: *thalassa* means sea (the Mediterranean) and *aneimia* means bloodlessness. Originally the term was applied to Mediterranean anemia, also known as Cooley's anemia or β-thalassemia major, because it was described in persons of Mediterranean origin, primarily Italians and Greeks (Weatherall and Clegg 1981). Today, thalassemia is classified by the globin chain, the synthesis of which is decreased or absent, including α-thalassemias, β-thalassemias, γ-thalassemias, δ-thalassemias, δβ-thalassemias, and so on.

α-Thalassemia

The most common form of α-thalassemia, especially in African Americans, is α-gene deletion. Because the α gene is duplicated, the normal α genotype is αα/αα in which two α genes are inherited from each parent.

Table X
Alpha thalassemias

Common Name	No. of Functional Genes	Phenotype	Genotype
Normal	4	Normal	$\alpha\alpha/\alpha\alpha$
Silent carrier	3	α-Thal 1	$-\alpha/\alpha\alpha$ *or* $\alpha^*\alpha/\alpha\alpha$
α-Thal trait	2	α-Thal 2	$-\alpha/-\alpha$ *or* $--/\alpha\alpha$ *or* $\alpha^*\alpha^*/\alpha\alpha$ *or* $\alpha^*\alpha/\alpha^*\alpha$
Hb H disease	1	α-Thal 3	$--/-\alpha$ *or* $\alpha^*\alpha^*/\alpha^*\alpha$
Hydrops fetalis	0	α-Thal 4	$--/--$ *or* $\alpha^*\alpha^*/\alpha^*\alpha^*$

Note: α^* Indicates that α gene is structurally present but not functional.

Deletion of one or more α genes results in the various forms of α-thalassemia (Table X) (Higgs et al. 1989). About 65% of African Americans, whether they carry the sickle gene or not, have normal α genotype ($\alpha\alpha/\alpha\alpha$), about 30% have one α-gene deletion ($-\alpha/\alpha\alpha$ genotype), and the remaining 5% have two α-gene deletions ($-\alpha/-\alpha$) in trans, i.e., one α gene is deleted from each allelic chromosome. This form contrasts with the α-thalassemia that occurs in Asians where the α-gene deletion is in cis ($--/\alpha\alpha$), i.e., two a genes are deleted from one chromosome.

Because these α-gene deletions are relatively common in African Americans, they play an important role when they are associated with the sickle mutation as will be discussed below. Nondeletional acquired forms of the α-thalassemia phenotype (Hb H disease) have been reported in association with mental retardation and with myeloproliferative disorders (Weatherall 1994). This observation suggests that transacting factors may be involved in the expression of α-globin genes.

β-Thalassemia

Unlike α-thalassemias, β-thalassemias are usually the result of point mutations of the β-globin gene and rarely due to gene deletion. A notable exception is the syndrome of hereditary persistence of fetal hemoglobin (HPFH) where the β and/or the δ genes are deleted. Defects of the globin gene cluster that result in thalassemia are broadly divided into two groups: β^+-thalassemia in which the affected gene produces β globin but in reduced amounts, and, β^o- thalassemia, in which the affected gene produces no β globin. More than 175 different nondeletional mutations (Huisman et al. 1997) resulting in either β^+ or β^o thalassemia have been described.

β⁺-Thalassemia

Single base substitutions involving certain regions within and flanking the β gene affect the rate of transcription of the gene and result in mildly or severely decreased β-globin synthesis. For example, mutations at -88 and -87 from the cap site result in mildly depressed transcription. Mutations near the splice junctions may interfere with normal splicing and result in defective mRNA processing and decreased normal mRNA for translation. Examples of these mutations have been described in persons of African, Asian, and Mediterranean origins.

Hb E, the most common β-globin variant in Asians, results from a mutation in codon 26, which is close to codon 30, the junctional codon between axon 1 and intron 1. Hb E is associated with a mild β-thalassemia phenotype.

β°-Thalassemia

Some mutations surrounding and within the β gene result in complete absence of β-globin synthesis. Nonsense and frameshift mutations within the axons either cause in-phase premature termination of transcription or the transcription of anomalous sequences into abnormal and unstable proteins. Mutations at or near splice junctions that completely block normal splicing have also been described. Again, examples of all these mutations have been found in persons of African, Asian, and Mediterranean origin.

Another group of β°-thalassemia syndromes involves gene deletions similar to the deletions seen in a thalassemia. The largest of these deletions removes all the β-like gene cluster and results in (γδβ)-thalassemia. Other less extensive deletions spare one or more of these genes and create clinical syndromes such a Gγ(δβ)°-thalassemia, GγAγHPFH (hereditary persistence of fetal hemoglobin), GγAγ(δβ)°-thalassemia, and the Lepore hemoglobin syndromes.

SICKLE CELL SYNDROMES

MALARIAL HYPOTHESIS

A common feature among all sickle cell syndromes is their association with the sickle gene either in a heterozygous or homozygous manner. Ample indirect evidence indicates that the sickle gene arose in Africa where cerebral malaria is hyperendemic (Allison 1954). The introduction of slash-and-burn agriculture about 2000 years ago destroyed the root structure of tropical jungles that drained brackish water and thus introduced sunlight into these previously shadowy areas (Livingstone 1958; Eaton 1994). This change provided a favorable breeding ground for the mosquito vector *Anopheles gambiae* and the spread of malaria in tropical Africa. Hemoglobin S in heterozygotes seems to confer a biological advantage through partial protection against *Plasmodium falciparum*, the parasite that causes cerebral malaria, the most severe form of the disease. The following lines of evidence support this hypothesis: (1) parallel distribution between the sickle gene and falciparum malaria (Allison 1957; Wiesenfeld 1967; Nagel 1984); (2) in hyperendemic areas reduced morbidity and mortality in persons with sickle trait compared to normal persons and patients with sickle cell anemia; (3) a significantly lower prevalence of cerebral malaria (Vandepitte et al. 1957; Livingstone 1971; Fleming et al. 1979) and of parasitemia (Vandepitte et al. 1957) in children with sickle cell trait compared to normal controls.

The mechanisms by which the sickle gene provide protection against malaria are not well understood. Suffice to say that a red cell from a person with sickle trait seems to be a graveyard for the invading parasite due to possible factors consequent to the invasion such as cellular dehydration, hyperkalemia, reduced pH values, release of oxygen radicals, and decreased intracellular oxygen tension. The resultant sickling and destruction of the red cell containing the parasite thus disrupts the malarial cycle (Luzzato et al. 1970; Roth et al. 1978).

β HAPLOTYPES

In recent years restriction endonuclease analysis of the DNA from various populations with sickle cell anemia has demonstrated distinct polymorphisms within and around the β-globin gene (Wainscoat et al. 1983; Pagnier et al. 1984). Collectively, these polymorphisms are referred to as β haplotypes that have specific ethnogeographic origins. Simply stated, all $β^S$ haplotypes carry the same sickle mutation but the nucleotide sequence around it differs among populations. Thus, a $β^S$ haplotype may be considered as a fingerprint of a certain population. To date, five major β haplotypes have been described (Fig. 5): Benin, Senegal, Central African Republic (also called Bantu), Cameroon, and Arab-Indian. The role of β haplotypes in the clinical expression of sickle cell disease is a subject of significant controversy (Nagel et al. 1985, 1987, 1991; Rieder et al. 1991). Some studies suggest that those associated with elevated Hb F level, such as the Senegal haplotype, may have a salutary effect on sickle cell disease. The presence of these haplotypes, however, provides evidence that the sickle mutation arose at least five times during the course of its evolution, four times within Africa and once in Arabia-India.

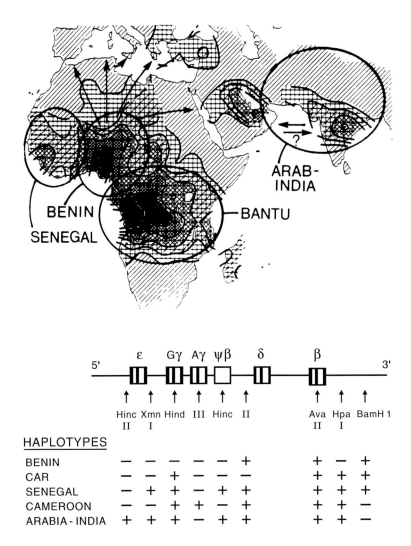

Fig. 5. β Haplotypes of the sickle gene. **Top:** Distribution of the sickle gene in Africa and Asia with known haplotypes superimposed (from Ragusa et al. 1988, with permission). **Bottom:** Classification of β^S haplotypes associated with sickle cell disease based on restriction endonuclease fragment length polymorphism.

CLASSIFICATION OF SICKLE CELL SYNDROMES

Sickle cell disease is a generic term for a group of chronic inherited disorders of hemoglobin structure in which the affected person inherits two mutant globin genes (one from each parent), at least one of which is always the sickle mutation. The latter results from a single nucleotide change (GAT→GTT) in the sixth codon of axon 1 of the β-globin gene responsible for the synthesis of the β-globin chain. The resulting replacement of the normal glutamic acid by valine at position 6 in the β chain leads to the formation of sickle hemoglobin (Hb S). Sickle cell anemia (SS) is the homozygous state, in which the sickle gene is inherited from both parents. Other sickle cell syndromes result from the co-inheritance of the sickle gene and a nonsickle gene, such as Hb C, Hb O^{Arab}, Hb D, β$^+$-thalassemia, or β^o-thalassemia. Table XI lists the common sickle cell syndromes and their typical hematological parameters. The prevalence of these sickle cell syndromes among African Americans in decreasing order is: sickle trait, sickle cell anemia, Hb SC disease, sickle-β$^+$-thalassemia, sickle-β^o-thalassemia, and other combinations such as Hb SO^{Arab} and Hb SD. Moreover, deletion of one or more of the α-globin genes affects the hematological and clinical picture of sickle cell anemia (Serjeant 1992). Thus, patients with SS and two α-gene deletions (β^S/β^S; −α/−α) have a higher incidence of avascular necrosis (Ballas et al. 1989b, 1997; Milner et al. 1991) than do patients with no deletion (β^S/β^S; αα/αα).

Sickle cell trait, however, is essentially a benign condition. Persons with sickle trait are not anemic and do not experience recurrent attacks of acute painful episodes or organ failure due to sickling. Hematuria, hyposthenuria, and sudden death in military recruits have been reported in persons with sickle cell trait (Jones and Binder 1970; Sears 1978). The factors that contribute to the increased risk of sudden death with strenuous exercise in sickle cell trait are unknown. Together, the data in the literature indicate that sickle cell trait is benign with few identifiable complications and no clinically significant hematological abnormalities (Sears 1994). Those with sickle cell trait can experience other medical problems that are coexistent disorders and not due to sickle trait.

The hematological and clinical picture varies among the sickle cell syndromes. Patients with S-β^o-thalassemia have microcytosis, hypochromia, high Hb A2 levels, and variable Hb F values. Smears prepared from their peripheral blood show variable number of sickle cells, target cells, basophilic stippling, and variation in the size and shape of their RBC (anisopoikilocytosis). The anemia in Hb S-β$^+$-thalassemia is mild and usually with an Hb level greater than 10 g/dl. Peripheral smears from their blood show similar findings to those seen in Hb S-β^o-thalassemia. Hb SC disease is typically characterized by microcytic and hyperchromic RBC indices (Ballas and Kocher 1988). Peripheral smears from patients with Hb SC disease show "boat-shaped" or "fat" sickle cells, microspherocytosis, and target cells. Fig. 6 shows typical peripheral smears from patients with various sickle cell syndromes.

Acute painful episodes are most common in patients with sickle cell anemia. Retinopathy occurs most frequently in Hb SC disease (Ballas et al. 1982).

Table XI

Major types of sickle cell syndromes and their typical hematological parameters

Syndrome	Abbrev.	Genotype	Hb g/dl	Reticulocyte Count (%)	MCV* fl	Hemoglobin Composition (%)			
						Hb A	Hb A2	Hb S	Hb F
Sickle cell anemia	SS	β^S/β^S; $\alpha\alpha/\alpha\alpha$	7.0–8.0	10–20	85–110	0	2.5–3.5	75–96	1–20
Sickle-β°-thalassemia	S-β°-Thal	$\beta^S/\beta^{\circ thal}$	7-0–10.0	6–15	60–70	0	4.0–6.0	70–90	1–20
Sickle-β^+-thalassemia	S-β^+-Thal	$\beta^S/\beta^{+ thal}$	>10.0	5–10	60–70	10–20	4.0–6.0	65–85	1–15
Hb SC disease	SC	β^S/β^C; $\alpha\alpha/\alpha\alpha$	>10.0	5–10	75–85	0	45–50[†]	50	1–6
Sickle trait	AS	β^S/β^A; $\alpha\alpha/\alpha\alpha$	12–16	1.0–2.0	>82	60	2.5–3.5	40	<1.0
None (normal)	AA	β^A/β^A; $\alpha\alpha/\alpha\alpha$	>12	<2.0	82–94	>95	2.5–3.5	0	<1.0

Note: All disorders listed may be associated with variable degrees of deletion of α-genes and different types of β^S haplotypes.

*Mean corpuscular volume.

[†]Hb A$_2$ and Hb C have the same electrophoretic mobility and are not separable on routine analysis.

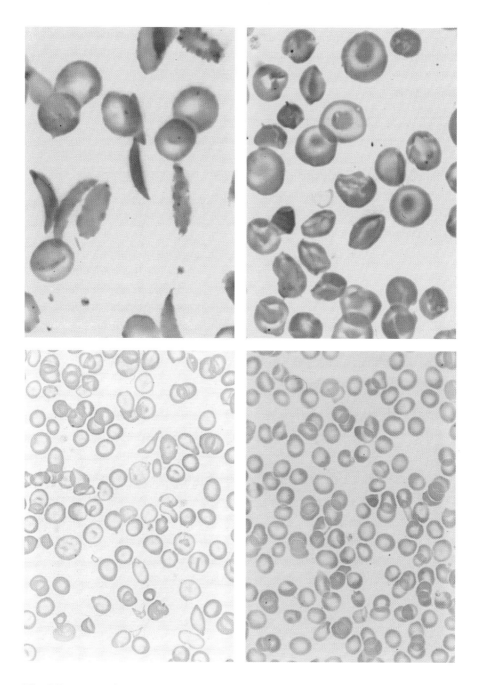

Fig. 6. Representative morphological picture in peripheral smears from patients with sickle cell syndromes. **Top left:** Sickle cell anemia. **Top right:** Hb SC disease. **Bottom left:** Sickle-β^o-thalassemia. **Bottom right:** Sickle-β^+-thalassemia.

Those sickle cell syndromes that have relatively high level of Hb (such as SS with two α-gene deletions, Hb SC disease, and Hb S-β$^+$-thalassemia) seem to have higher incidence of avascular necrosis of the humeral and femoral heads.

Table XI lists only clinical entities with no α-gene deletion. Each category, however, may be divided into three subclasses with four, three, or two α genes. Inclusion of the β^S haplotypes increases the degree of molecular heterogeneity by at least six-fold for each entity. This vast heterogeneity at the molecular level may explain the similarly vast heterogeneity at the clinical level seen in these disorders.

INHERITANCE

Sickle cell syndromes are inherited in an autosomal co-dominant manner according to simple Mendelian principles. Table XII lists possible outcomes of pregnancy among parents who carry different combinations of normal and abnormal genes. In genetic counseling and prenatal diagnosis it is important to emphasize that these probabilities are for each pregnancy and not for the family as a whole. Thus, two parents with sickle cell trait may have normal children after subsequent pregnancies. Only in certain pairings is the outcome of pregnancy predicted in 100% of cases (Table XII).

Table XII
Probable genotype of offspring according
to the genotypes of parents

Genotypes of Parents	Probability of Genotypes Among Zygotes
SS × AA	100% AS
SS × AS	50% AS, 50% SS
AS × AS	50% AS, 25% SS, 25% AA
SS × SS	100% SS
SS × AC	50% AS, 50% SC
SS × CC	100% SC
SS × Aβ$^{o\ thal}$	50% AS, 50% Sβ$^{o\ thal}$
SS × Aβ$^{+\ thal}$	50% AS, 50% Sβ$^{+\ thal}$
SS × β$^{o\ thal}$β$^{o\ thal}$	100% Sβ$^{o\ thal}$
SS × β$^{+\ thal}$β$^{+\ thal}$	100% Sβ$^{+\ thal}$

Abbreviations: AA, normal adult hemoglobin; SS, sickle cell anemia; AS, sickle trait; AC, Hb C trait; CC, Hb C disease.

Part II
Sickle Cell Pain Syndromes

3

Classification of Sickle Cell Pain

English, which can express the thoughts of Hamlet and the tragedy of Lear, has no words for the shiver and the headache. . . . The merest schoolgirl, when she falls in love, has Shakespeare and Keats to speak for her; but let a sufferer try to describe a pain in his head to a doctor and language at once runs dry.
— Virginia Woolf, 1882–1941

Those who do not feel pain, seldom think that it is felt.
— Johnson, 1709–1784

Painful episodes in sickle cell disease are unpredictable in location and timing. They are repetitive, intermittent, and may start as early as 6 months of age (Shapiro 1989; Serjeant 1992; Ballas 1994b). As with other types of pain (Bonica 1990a), sickle pain can be classified according to different schemes (Ballas et al. 1995b). To date, however, sickle pain has not been classified into a unified and comprehensive scheme that is accepted by providers and researchers. Some large studies have reported the characteristics of certain types of sickle cell pain such as acute painful crises or episodes (Platt et al. 1991), acute chest syndrome (Castro et al. 1994; Vichinsky et al. 1994), leg ulcers (Koshy et al. 1989), and osteonecrosis (Ballas et al. 1989b; Milner et al. 1991). Other types of pain have been the subject of smaller studies, most of which are anecdotal. To the best of my knowledge there are no major longitudinal studies to document and classify the types of pain experienced by a large group of patients followed over five or more years. The study by Platt et al. (1991) addressed the rates and risk factors of acute sickle cell painful episodes but did not delve into such details as the location, etiology, quality, severity scores, opioid consumption, and response to management. One difficulty is that over time the same patient may experience different types of pain syndromes, and the features of one painful episode may differ considerably from others. Nevertheless, an accepted scheme of classification of sickle cell pain would facilitate communication and transfer of information pertinent to pain research, therapy, and clinical records. Table I lists the methods that could be used to classify sickle cell pain as discussed below.

43

Table I
Methods of classification of sickle cell pain

Pathophysiologic	Severity
Nociceptive	Mild
Neuropathic	Moderate
Psychogenic	Severe
Any combination of the above	*Etiologic*
Temporal	Secondary to the disease itself
Acute	Secondary to therapy
Chronic	Unrelated to sickle cell
Both	*Regional*
Anatomic	Head and neck pain
Somatic	Chest pain
Visceral	Abdominal pain
Deafferentation	Extremities
	Other regions

PATHOPHYSIOLOGIC CLASSIFICATION

Pathophysiologically, pain may be secondary to tissue damage (nociceptive), to aberrant somatosensory processing in the central or peripheral nervous system (neuropathic), to psychological factors such as anxiety, depression, disturbed affect (psychogenic), or to any combination of these three types. Sickle cell pain is primarily nociceptive due to tissue damage secondary to vaso-occlusion of the microcirculation by sickled red cells as will be described in Chapter 4. Neuropathic pain rarely occurs in sickle cell disease. Although the etiology of sickle pain is not psychogenic, psychological factors resulting from chronic pain contribute significantly to its onset, severity, and chronicity in a manner similar to other pain syndromes (American Psychiatric Association 1994).

TEMPORAL CLASSIFICATION

Pain syndromes may be acute or chronic. Acute pain has a duration of less than six months, while pain that continues uninterrupted for more than six months is chronic (American Psychiatric Association 1994). Patients with sickle cell anemia experience both. The sickle cell painful crisis is the prototype of acute pain, whereas leg ulcers, avascular necrosis of humeral or femoral heads, and bone infarcts cause chronic pain.

Major characteristics of acute pain include fear and anxiety, which are especially pronounced when associated with fear of death. A vicious cycle of pain, anxiety, fear, helplessness, and sleep deprivation accompanies acute painful episodes (Ballas 1990b). Some patients hardly sleep during the early phase of a sickle cell painful crisis despite large doses of hypnotics and opioid analgesics. Sedation is an important salutary effect of the use of narcotic analgesics for acute pain, a fact not always appreciated by health care providers, as discussed below. Rebound somnolence is often observed as the acute painful episode wanes. When acute pain persists for several days the patient may express anger, depression, and resentment, especially if the patient perceives that health care providers are withholding pain relief. These factors contribute to a vicious circle of pain, depression, and diminished confidence in the ability and interest of medical providers to relieve pain.

Major characteristics of chronic pain include emotional, behavioral, affective, and physiological responses that differ from those of acute pain. Patients with chronic pain frequently suffer from a combination of nociceptive and psychogenic pain; the latter includes depression, paranoia, feeling of hopelessness, and despair. Many patients with chronic sickle cell pain become preoccupied with their pain and gradually withdraw from social activities. Their existence becomes a circuitous journey from home, to the doctor's office, to the pharmacy, back to home.

Patients with sickle cell disease who suffer from both acute and chronic pain syndromes, such as avascular necrosis, and frequent acute painful crises are seriously disadvantaged. Their management commands infinite patience, understanding, empathy, and long-term follow-up by their medical attendants.

ANATOMIC CLASSIFICATION

Depending on the site and mechanism of activation of nociceptors, pain syndromes may be classified into three categories: somatic, visceral, and de-afferentation (Payne 1987). Somatic pain results from activation of nociceptors in cutaneous, subcutaneous, and deep tissues. It is usually well localized and often described as constant, gnawing, aching, sharp, or throbbing. Painful episodes involving the musculoskeletal system are the prototypes of somatic pain in sickle cell anemia.

Visceral pain results from activation of nociceptors by inflammation, stretching, or distention of thoracic and abdominal viscera. This type of pain is not well localized and is often described as constant, dull, deep, or squeezing and may be accompanied by nausea, vomiting, hypertension, tachycardia, tachypnea, and diaphoresis. Acute splenic sequestration, right upper quadrant syndrome (especially hepatic crisis), and acute chest syndrome are examples of visceral pain in sickle cell anemia. Patients with generalized sickle cell painful episodes usually have both somatic and visceral types of pain. Moreover, visceral pain may be referred to superficial cutaneous sites distant from the primary site of pain and may be accompanied by tenderness at the referred site, e.g., chest pain secondary to splenic infarction.

Deafferentation pain is usually described as a severe, constant, dull ache with superimposed paroxysms of burning, shooting, or electric shock-like sensations. This type of pain is not usually seen in sickle cell disease, but is characteristic of the cancer patient with injury to the central or peripheral nervous system from tumor compression, infiltration, surgery, chemotherapy, or irradiation. Brachial or lumbosacral plexopathies due to metastasis are typical examples of this type of pain. Although patients with β-thalassemia may experience deafferentation pain as a result of spinal nerve compression by extramedullary myeloid masses, this event is rare in sickle cell disease.

CLASSIFICATION BY FREQUENCY AND SEVERITY

Sickle cell disease may be mild or severe depending on the frequency and severity of acute painful episodes. Patients who experience three or more acute painful episodes per year that require treatment with parenteral opioid analgesics in a medical facility for four or more hours are considered to have severe disease (Charache et al. 1995). Patients who experience fewer than three such episodes per year are considered to have mild disease. This definition is useful in that it allows the prospective collection and computerization of data for analysis. The definition is limited, however, in that it confounds frequency and severity and excludes the stoic patient who endures and treats severe pain at home while it includes the anxious patient with relatively mild pain who rushes to a medical facility for therapy.

The above scheme classifies sickle cell disease as a whole into mild and severe categories. Some studies have shown that pain episodes, whether mild, moderate, or severe, are often treated at home (Shapiro 1989; Shapiro et al. 1990). Another type of classification considers place of therapy in addition to pain severity and duration (Table II). Thus, a pain scored less than 4 on a

Table II
Classification of painful crisis by severity of pain, duration,
and usual place of analgesic therapy

| Severity | Pain Score | Duration and Usual Place of Treatment | |
		< 4 hours	> 4 hours
Mild	< 4	Home/outpatient facility	Home/outpatient facility
Moderate	4–6	Home/outpatient facility	Home/outpatient facility/ED
Severe	> 6	Home/ED	ED/hospital

ED = emergency department.

scale of 0 to 10 is considered mild irrespective of its duration and is usually treated with oral analgesics at home or in an outpatient facility. Moderate pain, scored between 4 and 6, is usually treated like mild pain but with higher doses of analgesics. Severe pain usually has a score greater than 6, lasts more than four hours, and is usually treated in a medical facility with parenteral opioids. As mentioned above, some patients may manage even very severe pain episodes at home.

ETIOLOGIC CLASSIFICATION

Table III lists the major pain syndromes of sickle cell disease, which also are divided into those due to the disease itself, those associated with therapy,

Table III
Etiologic classification of sickle pain

Pain Secondary to the Disease Itself
Acute Pain
    Painful crisis
    Acute chest syndrome
    Hepatic crisis
    Bowel infarction and necrosis
    Priapism
    Calculous cholecystitis
    Hand-foot syndrome*
    Splenic sequestration*

Chronic Pain
    Aseptic necrosis
    Arthropathies
    Vertebral body collapse
    Leg ulcers
    Impaction
    Intractable painful crisis

Pain Secondary to Therapy
    Postoperative pain (surgery to treat complications of the disease itself)
    Withdrawal
    Loose prosthesis (hip or shoulder)
    Iron overload due to chronic transfusion

Pain Unrelated to Sickle Cell Disease or Its Therapy
    Infection (except disease-related infection)
    Trauma
    Arthritis (septic, degenerative, collagen disease)
    Peptic ulcer disease
    Postoperative pain (surgery not related to the disease itself)

*Occurs in infants and children, rarely in adults.

and those that are independent of the disease or its therapy. The acute painful crisis that is the hallmark of sickle cell disease is unpredictable. It may be precipitated by known stress or have no apparent precipitant, involve any part of the body, and vary in severity, location, and duration. In contrast, chronic sickle cell pain seems to be similar in many aspects to cancer pain.

REGIONAL CLASSIFICATION

Sickle pain may involve any part of the body and often can be generalized and involve multiple sites. An advantage of regional classification of pain is that it potentially can clarify the pathophysiology, clinical picture, and outcome of the painful episode. Recent studies on acute chest syndrome in sickle cell disease, for example, have described pathophysiological events, clinical course, complications, and recommended therapy. Regional types of sickle pain will be discussed in detail in Chapter 5.

ILLUSTRATIVE CASE

CASE 3.1

A 34-year-old African American man who has been followed in our sickle cell program for nine years was diagnosed with sickle cell anemia at the age of 6 months when he presented with acute and painful swelling of both hands and feet (hand-foot syndrome). At the age of 4 years he developed acute splenic sequestration that required splenectomy. Since childhood he has experienced recurrent attacks of acute pain that increased in frequency and severity with age. During the last 10 years these attacks involved his low back, abdomen, chest, and knees. The pain was throbbing in the knees and sharp in the other regions. He treated these episodes with oral opioid analgesics (oxycodone initially and meperidine later) at home if the pain was mildly or moderately severe (pain score <6). He sought treatment in the emergency department/hospital for severe pain (score >6) and was given parenteral meperidine. Between 1990 and 1995 he was admitted 39 times to our facility (6.5 admissions/year) and required a total of 424 hospitalization days with an average length of stay of 10.9 days per admission. During the same period he was treated 57 times in the emergency department for acute painful episodes and was seen 187 times in the outpatient office.

Besides the recurrent acute painful episodes, he experienced other painful complications of his disease. He reported several episodes of acute chest syndrome (mostly pneumonia) characterized by fever, chest pain, and pulmonary infiltrates on chest X-ray. The pain associated with this syndrome was deep and differed from that of his acute painful episodes. He also had complained of recurrent episodes of priapism since adolescence. They usually woke him before dawn, lasted for 30 minutes to two hours, and were treated symptomatically with meperidine and benzodiazepine. At age 25 he was diagnosed with asymptomatic cholelithiasis. Nevertheless, he had cholecystectomy at age 33 following an episode of calculous cholecystitis. In 1993 he developed pain in both hips (more severe on the left side) that was deep, achy, constant, and different from the acute episodes of pain. Evaluation of this new type of pain revealed avascular necrosis of both femoral heads. He continues to complain of this chronic pain.

Other pain syndromes experienced by this patient included postoperative pain following cholecystectomy and the surgical extraction of 12 carious and unrestorable teeth with four quadrants of alveoplasty, and severe headache following a motor vehicle accident in 1993. The work-up for the headache included computed tomography, which revealed no cerebral hemorrhage or other neurological complications. The headache resolved within a few weeks after the accident but was associated with a typical acute painful episode involving his low back, chest, and upper extremities that, apparently, was precipitated by the trauma. In 1995 he complained of numbness and tingling of the left hand associated with spontaneous and locked flexion of the wrist following the intramuscular injection of meperidine in the left deltoid muscle. He could unlock the flexion forcibly with his right hand. Physical examination showed decreased pin sensation over the left hand and reproduced the spontaneous flexion described by the patient. These signs and symptoms disappeared within a few weeks and were thought to be due to iatrogenic peripheral neuropathy secondary to the intramuscular injection.

Comment on case 3.1

This case demonstrates the different types of pain syndromes that a patient with sickle cell disease may experience over the years (Table I). This patient experienced most of the types with the possible exception of psychogenic pain, although the latter could not be completely ruled out because he refused any psychiatric consultation. Thus, he had both acute painful episodes and chronic pain from avascular necrosis, and pain that ranged from mild to severe. Most of his pain was musculoskeletal and somatic, except for the pain associated with the acute chest syndrome that seemed visceral. The pain of acute episodes, avascular necrosis, acute chest, and priapism were all secondary to tissue damage due to sickling. The postoperative pain of cholecystectomy and the neuropathic pain were secondary to therapeutic modalities and their complications. The headache following the motor vehicle accident and the postoperative pain following dental surgery were incidental and not primarily related to sickle cell disease.

Although for years this patient has been taking relatively high doses of meperidine, he has experienced no myoclonus or seizures to date. He consumes about 4000 mg of meperidine orally at home each week and requires up to 150 mg of meperidine parenterally every two hours when treated in the emergency department or hospital for acute painful episodes. He reported severe allergic side effects to morphine and refused to try opioids other than meperidine despite explanation of its potential neurological side effects.

Although acute painful episodes are the most common manifestations of sickle cell disease, it is important to keep in mind that patients are prone to develop other pain syndromes. The clinician should not assume that the complaints of a patient with sickle cell disease are just another painful crisis. Careful evaluation may reveal other complications that require different therapy, future monitoring, observation, and patient education and counseling.

4

The Acute Painful Episode

Pleasure is oft a visitant
But pain clings cruelly to us.
—John Keats, 1795–1821

Pleasure is an interval between two pains
—Sri Satya Sai Baba, 1926–

Although sickle cell disease is characterized by a myriad of complications (including cerebral vascular accidents, retinopathy, acute chest syndrome, septicemia, splenic sequestration, osteomyelitis, cholecystitis, priapism, and renal failure), the most common manifestation and the hallmark of the disease is the acute painful crisis or vaso-occlusive episode. About 90% of hospital admissions of patients with sickle cell disease are for the treatment of acute pain (Ballas 1995a; Brozovic et al. 1987). Children and adolescents experience pain and miss school because of painful episodes surprisingly often, and nearly 90% of their painful episodes are managed at home (Shapiro et al. 1995). Furthermore, an increased frequency and severity of painful episodes is associated with shortened survival (Platt et al. 1991). We thus would expect that acute sickle pain would be the target of active basic and clinical research to elucidate its pathophysiology and clinical syndromes. Unfortunately, although pain and its management is a major concern for patients and their families, it has not been a major focus for investigation by hematologists. Consequently, the molecular mechanisms that underlie the various clinical manifestations of acute sickle cell painful episodes are not well understood. Moreover, the frequency and severity of the various pain syndromes that complicate sickle cell disease are not well documented and have not been studied longitudinally.

It is generally believed that acute sickle pain is the result of vaso-occlusion that leads to local hypoxia, ischemia, and eventually tissue damage. Recent studies in animals and to a lesser extent in humans (suffering from postoperative pain, cancer pain, or neuropathic pain) have shown that tissue damage generates a variety of inflammatory mediators that activate or sensitize afferent nerve fibers and posterior horn cells of the spinal cord by different mechanisms that affect pain perception. This chapter will systematically review what is known about factors that emerge following tissue damage and might affect the severity, perception, clinical manifestations, and the signs and symptoms of pain during the evolution of acute sickle cell painful episodes.

PATHOPHYSIOLOGY

MOLECULAR MECHANISMS OF VASO-OCCLUSION

Vascular occlusion plays a pivotal role in explaining the clinical course of sickle cell disease (Powars 1990; Francis and Johnson 1991; Hebbel 1991; Serjeant 1992; Embury et al. 1994b; Kaul et al. 1996). It may involve both the microcirculation and the macrocirculation. The former underlies the acute sickle cell painful episode and the latter is associated with organ failure (Boros et al. 1976; Powars et al. 1978; Powars 1990; Serjeant 1992; Embury et al. 1994b; Reid et al. 1995).

The major pathophysiologic events that lead to microvascular occlusion (Fig. 1) are: (1) polymerization of deoxy Hb S, (2) generation of dense

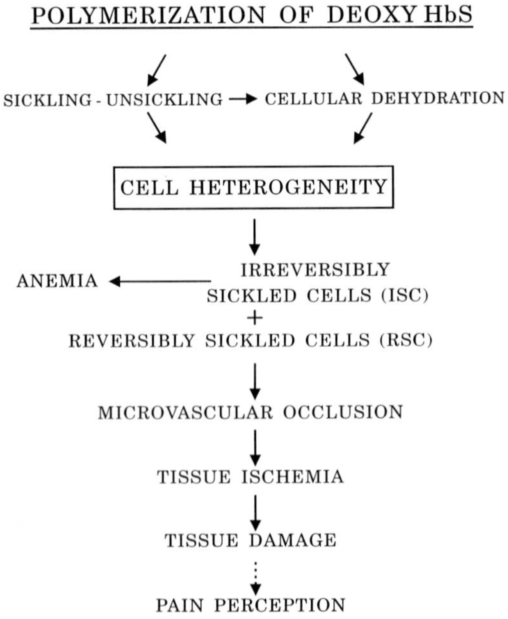

POLYMERIZATION OF DEOXY HbS

SICKLING - UNSICKLING → CELLULAR DEHYDRATION

CELL HETEROGENEITY

ANEMIA ◄——— IRREVERSIBLY SICKLED CELLS (ISC) + REVERSIBLY SICKLED CELLS (RSC)

MICROVASCULAR OCCLUSION

TISSUE ISCHEMIA

TISSUE DAMAGE

PAIN PERCEPTION

Fig. 1. Sequence of pathophysiologic events that lead to vaso-occlusion and consequent pain perception.

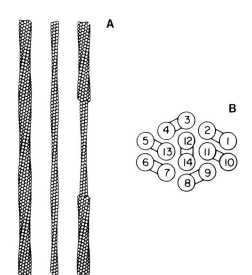

Fig. 2. A: Three-dimensional image reconstruction of deoxy Hb S fiber, a structure with a solid core, an inner core of four strands, and an outer sheath of 10 strands. Each sphere represents a tetramer of Hb S (Dykes et al. 1979 with permission). **B:** Schematic cross-section of the deoxy Hb S fiber showing the orientation of the 14 strands as described in A (Crepeau et al. 1981 with permission).

sickled cells, both reversibly and irreversibly sickled (RSC and ISC), (3) microvascular occlusion, (4) tissue ischemia, (5) tissue damage secondary to hypoxia, and (6) stimulation of peripheral nerve endings leading to pain perception (Powars 1990; Francis and Johnson 1991; Hebbel 1991; Embury et al. 1994b). Precise dynamics of these events and their interrelationships are complex and poorly understood.

The primary process responsible for microvascular occlusion is the polymerization of Hb S upon deoxygenation (Hofrichter et al. 1976; Edelstein 1981; Ferrone et al. 1985; Perutz 1976). Each polymerized strand consists of 14 fibers (Fig. 2) arranged in a helical fashion with an inner core of four strands surrounded by a sheath of 10 strands (Dykes et al. 1979; Crepeau et al. 1981). Upon deoxygenation an important hydrophobic bond forms between the β-6 valine of one tetramer and β-85 phenylalanine and β-88 leucine of the adjacent tetramer (Fig. 3), which leads to the generation of a nidus of polymerized Hb S (homogeneous nucleation). When 30 tetramers of deoxy Hb S aggregate, they generate a "critical nucleus" to which additional tetramers are added to produce stable polymer. This stable polymer provides the surface area necessary for the initiation of a second nucleation phase (heterogeneous nucleation) from which additional fiber formation can proceed (Fig. 4). As polymerization progresses more surface area becomes available for heterogeneous nucleation and the process becomes autocatalyic (Samuel et al. 1990). This double nucleation mechanism is responsible for shortening the lag time between the initiation of polymer nucleation and the exponential rise in polymer formation. The lag time is extremely sensitive to Hb concentration and is inversely proportional to the thirtieth power of Hb

Fig. 3. A schematic diagram of the deoxy Hb S crystal structure. The hemoglobin molecules consisting of two α-globin and two β-globin polypeptides are represented as circles. Some of the amino acid residues within an intermolecular contact region are indicated by arrows. Only one of the two mutant β6Val residues on each Hb S molecule is located within an intermolecular contact region. The middle right circle shows the mutant β6Val forming hydrophobic bonds with the β-85 phenylalanine and β-88 leucine of an adjacent tetramer (from Schecter et al. 1987 with permission).

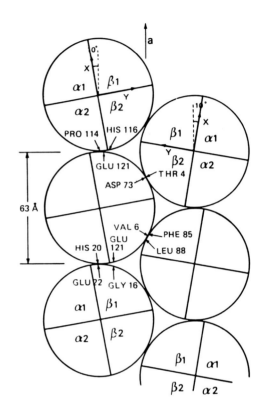

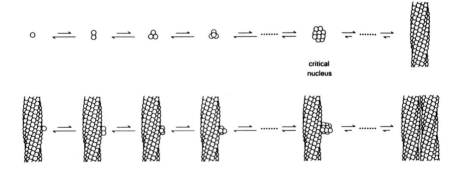

HOMOGENEOUS NUCLEATION

critical
nucleus

HETEROGENEOUS NUCLEATION

Fig. 4. Schematic model showing the polymerization and alignment of deoxy Hb S via homogenous and heterogeneous nucleation (Ferrone et al. 1985 with permission).

concentration (Samuel et al. 1990). Nevertheless, the lag time has to be shorter than the transit time of SS RBC through the microcirculation for sufficient Hb S polymer to form and rigidify the red cell during its transit through the capillaries to result in the occlusion by sickled RBC.

The rate and extent of intracellular polymerization of deoxy Hb S is a complex process and depends on several factors including the intracellular concentrations of Hb, the intracellular composition of Hb (percentage of other hemoglobin species such as Hb F, Hb C) the percentage of oxygen saturation, temperature, pH, ionic strength, and 2,3 diphosphoglycerate (DPG) (Briehl et al. 1973; Ross et al. 1975; Magdoff-Fairchild et al. 1976; Goldberg et al. 1977; Ross et al. 1977; Briehl 1978; Poillon and Bertles 1979; Gill et al. 1980; Sunshine et al. 1981). The generation of dense sickle cells seems to proceed via two mechanisms. The first involves repeated cycles of sickling-unsickling with deoxygenation and reoxygenation, respectively (Joiner 1993). With each cycle the red cell loses membrane, becomes dehydrated, rigid, fragmented, less deformable, and eventually assumes an irreversibly sickled shape (ISC). Cells generated by this mechanism show great heterogenicity in size, shape, and Hb concentration. These cells are rigid, have decreased life span, show positive correlation with the severity of the anemia, and may contribute to vaso-occlusion. The second mechanism by which dense cells are produced postulates that these cells can be generated directly from sickle reticulocytes without going through repeated cycles of deoxygenation and reoxygenation (Lew et al. 1991). Cells generated by this mechanism tend to be reversibly sickled (RSC) and do not exhibit the morphological abnormalities associated with the ISC. In most patients both mechanisms seem to be operative.

The above sequence of events is supported by in vitro experiments showing that slow deoxygenation of sickle cells generates the classic crescent shape, while rapid deoxygenation results in a granular appearance with no projections from the cell surface (Fig. 5).

Microvascular occlusion will occur whenever intracellular and extracellular conditions promote the generation of sufficient numbers of dense sickle cells with polymerized hemoglobin capable of blocking capillaries. These conditions include, but are not limited to: (1) increased numbers of dense SS RBC that contain polymerized Hb S even at arterial oxygen saturation (Noguchi and Schechter 1981) and thus reduce the lag time for Hb S polymerization during their transit through the microcirculation (Eaton and Hofrichter 1987); (2) rapid deoxygenation that results in the formation of extensive Hb S polymer without classic morphologic sickling (which may explain the selective trapping of dense SS RBC containing Hb S polymers but without morphologic sickling; Kaul et al. 1989); and (3) situations that

Fibers   **Cells**

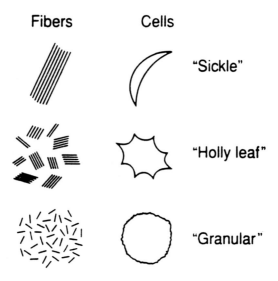

"Sickle"

"Holly leaf"

"Granular"

Fig. 5. Effect of the rate of deoxygenation on the shape of sickled cells. Slow deoxygenation (top) generates the classic sickle cell morphology due to the formation of single domain of well-aligned fibers. Intermediate rates of deoxygenation (middle) result in the formation of smaller domains of shorter aligned fibers and the "holly leaf" morphology of sickle cells. Rapid deoxygenation (bottom) generates multiple domains with randomly oriented fibers resulting in a granular appearance with no projections from the cell surface (Eaton and Hofrichter 1987 with permission).

prolong the transit time through the microcirculation such as increased SS RBC adhesion to the endothelium and altered vascular tone.

MOLECULAR MECHANISMS OF PAIN

Noxious stimuli elicited by tissue damage initiate a complex series of biochemical, neurological, and electrochemical events collectively referred to as nociception (Fields 1987; Katz and Ferrante 1993; Wall and Melzack 1994). Nociceptors are primary afferent nerves with peripheral terminals that can respond differentially to tissue-damaging stimuli. Although the pathophysiologic events that lead to the sensation of pain in sickle cell disease have not been directly studied, circumstantial evidence implicates the noxious stimuli that activate nociceptors after ischemic tissue injury and the consequent microinfarcts resultant from vaso-occlusion due to sickling (Fig. 1). Nociception involves four major pathophysiologic processes (Fields 1987; Katz and Ferrante 1993): transduction, transmission, modulation, and perception. Major features of these processes and their probable relevance to sickle cell disease are described below and illustrated in Fig. 6.

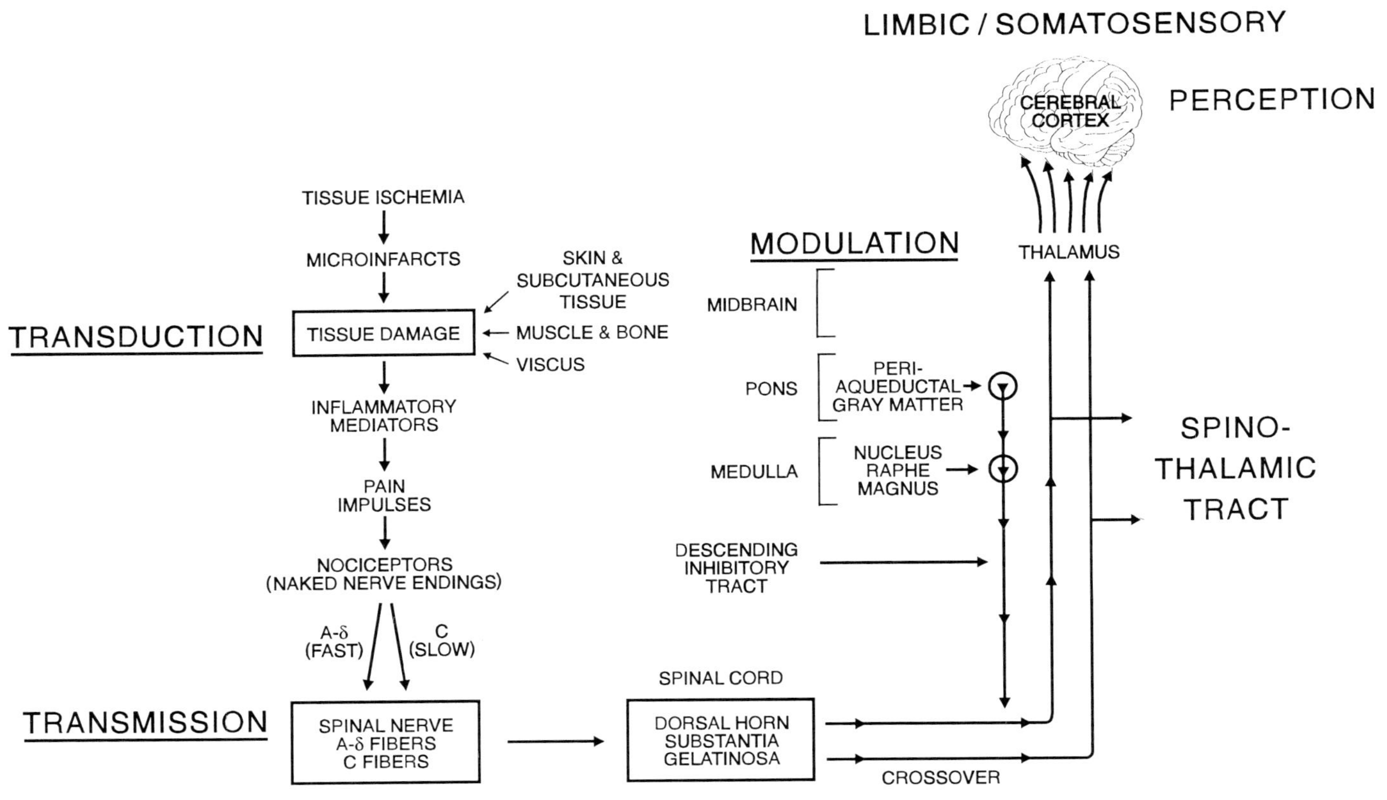

Fig. 6. Anatomic pathways of pain in sickle cell disease (modified from Ballas 1994b with permission).

Transduction

Transduction is the process whereby noxious stimuli activate nociceptors by converting one form of energy (chemical, mechanical, or thermal) to an electrochemical impulse in the primary afferents. Information about the noxious stimulus is coded by impulse frequency, a form that is accessible to the brain for decoding and interpreting the message as a painful experience. Fig. 7 is an oversimplified scheme showing vascular occlusion due to sickling with consequent microinfarcts and pain (Ballas 1995b). Tissue infarction secondary to sickling initiates a secondary inflammatory response. The latter may enhance sympathetic activity and trigger release of norepinephrine (Levine and Taiwo 1994), which causes more pain and creates a vicious circle. This combination of ischemic tissue damage and secondary inflammatory response may explain the acuteness and severity of the pain of sickle cell disease.

Fig. 8 illustrates the major pain modulators that are generated by tissue injury and the consequent inflammatory response. Tissue ischemia and associated inflammation cause the release of algesic chemical mediators that activate and sensitize nociceptors (Fields 1987; Cousins 1989, 1994; Katz and Ferrente 1993; Levin and Taiwo 1994; Wall and Melzack 1994). Interleukin-1 (IL-1) is an endogenous pyrogen and also activates the cyclooxygenase gene, which leads to synthesis of prostaglandins E_2 and I_2. Bradykinin, potassium and hydrogen ions, and serotonin activate nociceptive afferent nerve fibers and evoke a pain response. Prostaglandins, leukotrienes, nerve growth factor, and bradykinin sensitize peripheral nerve end-

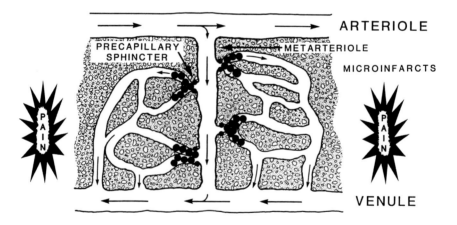

Fig. 7. Impairment of microcirculation by sickle RBC. Adhesion of sickle RBC causes vascular occlusion with consequent hypoxia and tissue damage secondary to microinfarcts that initiate the acute painful episode. Arrows indicate the direction of blood flow (Ballas 1995a with permission).

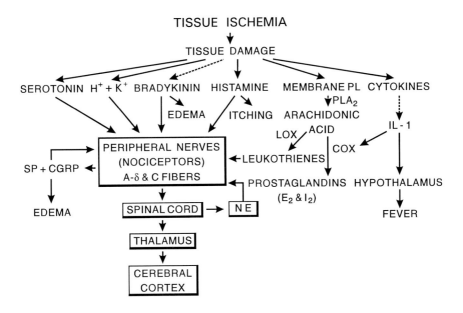

Fig. 8. Pain pathways. Tissue damage results in the release of numerous inflammatory mediators that initiate the production of noxious stimuli. These activate peripheral nerves which, in turn, transmit painful stimuli to the central nervous system (modified from Ballas 1995a with permission).

ings and facilitate the transmission of painful stimuli that reach the cerebral cortex via the spinal cord and the thalamus. Moreover, activated nociceptors release stored substance P in peripheral nerves and in the spinal cord, which itself facilitates the transmission of painful stimuli. Bradykinin and substance P also cause vasodilation with extravasation of fluids that can lead to local swelling and tenderness.

Transmission

Transmission is the process by which electrical impulses, carrying coded information about noxious stimuli, are relayed to and through the central nervous system to brain regions where pain sensation is generated. The neural pathways established in transmission include primary afferent nociceptor nerves, the dorsal horn cells giving rise to spinothalamic tracts, and thalamocortical projections.

Primary afferent nociceptors (PANS) are involved in both transduction and transmission. Several subtypes of somatic PANS are located in skin, subcutaneous tissue, muscles, and joints. These subtypes are defined by their microscopic appearance, conduction velocity, and pattern of response to chemical, thermal, and mechanical stimuli. Visceral PANS are found in the gastrointestinal tract, cardiopulmonary system, and genitourinary tract and are activated by irritation, torsion, traction, and distention, particularly in conjunction with inflammation. Impulses generated by visceral nociceptors are conducted via splanchnic nerve fibers.

Impulses generated by activation of nociceptors are conducted by specific fibers within peripheral nerves, as shown in Fig. 6 (Fields 1987; Wall and Melzack 1994). Table I summarizes the characteristics of these nerve fibers, which are classified into three major types (A, B, and C) according to size and conduction velocity of noxious stimuli. The $A\delta$ and C fibers are most important in transmitting the painful stimuli of sickle cell pain crises.

The $A\delta$ fibers are thin myelinated fibers, about 50% of which respond to noxious mechanical, thermal, or chemical stimuli. The $A\delta$ fibers elicit sharp, localized pain. In contrast, C fibers, conducting at less than 2 m/sec, are unmyelinated, respond to mechanical, thermal, and chemical stimuli, and elicit dull, diffuse pain sensation.

Nociceptive stimuli from the neck and below are transmitted along afferent neurons of the spinal nerves; pain stimuli above the second cervical segment are transmitted by sensory fibers in the Vth, VIIth, IXth, and Xth cranial nerves. These nerves enter the brain stem, become associated with the sensory nucleus of the trigeminal nerve, and synapse with second-order neurons in the dorsal horn of the upper cervical spinal cord (Bonica 1977; Payne 1987). Subsequent transmission of these stimuli is similar to that described below.

Central pain mechanisms involve the dorsal horn of the spinal cord, ascending spinothalamic tracts, and the cerebral cortex. The dorsal horn region of the spinal cord receives pain stimuli from the $A\delta$ and C fibers of the spinal nerves (and cranial nerves as described above) via the dorsal root

Table I
Characteristics of primary afferent nociceptors

Type	Stimulus	Conduction Velocity (m/sec)	Diameter (µm)	Sensation
Aβ	Mechanical, motor, pressure, proprioception	30–70	5–15	Sharp pain, allodynia
Aδ	Mechanical, thermal, nociception	5–30	1–4	Sharp, localized pain
C	Mechanical, thermal, chemical	0.2–1.5	0.5–1.5	Dull, diffuse pain

ganglion (Fig. 6). Afferent fibers that enter the spinal cord laterally in the dorsal root bifurcate, ascend and descend in the Lissauer's tract, and synapse in the dorsal horn, a complex structure consisting of six laminae, with lamina I the most dorsal. Each lamina corresponds to some of the horn's anatomic and functional characteristics. Cells in laminae I, II, and V respond preferentially to noxious stimuli. Laminae II and III constitute the substantia gelatinosa, where nociceptive and non-nociceptive input into the spinal cord are integrated (Melzack and Wall 1965, Wall and Melzack 1994).

Primary afferent nociceptors form synaptic connections with neurons in laminae I, II, and V in the dorsal horn. Some of these dorsal horn neurons cross over to form the contralateral spinothalamic tract. This tract sends connections to the brain stem, hypothalamus, and the thalamus. Some thalamic relay neurons connect to limbic forebrain structures associated with the emotional aspect of pain (Fig. 6). Besides the spinothalamic tract, other afferent systems such as the spinoreticular and spinomesencephalic tracts provide ascending pathways for noxious stimuli.

The role of the cerebral cortex in pain perception is controversial. Some reports indicate that large lesions of the somatosensory cortex do not alter pain, while others state that small cortical lesions ablate pain perception. Recent functional imaging studies have clearly implicated somatosensory and limbic system-related neocortex in human pain perception (Casey 1994).

Modulation

Modulation is the process by which several neural mechanisms modify the transmission of nociceptive stimuli. These mechanisms may enhance or inhibit the transmission of noxious stimuli (Table II). Pain modulation occurs at the level of the dorsal horn of the spinal cord. Proposed neural mechanisms include segmental sensory inputs and the descending inhibitory tract.

According to the gate control theory introduced by Melzack and Wall (1965), transmission of nerve impulses from afferent fibers to the transmission cells of the spinal cord is controlled by a gating mechanism located in the dorsal horn. The closing and opening of the gate is determined by the relative amount of activity in small (C, Aδ) and large (Aβ) fibers. When the effects of activity of the large (Aβ) fibers is greater than that of the small C and Aβ fibers, the gate closes and inhibits further transmission of afferent pain impulses. Conversely, when small-fiber activity predominates, the gates open and facilitate transmission of pain impulses.

The supraspinal descending neural systems have a considerable modulating influence on dorsal horn pain transmission neurons (Basbaum 1983;

Table II
Major endogenous neurotransmitters and their
effect on pain transmission

Neurotransmitter	Effect on Pain Transmission
Substance P	Excitation
L-Glutamate	Excitation
Somatostatin	Excitation
Norepinephrine	Inhibition (central)
	Excitation (peripheral?)
Serotonin	Inhibition (central)
Opioid peptides	
Enkephalin	Inhibition
β-Endorphin	Inhibition
Dynorphin	Inhibition

Basbaum and Fields 1984). One such pathway begins in the periaqueductal gray matter (Fig. 6) of the midbrain and descends to the nucleus raphe magnus, from which long fibers descend via the dorsolateral funiculus to terminate in laminae I, II, and V of the dorsal horn, where they modulate afferent nociceptive impulses. Both electrical stimulation and opiate micro-injection of the periaqueductal gray matter result in analgesia; both of these forms of analgesia are abolished by naloxone.

PREDISPOSING FACTORS

The clinical manifestations of sickle cell syndromes vary widely from one patient to another and in the same patient over time. Some patients with sickle cell anemia, for example, have mild disease while others suffer from a severe form and die at a relatively young age. Some patients may have a clinical picture characterized by waxing and waning of the frequency and severity of painful episodes. Francis and Johnson (1991) have reviewed the following factors proposed as indicators of the severity and frequency of the vaso-occlusive episodes.

GENETIC FACTORS

Fetal hemoglobin (Hb F)

There is a reasonable consensus that a very high level of fetal hemoglobin (Hb F) and its pancellular distribution is associated with a milder clinical picture of sickle cell anemia. Patients from eastern Saudi Arabia who had markedly elevated Hb F (18–25% of total Hb) had a relatively mild disease course (Perrine et al. 1972, 1978). Even small increments of Hb F level have an ameliorating effect on the frequency of painful crises and may ultimately improve survival (Platt et al. 1991). High levels may decrease the severity of certain sickle cell syndromes (Jackson et al. 1961; Perrine et al. 1972, 1978; Wrightstone and Huisman 1974; Serjeant 1975; Wood et al. 1980) because Hb F inhibits polymerization of Hb S during the sickling process (Cheetham et al. 1979; Nagel et al. 1979; Nibu and Adachi 1985). In vitro polymer studies of Hb S and F demonstrated that FS hybrids are excluded from nuclei formation and possibly from the sickling process in vivo (Goldberg et al. 1977; Nagel et al. 1979; Nibu and Adachi: 1985). To exert maximal beneficial effect on the painful crisis, Hb F level must be very high, usually above 20% of total hemoglobin (Powars et al. 1984; Steinberg and Hebbel 1984).

These encouraging findings have paved the way for identification of pharmacologic agents to increase the synthesis of Hb F in vivo. Hydroxy-urea is one such agent that has effectively decreased the frequency of painful episodes (see Chapter 12). It must be emphasized, however, that these are patients with very low Hb F level (< 2%) with mild disease and patients with high Hb F level (> 20%) and severe disease (Ballas et al. 1988; Ballas 1991). Other factors, therefore, must be involved in determining the final outcome of the clinical picture in certain patients with sickle cell anemia.

α-Thalassemia

The effect of α-gene deletion on the clinical expression of sickle cell anemia has attracted much interest in recent years. Table III lists the effects of α-thalassemia on certain aspects of sickle cell anemia. Undoubtedly, the coexistence of α-thalassemia with sickle cell anemia in adults has a beneficial effect on the anemia itself (Embury et al. 1982; Higgs et al. 1982; De Ceulaer et al. 1983; Ballas et al. 1988). In addition, there is some agreement that α-gene deletion does not affect the frequency and severity of the painful

Table III
Effect of α-thalassemia on the clinical
expression of sickle cell anemia

Higher Hb and hematocrit levels
Higher incidence of avascular necrosis
Higher incidence of retinopathy
Splenomegaly
No effect on frequency of painful crises
Less tissue damage

sickle cell crisis (Steinberg and Hebbel 1984; Steinberg et al. 1984; Ballas et al. 1988; Mukherjee et al. 1997). Other investigators (Billet et al. 1986; Bailey et al. 1991; Gill et al. 1995), however, reported paradoxical increase of painful crises in patients with SS and α-thalassemia.

A significant positive correlation exists between α-gene deletion and the prevalence and extent of avascular necrosis in patients with sickle cell anemia (Ballas et al. 1989b, 1997; Milner et al. 1991). Thus, patients with sickle cell anemia who are also homozygous for α-thal 2 thalassemia (–α/–α) have the highest incidence of avascular necrosis (Fig. 9). Similarly, the incidence of retinopathy may be increased in this subset of patients (Steinberg et al. 1984). The effect of α-gene deletion on tissue damage, however, remains controversial. Higgs and colleagues (1982) found less frequent acute chest syndrome and leg ulcers in Jamaican children with homozygous α-thal-2 (–α/–α). This finding, however, could not be confirmed by Steinberg and associates (1984) in a subset of their African American patients. Koshy et al. (1989) reported decreased incidence of leg ulcers with α-gene deletion. Powars and colleagues (1990b) reported decreased incidence of tissue damage (cerebrovascular complications, acute chest syndrome, nephropathy, and leg ulcers) in patients with sickle cell anemia and α-thalassemia.

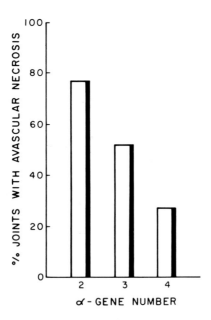

Fig. 9. Effect of α-globin gene number on avascular necrosis in sickle cell anemia. Patients with two α genes have the highest prevalence of avascular necrosis. There is significant negative correlation between the α-gene number and the prevalence of avascular necrosis (Ballas et al. 1989b with permission).

β-Thalassemia

The co-inheritance of a gene for β-thalassemia with one for Hb S results in the compound heterozygous state of Hb S-β-thalassemia. It is generally believed that Hb S-β°-thalassemia (with no Hb A) and Hb S-β⁺-thalassemia (with some Hb A) are less severe than sickle cell anemia alone. The report of the Cooperative Study of Sickle Cell Disease (CSSCD; Platt et al. 1991), however, indicated that patients with Hb S-β°-thalassemia had, on the average, similar frequency of painful episodes as patients with sickle cell anemia. Some patients with Hb S-β⁺-thalassemia may have more frequent painful crises than do some patients with sickle cell anemia or Hb S-β°-thalassemia.

Double heterozygosity

The co-inheritance of a gene for Hb C with a gene for Hb S results in the compound heterozygous state of Hb SC disease. Table IV lists major differences between sickle cell anemia and Hb SC disease. Erythrocytes in Hb SC disease (in the absence of α-thalassemia) are unique in that they are microcytic and hyperchromic (Ballas and Kocher 1988). A possible cause is cellular dehydration resulting from the interaction of Hb C with the inner surface of the red cell membrane. Patients with Hb SC disease have milder anemia, fewer painful crises, more splenomegaly, less priapism, less renal failure, and fewer leg ulcers than do patients with sickle cell anemia. Hb SC disease, however, increases the risk of retinopathy, thromboembolic disease, and renal papillary necrosis (Ballas et al. 1982). Occasionally, some patients with Hb SC disease may have a higher incidence of painful crises than do some patients with sickle cell anemia.

Table IV
Characteristics of Hb SC disease
in comparison to sickle cell anemia

Features that are milder in Hb SC
Anemia and its sequelae
Frequency of painful crisis
Asplenia
Priapism
Renal failure
Leg ulcers
Features that are more severe in Hb SC
Retinopathy
Thromboembolic complications
Renal papillary necrosis

Other doubly heterozygous states such as Hb SO Arab and Hb SD generally seem to have a milder clinical expression than sickle cell anemia, with a few exceptions. One exception is Hb S Antilles, which is characterized by a double mutation in the β chain ($\beta^{6\ Glu \rightarrow val,\ 23\ val \rightarrow Ile}$) and the same electrophoretic mobility as Hb S but a distinct pattern shown by isoelectric focusing. This Hb has lower solubility than Hb S and produces a sickling disorder in the carriers of the Hb A/S Antilles trait (Monplaisir et al. 1986).

β-Haplotypes

Kan and Dozy (1978) described a polymorphism in the DNA sequence in an Hpa 1 restriction enzyme site 3′ to the β-globin locus and showed that it is associated with the β^S gene. Their report was followed by the discovery of multiple-sequence polymorphisms within and around the β-globin gene cluster (Antonarakis et al. 1982). Linked groups of these polymorphisms, called haplotypes, are useful markers for genetic analysis and allow the identification and tracing of gene flow within populations (Kan and Dozy 1980; Antonarakis et al. 1982; Orkin et al. 1982). Nagel et al. (1985) studied subjects with sickle cell anemia from Atlantic West Africa (Senegal), Central West Africa (Benin), and the Central African Republic (CAR) and found that different β haplotypes, which they called Senegal, Benin, and Bantu (or CAR), were predominant in these areas. The effect of these β haplotypes on the clinical expression of sickle cell anemia remains highly controversial. According to one study Senegalese subjects had higher levels of Hb F and Gγ chains and fewer dense and irreversibly sickled red blood cells compared to subjects from Benin (Labie et al. 1985). These investigators proposed that the level of Hb F and the proportion of Gγ chains in Hb F were linked to specific haplotypes. Others (Gilman and Huisman 1985; Hattori et al. 1986; Ballas et al. 1991), however, showed that the correlation between the Senegalese haplotype and Hb F level is weak and that the presence of a polymorphic site for the restriction enzyme XmnI, 5′ to the Gγ gene, was associated with positive and significant correlation with the expression of Gγ chains. Moreover, the Senegalese haplotype is almost always associated with the presence of the XmnI polymorphic site. Rieder et al. (1991), in a retrospective study, found that β haplotypes had no effect on the hematological and clinical features of sickle cell anemia. In another prospective study, Powars et al. (1991) found that the risk for sickle cell renal failure increased in patients who had inherited the CAR β haplotype. Steinberg et al. (1995) found that gender and β haplotypes together affect the hematological manifestation of adult sickle cell anemia. Thus, women had higher levels of Hb F than did men with the same haplotype and females who were homozygous for the

Senegalese haplotype had the highest values of Hb F. This study, however, did not explore the effect of haplotypes on the clinical picture.

CELLULAR FACTORS

Degree of anemia

As mentioned above, the coexistence of α-thalassemia with sickle cell anemia results in milder anemia than otherwise but does not affect the frequency of painful crises. Moreover, there is a direct relation between the frequency of painful crises and the hematocrit value irrespective of the presence or absence of α-thalassemia (Baum et al. 1987; Platt et al. 1991). Thus, painful episodes are more frequent in patients with relatively mild anemia than in those with severe anemia. This association indicates a dichotomy between clinical severity and hematological severity. The higher blood viscosity of the patients with milder anemia may accentuate the severity of vaso-occlusion, and hence, frequency of painful crises.

Adhesion

Adhesion of sickle erythrocytes to the endothelium, a phenomenon first suggested by Hebbel et al. (1980a,b), also seems to contribute to vaso-occlusive crises. Sickle erythrocytes adhere to cultured endothelial cell layers, while normal red cells do not. This property of sickle cells may be related to an abnormal distribution of negative charges on the surface of sickle erythrocytes (Hebbel et al. 1980b), although other investigators have found no abnormality in the distribution of surface charge (Clark et al. 1981). Both cellular and plasma factors affect the property of adhesion of sickle red cells to vascular endothelium. Thus, young deformable sickle erythrocytes are more adherent to vascular endothelium than are dense, rigid, irreversibly sickled cells (Mohandas and Evans 1984; Barbarino et al. 1987; Kaul et al. 1989). Plasma factors that enhance adhesion include fibrinogen, Factor VIII, fibronectin, hyperosmolarity, and von Willebrand's factor. Moreover, endothelial injury facilitates cell adherence.

Given that fibrinogen is an acute phase reactant, it is reasonable to postulate that changes in the plasma environment of sickle erythrocytes, such as occur during infection, may precipitate vaso-occlusive crises. Moreover, endothelial cells infected with herpes simplex virus type I express Fc receptor glycoprotein that recognizes the increased amounts of IgG on sickled red cells with consequent enhancement of erythrocyte adherence to the infected endothelium (Hebbel et al. 1987). This sequence of events may explain the precipitation of painful crises by viral infection. According to

Hebbel et al. (1980a, 1981) the adherence of sickle red cells to endothelium correlates with the clinical vaso-occlusive severity of the disease, and changes in the extracellular environment may precipitate painful episodes by the sudden facilitation of erythrocyte/endothelial interactions. However, there is no consensus that adhesiveness of sickle red cells to vascular endothelium contributes to the clinical picture of the disease.

Rheology

Determinants of RBC rheological properties include the number of dense cells, the number of irreversibly sickled cells (ISC), and RBC deformability. These three factors seem to be interdependent. Thus, the higher the number of dense cells (or ISC) the lower the RBC deformability and vice versa. Recent reports have indicated a paradoxical effect of the rheological properties of RBC on the clinical picture of sickle cell anemia. Traditionally, it has been thought that a low percentage of ISC, a low percentage of dense cells, and a high degree of deformability are beneficial factors and should ameliorate the severity of sickle cell anemia. It turns out that these factors have the opposite effect. Thus, Billet et al. (1986) found that the percentage of dense red cells does not predict the incidence of sickle cell painful crises. Patients (both adults and children) who have decreased cell deformability and increased number of ISC and dense cells have mild disease in respect to the painful crisis (Ballas et al. 1988; Lande et al. 1988). In a recent study (Ballas 1991) patients whose RBC deformability averaged 37% or less of control values and whose dense cells averaged 22% of total circulating cells had fewer painful crises, less mortality, higher incidence of leg ulcers, and lower incidence of urinary tract infection although their Hb F was relatively low. Moreover, this group of patients with low RBC deformability had lower hematocrit than did the group with high deformability, which confirmed the finding by others that the frequency of painful crises varies directly with the hematocrit. This subset of patients with relatively mild clinical expression of sickle cell anemia was given the acronym MIDDD Syndrome: Mild disease in respect to painful crises, Increased number of Dense cells, and Decreased red cell Deformability.

PRECIPITATING FACTORS

Similar to other acute episodes of illness, the sickle cell painful crisis has predisposing and precipitating factors. Table V lists the major factors that precipitate vaso-occlusive crises and their reported clinical effect on the

Table V
Precipitating factors of painful episodes

Factor	Reported Clinical Effect	References
Cold, including cold weather, air conditioning, and swimming in cold water	Associated with increased frequency of pain crises	Baum et al. 1987; Addae 1971; Ibrahim 1980; Amjad et al. 1974; Serjeant et al. 1978; Stevens et al. 1981.
	No relationship between weather and crises	Diggs and Flowers 1971; Slovis et al. 1986; Seeler 1973b
Infection	Often precedes painful crises	Paterson and Sprague 1959; Margolis 1951; Wright and Gardner 1960
Metabolic acidosis	Associated with painful crises	Barreras and Diggs 1964
Physical stress	Associated with painful crises	Diggs 1965
Emotional stress	Associated with painful crises	Nadel and Portadin 1977
Menstruation	No clear relationship	Samuels-Reid and Scott 1985
Pregnancy and postpartum	Associated with increased incidence of vaso-occlusive episodes	Baum et al. 1987; Anderson et al. 1960; Hendrickse et al. 1972
Sleep apnea	Associated with painful crises	Scharf et al. 1983; Sidman and Fry 1988

frequency of acute painful episodes. Stress (physical or emotional), infection, acidosis, sleep apnea, and pregnancy are associated with an increased incidence of painful episodes. Nevertheless, most painful episodes are not preceded by an obvious precipitating factor.

CLINICAL ANATOMY OF THE ACUTE PAINFUL EPISODE

CLINICAL FEATURES

The clinical features of the acute sickle cell painful episode vary with age and sex. The frequency of painful crises increases significantly in males aged 15 to 25 years (Serjeant 1992), whereas nonpregnant females show no age-related change (Baum et al. 1987). In Jamaican patients with sickle cell anemia the frequency and severity of painful crises decrease after age 30 and are rare after age 40 (Serjeant 1992). This change seems due to a true amelioration of disease and not simply the prolonged survival of mildly affected patients. In one large study of more than 3000 patients with sickle cell disease (Platt et al. 1991), pain occurred twice as often in sickle cell anemia than in Hb SC disease or sickle $-\beta^+$-thalassemia. In those who had between three and 10 painful episodes per year, 5% of patients accounted for 30% of crises. Nearly 40% of patients did not have a pain episode in any given year (Platt et al. 1991). In another patient population, approximately 20% experienced frequent pain episodes that occurred weekly or monthly; about 50% had occasional painful events, while the remainder rarely or never had pain (Vichinsky et al. 1982). Some adults have pain daily with acute exacerbations, but the causes are not well understood. Pain rates are highest between ages 19 to 39 years; in persons over 20 years mortality was highest in those with the most painful episodes (Platt et al. 1991). Children may experience painful episodes as early as 6 to 9 months of age, perhaps related to the rate of decline of the Hb F level (Serjeant 1992). Sickle cell dactylitis occurs in children under the age of 5 years and may be among the first signs of disease, but for some patients painful episodes do not commence until adolescence or early adulthood. The rate of pain varies directly with the hemoglobin level and inversely with the percentage of Hb F (Platt et al. 1991).

Despite extensive reports on basic aspects of sickle cell disease, there has been an embarrassing dearth of information on clinical details of acute painful episodes. Diggs (1965) briefly but accurately described the clinical features of a typical painful crisis. He reported that patients are awakened early in the morning with severe pain in the low back or in one or more joints or bones of the extremities. The pain may be localized or migratory, and is continuous and throbbing. Severe pain causes patients to grunt, groan, cry, twist and turn, and to assume abnormal postures in the futile attempt to obtain relief; descriptors of pain include "gnawing me down," "cutting me to pieces," or "like a toothache."

Serjeant et al. (1994) conducted a prospective study of the onset of perceived precipitating factors, associated symptoms, and pain associated in sickle cell anemia in 183 painful episodes in 118 patients admitted to a day care center in Kingston, Jamaica. Painful crises developed most frequently between 3 P.M. and midnight, most commonly affected patients aged 15–29 years, affected the sexes equally, and were not obviously influenced by the menstrual cycle. Of the perceived precipitating factors, skin cooling was reported by one-third of the patients, a finding consistent with the steal syndrome (Serjeant and Chalmers 1990; steal syndrome is defined as a reflex shunting of blood away from the bone marrow in response to cutaneous cooling, thus explaining the commonly observed bilateral and symmetrical distribution of acute sickle cell painful episodes). Pain affected the lumbar spine in 49%, abdomen in 32%, femoral shaft in 30%, and knees in 21%. Limb and rib pain occurred with a highly significant excess of bilateral involvement. Contrary to previous impressions, recurrent episodes of pain usually do not involve the same anatomic sites.

Ballas and Delengowski (1993) prospectively followed 23 adult African American patients (9 women and 14 men) with sickle cell anemia who were hospitalized during 60 acute painful episodes. Men accounted for 49 hospital admissions (82%). Painful areas of the body most frequently affected included the back, legs, knees, arms, chest, and abdomen in descending order. The words most often selected to describe the pain were throbbing, sharp, dull, and stabbing.

More studies are needed to characterize clinical details of the sickle cell acute painful episode. Unfortunately, the term painful episode or painful crisis is often used without further description, which erroneously implies that the episode is a constant and uniform clinical entity.

OBJECTIVE SIGNS

Table VI lists the most commonly reported objective signs. It should be noted, however, that published reports about the sickle cell painful crisis suffer, in general, from at least four limitations: (1) most reports are not comprehensive but are focused on a limited number of laboratory parameters; (2) some studies were not longitudinal but compared findings from a

Table VI
Reported objective signs of the sickle cell painful crisis

Clinical Signs	*Changes in Plasma Factors*
Fever	Coagulation/thrombosis parameters
Swelling and tenderness	Fibrinogen
Joint effusions	Factor VIII
Cellular Changes	Vw Factor
Red blood cells	Antithrombin III
Hyperhemolysis	Protein C
Irreversibly sickled cells (ISC)	Protein S
Dense cells	Fibrinopeptide A
Red cell distribution width (RDW)	D-dimer
Hemoglobin distribution width (HDW)	Acute-phase reactants
Red blood cell deformability	C-reactive protein
White blood cells	Serum amyloid A
Leukocytosis	Fibrinogen
Impairment of leukocyte function	Orosomucoid (α_1-acid glycoprotein)
Leukocyte alkaline phosphatase (LAP)	Serum enzymes
score	Lactic dehydrogenase
Changes in platelet count	Creatinine phosphokinase
Platelet activation	*Other Changes*
Decreased lifespan	Plasma viscosity
Platelet aggregation	Erythrocyte sedimentation rate (ESR)
	Endothelial cells

Note: The laboratory parameters listed increase, decrease, or demonstrate bimodal change during the evolution of the painful crisis, as illustrated in Fig. 10 and Table VIII.

cohort of patients in crisis to a different cohort in periods between crises; (3) lack of reliable intercrisis data prevented comparison with the findings during the crisis; and (4) not all investigators specified when during the crisis the observation was made. These problems may explain some of the apparently contradictory laboratory findings reported to be associated with the painful crisis.

Clinical signs

Severe painful crises usually involve mild to severe pyrexia up to 101°F (38.3°C), and sometimes higher. Pyrexia develops after the onset of pain and gradually declines as the severity decreases (Diggs 1965; Ballas et al. 1988; Serjeant 1992). In one study (Ballas et al. 1988) 21% of the painful episodes that required hospitalization were accompanied by fever of 100°F (37.8°C) or higher in the absence of infection, and another nearly 15% of the crises were associated with other objective signs such as swelling, tenderness, or vomiting. Passage of dark urine is a common complaint and may reflect increased urinary porphyrin excretion (Neuman et al. 1966). Painful crises may also be associated with joint effusions (Schumacher et al. 1973; Schumacher 1975; De Ceulaer et al. 1984; Serjeant 1992). Aspirates from these joints are usually sterile and noninflammatory and are thought to result from necrosis of marrow that is adjacent to the synovial membranes or from congestion and vascular thrombosis of the small vessels of the synovium. Joint effusions may be mild and unilateral or severe and migratory (Mallory 1941; Brugsch 1944; Espinoza 1974). These signs of the painful crisis reflect the accumulation of inflammatory mediators such as bradykinin and substance P that are known to cause local pain, vasodilatation, extravastion of fluids, and edema (Miller 1975). A controlled longitudinal study that documents the clinical sequence of events that occur during the painful crisis is needed to clarify the relation of tissue ischemia to the progression of the inflammatory response.

Other clinical signs include tenderness or pressure over affected sites, usually over bone rather than joints (Dorwart and Gebuzda 1985; Schumacher et al. 1990; Valeriano-Marcet and Kerr 1991). Acute urinary retention (Walker et al. 1980) and muscle swelling and tenderness due to myonecrosis may also occur.

Red cell changes

Reported red blood cell changes during the acute sickle cell painful episode have centered around the severity of the hemolytic anemia (total Hb levels), the percentages of irreversibly sickled cells (ISC) and dense cells, red cell distribution width (RDW), hemoglobin distribution width (HDW), and red cell deformability.

Hyperhemolyis

The combination of pain, jaundice, and increased urobilin content of the urine that is associated with sickle cell anemia is similar to the crises seen in congenital hemolytic anemia. Consequently, the recurrent episodes of illness that characterize sickle cell anemia are often referred to as hemolytic crises with the implication that these episodes are characterized by a drop in the level of total hemoglobin that accompanies pain. Sydenstricker (1924a,b,c, 1929) implied the presence of hyperhemolysis by noting that the anemia worsens and the reticulocyte count increases during the "active" phase of the disease. It was Diggs (1956), however, who observed that it is the "painful crisis" and not the hemolytic crisis that is the hallmark of the disease. Initially Diggs (1956) found no change in the total hemoglobin level during painful crises but later he (1965) indicated that hemolytic crises do complicate the clinical picture of sickle cell anemia and may be associated with painful crises. Sickle cell anemia is characterized by chronic hemolysis in the steady state, and most evidence suggests that hyperhemolysis characterized by decreased total Hb levels and increased reticulocyte count occurs in some patients during the evolution of the painful episode (Fabry et al. 1984). Ballas and Smith (1992) determined hematological parameters during 117 painful crises affecting 36 patients over five years and found that the Hb level decreased to a minimum on days five to six and the reticulocyte count reached a maximum on days six to seven. However, the report did not include concomitant values of other parameters of hemolysis such as bilirubin and serum lactate dehydrogenase (LDH).

Changes in dense cells and ISC

These two parametersISC and dense cellswill be discussed together because they vary directly (Clark et al. 1982; Ballas et al. 1988). The presence of irreversibly sickled cells in the peripheral blood of patients with sickle cell anemia is a hallmark of the disease. The percentage of these cells varies in different persons in the steady state (at least 2–4 weeks without a painful episode) but tends to remain constant in a given patient over time (Diggs 1965). Sydenstricker (1924a,b,c) noted that the "blood picture changes with considerable rapidity as the disease fluctuates" and that during crisis sickled cells may increase to 40% of the total RBC count and that, as the crisis resolves, sickled cells may disappear almost completely. Barreras and

Diggs (1964) noted that the percentage of multipointed sickled cells in venous blood increased with onset of pain and decreased as the pain subsided. Warth and Rucknagel (1984) used the technique of discontinuous Stractan density gradient ultracentrifugation of whole blood to compare ISC during episodes of painful crisis to pain-free episodes. They found an increased percentage of echinocytic ISC and echinocytic cells that were not ISC during crisis, and their replacement by normal-appearing dicocytes in the pain-free state. Fabry et al. (1984) noted a striking decrease in dense cells that was later found (Lawrence et al. 1985) to parallel a decrease in the RDW during painful crises. Careful examination of the data reported by Lawrence et al. (1985), however, reveals that in at least two patients an initial increase in the number of dense cells was followed by reduction as the painful crisis evolved. Our own experience (Ballas and Smith 1992) is that dense cells and ISC increase early, reach a maximum on day three of the painful episodes, and then decrease gradually to reach a minimum on day nine of the crisis (See also, Akinola et al. 1992). Both these studies indicate that the increase in dense cells typically precedes the onset of painful crisis by one or more days.

Other RBC changes during the painful crisis include alterations in the RDW, HDW, and the erythrocyte sedimentation rate (ESR). Both the RDW and the HDW decrease during the evolution of the painful crisis (Lawrence et al. 1985; Billet et al. 1988a; Ballas and Smith 1992). These parameters increase early in the crisis compared to steady-state values and later decrease as the crisis evolves. Furthermore, these changes coincide with changes in the percentage of dense cells and ISC. The ESR, which is typically low in the steady state with sickle cell anemia (Bunting 1939; Winsor and Burch 1944; Serjeant 1992), increases during the evolution of the painful crisis and reaches a maximum by day six to 13 (Lawrence and Fabry 1986; Buchanen et al. 1988). Lawrence and Fabry (1986) found that the low ESR in the steady state was not increased by substituting plasma from healthy control subjects, which suggests that the low ESR is an RBC-related phenomenon. When RBC taken from patients at the end of the sickle cell crisis were suspended in normal plasma from control subjects, the ESR remained high. Thus, it seems that the low ESR in the steady state and its increase during crisis are primarily related to RBC changes most likely secondary to the disappearance of dense cells, although the increase in serum fibrinogen level (vide infra) may be a contributing factor.

Changes in RBC deformability

Unlike the percentage of sickle cells during the evolution of sickle cell painful crisis, which is somewhat controversial, there is consensus on changes in the rheological properties of sickle RBC as the crisis develops. Thus, Rieber et al. (1977) found a uniform pattern in RBC rheology during the evolution of crises in eight patients. Comparison of data on the first and last days of hospitalization showed increased RBC filtrability and decreased percentage of sickled cells with recovery from crises. Unfortunately, however, they did not determine these parameters in the steady state for comparison. Kenny et al. (1985) showed that erythrocyte deformability was significantly reduced on day one of crisis in nine patients and 24 hours before the onset of pain in one additional patient. RBC filtrability gradually returned to precrisis values by day eight to nine. Lucas et al. (1985) showed that sickle cells have impaired filtrability on the second day of painful crisis in eight patients with sickle cell anemia and that the filtrability improved as the crisis resolved. Ballas and Smith (1992) expanded these observations by conducting longitudinal studies on 36 patients over five years and found that deformability was reduced early in the crisis and increased to values higher in the steady state as the crisis resolved. Akinola et al. (1992) found similar bimodal change in RBC deformability with decreased RBC filtrability compared to the steady state early in the crisis, and increased deformability in the last phase. Given that RBC deformability varies inversely with the number of ISC and dense cells (Mohandas et al. 1980; Ballas 1991) and that RBC deformability first decreases and later increases during the evolution of the painful crisis, it is logical to conclude that reciprocal changes in the percentage of dense cells occur as the painful crisis evolves.

Thus, the available data show that the following RBC changes occur during the evolution of the painful crisis: (1) hyperhemolysis occurs in some patients; (2) the percentages of dense cells, ISC, RDW, and HDW increase early in the crisis and then decrease as the crisis progresses; (3) RBC deformability decreases early in the crisis and later increases; and (4) these changes in RBC may occur one to three days before the onset of a typical painful crisis.

Changes in white blood cells

The white blood cell count increases during painful episodes to levels higher than those seen in the steady state (Buchanan and Glader 1978). This increase occurs in the absence of overt infection and may be secondary to the inflammatory response to ischemic tissue damage. If an infectious process complicates the painful crisis, the white cell count will increase further and be associated with bandemia (an increase in the percentage of band cells that are young or immature neutrophils). Some reports (Buchanan and Glader 1978) did not specify on which day of the crisis the leukocytosis was noted, but listed the white blood cell count only on the initial day of presentation. Billett et al. (1988b) reported no significant change in WBC count from steady state to painful crisis but a decrease from days 1–3 to days 6–9 of hospitalization. Akinola et al. (1992) indicated that the white blood cell count was elevated on day 1 of the crisis, reached a peak on days 3–5, and then decreased toward steady state values after the sixth day.

Besides change in the white cell count during crises, a few studies report impaired leukocyte function during the painful crisis (Walters and Reddy 1974; Kaplan and Nardi 1977; Akenzua and Amiegheme 1981; Lachant and Oseas 1987). Parameters of leukocyte function that were studied included phagocytosis, phagocytosis-associated activation of the hexose monophosphate shunt (HMS), hydrogen peroxide formation, microbicidal activity against *Staphylococcus aureus*, nitroblue tetrazolium (NTB) reduction, and chemotaxis. H_2O_2 production, chemotaxis, HMS activation, and microbicidal activity against *S. aureus* were decreased during crisis whereas phagocytosis per se and NTB reduction were unchanged. The significance of these findings is unclear and whether they contribute to the development of bacterial infections during the painful crisis in some patients needs further investigation.

The nature of the changes in the leukocyte alkaline phosphates (LAP) during the painful crisis is not settled. Wajima and Kraus (1975) and Rosner and Karayalcin (1974) reported that the LAP scores remain unchanged during the uncomplicated painful crisis. Closer examination of the data reported by Wajima and Kraus (1975), however, shows that although the mean LAP score remains within normal during the painful crisis, it is nevertheless significantly higher than the mean score in the steady state. Another report (Janis 1976) also indicated that the LAP score increases during the painful crisis in the absence of overt infection. Although the LAP score has not been related to a specific day of the crisis, all agree that the score increases further in the presence of infection.

Changes in platelets

Patients with sickle cell anemia usually have significantly increased platelet counts in the steady state with a mean value of 320×10^3 to 473×10^3 per μl (Green et al. 1970; Haut et al. 1973; Kenny et al. 1980). Green et al. (1970) and Billet et al. (1988a,b) reported that platelet counts did not change during painful episodes irrespective of the presence or absence of infection. Van der Sar (1970), however, reported that the platelet count increases to levels greater than 1.0×10^6/μl in patients recovering from crises. Gordon et al. (1974) studied 38 children and reported that the platelet count fell during painful episodes. Haut et al. (1973) showed that: (1) the life span of autologous platelets in three adult patients in crisis was one-third of normal; (2) the platelet count decreased during crisis; (3) marked rebound thrombocytosis to levels above those of the steady state occurred postcrisis (during the second week of onset); and (4) platelet aggregation was normal during crisis but increased postcrisis during the period of thrombocytosis. Alkjaersig et al. (1976) also showed transient decreases in platelet counts in adults during the first few days of the crisis with rebound thrombocytosis greater than in the steady state about two weeks after crisis onset. Stuart et al. (1974) found an impairment in the rate and percentage of first-phase platelet aggregation with ADP in 10 children with sickle cell anemia during vaso-occlusive crises as compared to their own baseline values and those of normal control subjects. They also demonstrated a concomitant decrease in platelet adhesiveness during painful episodes. Beurling-Harbury and Schade (1989) showed significant platelet activation with ADP release during acute sickle cell painful crises. This finding seems to be associated with decreased first-phase platelet aggregation with ADP reported by Stuart et al. (1974) because others (Rozenberg and Holmsen 1968) have shown that platelets incubated with ADP aggregate poorly on addition of more ADP, an observation referred to as the "platelet refractory state."

Discrepancies may have occurred among these studies in part because they were not performed serially but were based on random sampling at different times during the progression of the painful crisis. Nevertheless, there is some consensus that the platelet count decreases below the steady state during the first few days of the crisis with rebound thrombocytosis to values above the steady state after the first week of onset of the painful event.

Changes in hemostasis/thrombosis parameters

Studies of hemostasis and thrombosis during the sickle cell crisis focused on three major areas: (1) determination of changes, if any, in the concentration of certain coagulation factors; (2) investigation of thrombosis-associated parameters; and (3) checking the fibrinolytic activity.

Coagulation factors. Fibrinogen is an acute phase reactant and usually increases in response to an inflammatory or infectious process. Although most authors report elevated fibrinogen levels (Diggs 1965; Gordon et al. 1974), others find that they are unchanged during the painful crisis in comparison to the steady state (Fenichel et al. 1950; Mahmood 1969; Green et al. 1970). Most reports (Alkjaersig et al. 1976; Lawrence and Fabry 1986; Buchanan et al. 1988) indicate that fibrinogen levels rise during the progression of the crisis and consistently peak around the sixth or seventh day. This increase in fibrinogen was observed in the absence of demonstrable infection.

Changes in the levels of other coagulation factors have been reported by some but not all investigators who studied these parameters during painful events. Abildgaard et al. (1967) and Green et al. (1970) found no change in other clotting factors during the painful crisis, and Mackie et al. (1980) reported altered Factor VIII complexes in some patients in crisis. Richardson et al. (1979) reported elevated levels of Factor VIII:C, Factor VIIIR, Ag, and antithrombin III in the plasma of eight patients in the steady state and further increases when the patients were in painful crisis. Karayalcin and Lanzkowsky (1989) reported that plasma levels of protein C were low in children with sickle cell anemia in the steady state and fell even lower during episodes of vaso-occlusion, but increased to initial levels or higher postcrisis. They postulated that this decrease in protein C predisposes sickle cell patients to thrombotic events. Their findings, however, are not well supported by other investigators. Green and Scott (1986) and Terkonda et al. (1989) did find that protein C activity was decreased in patients with sickle cell anemia in the steady state but found no statistically significant difference between steady-state levels and those measured during painful episodes. Francis (1988) found normal mean levels of protein C activity in patients with sickle cell anemia both in the steady state and during vaso-occlusive episodes, but reported decreased levels of protein S (both total and free) in the steady state with no further decrease during crises.

Thrombosis-associated parameters. Green and Scott (1986) and Billet et al. (1988b) found no evidence of increased thrombotic activity during the evolution of the painful crisis in comparison to the steady state. Other investigators, however, reported that patients in vaso-occlusive crisis have evidence of increased thrombotic activity. Thus, Alkjaersig et al. (1976) reported that the onset of vaso-occlusive crisis is accompanied by an increase in plasma high-molecular-weight fibrinogen complexes. Fibrinopeptide A (FPA) levels have been used to measure coagulation activity in patients in painful crisis. FPA is produced by the action of thrombin on the alpha chain of fibrinogen and is the first fragment produced in the transformation of fibrinogen into fibrin (Nossel 1976). FPA has been reported to be normal in uncomplicated sickle cell anemia in the steady state but elevated during painful crisis (Leichtman and Brewer 1978; Benjamin 1986; Benjamin et al. 1985). Levels of Factors V and XIII are reduced in the steady state, consistent with ongoing thrombin activity (Ittyerah et al. 1976; Richardson et al. 1979), but no further decrease has been reported during vaso-occlusive episodes.

Fibrinolytic activity. There is also disagreement on the activity of the fibrinolytic system during the painful crisis. Some investigators (Mahmood et al. 1967; Mahmood 1969) found decreased fibrinolytic activity measured by euglobulin lysis time during the painful episode. Kwaan and Green (1973) demonstrated the presence of inhibitors of fibrinolysis during the crisis, also by measuring euglobulin lysis time. Devine et al. (1986) and Francis (1989), however, reported elevated levels of fibrin D-dimer during the painful crisis, which indicates increased fibrinolytic activity. The fibrin D-dimer fragment is produced by plasmin degradation of cross-linked fibrin and is an indirect indication of increased thrombin activity and fibrin formation. D-dimer levels were measured either by a latex agglutination assay (Devine et al. 1986) or an ELISA assay (Francis 1989) sensitive to D-dimer levels of less than 50 ng/ml. These assays are much more sensitive than the cumbersome euglobulin lysis time.

Recent studies, using sensitive assays of thrombosis/fibrinolysis markers, suggest that increased activity of the coagulation system may be important in the pathogenesis of vascular occlusion in sickle cell disease (Peters et al. 1994; Hagger et al. 1995). Together, available data indicate significant activation of coagulation, which may in part be due to reduced levels of the inhibitor proteins C and S, with consequent increase in fibrinolysis both in the steady state and during the sickle cell painful episode (Peters et al. 1994; Hagger et al. 1995). Devine et al. (1986) reported an elevation in fibrin D-dimer in patients with other complications of sickle cell anemia (leg ulcers, aseptic necrosis, etc.) in the absence of painful episodes. Moreover, the increase in some coagulation factors (fibrinogen and Factor VIII) may represent a response to an acute phase reaction. It is not clear whether the reported changes in coagulation are the result of microvascular occlusion or the cause that precipitates the painful events, although the former hypothesis seems more likely.

When present, frank disseminated intravascular coagulation (DIC) with thrombocytopenia, decreased fibrinogen, increased fibrin degradation products, and prolonged prothrombin and partial thromboplastin times in association with painful episodes usually indicate the presence of other complications such as septicemia, fat embolism, or multiorgan failure (Evans and Symnes 1975; McDonald and Eichner 1978). Corvelli et al. (1979), however, reported the presence of DIC in uncomplicated painful crisis in a patient with Hb SC disease. More controlled studies conducted serially are needed to elucidate the nature of the abnormality of the hemostatic and thrombotic parameters during the evolution of the painful crisis.

Other changes

Serum lactate dehydrogenase (LDH). Serum LDH exists as five separable isoenzymes numbered 1 to 5 according to their electrophoretic mobility from the anode (Neely et al. 1969). In normal human plasma serum LDH

1 and 2 predominate. LDH may rise following tissue injury, with the iso-enzyme pattern indicative of the damaged tissue. LDH1 and LDH2 are predominant in erythropoietic tissue. Serum LDH is usually elevated in sickle cell anemia in the steady state (Neely et al. 1969; White et al. 1978; Karayalcin et al. 1981; Roth et al. 1981). This finding reflects the chronic hemolytic state and the degree of elevation correlates with disease severity. Further increase in serum LDH level that is limited to LDH1 and LDH2 indicates that RBC are the source of the increased enzyme level. Neely et al. (1969) found that the increase in serum LDH is not correlated with plasma Hb level (which fluctuated widely); this finding indicates that the source of the LDH is not secondary to hemolysis but to tissue damage, most likely bone marrow infarction. In such situations the LDH value is greater than 1000 units. Akinola et al. (1992) noted that LDH increased during the crisis to a maxi-mum value on days 3–5 and then decreased.

Creatinine phosphokinase and myoglobin. Creatinine phosphokinase (CPK) and myoglobin (Mb) are abundant in muscle and an increase in their values indicates muscle injury. Billet et al. (1988b) reported dramatic in-crease in CPK levels on days 5–8 of the crisis as compared to the level on days 1–3, but it is not clear whether this increase was the result of the frequent intramuscular injections usually given to patients in crisis or the result of muscle injury or both. Roth et al. (1981) noted that plasma Mb increased during the painful crisis, but did not evaluate this increase in relation to the frequency of i.m. injections.

Acute-phase reactants. Acute-phase reactants measured during painful episodes include plasma fibrinogen, serum C-reactive protein (CRP), serum orosomucoid (α1-acid glycoprotein), and serum amyloid A (Richardson et al. 1979; Lawrence and Fabry 1986; Becton et al. 1989; Akinola et al. 1992). CRP and SAA increase and reach a peak on days 3–5 of the crisis, whereas serum orosomucoid, like fibrinogen, reaches a peak on days 6–7. The increase in these parameters a few days after the onset of pain suggests that they are markers of the secondary inflammatory response that ensues following ischemic tissue damage.

Plasma viscosity. Plasma viscosity increases during the painful crisis and reaches a peak after the sixth day (Richardson et al. 1979; Lawrence and Fabry 1986; Akinola et al. 1992), which suggests that this increase is, at least in part, secondary to the increase in plasma fibrinogen and decrease in the number of ISC.

Endothelial cells. Sowemimo et al. (1989) noted that circulating endo-thelial cells significantly increase during the painful sickle cell crisis, which they concluded may be the result of acute endothelial injury (Bouvier et al. 1970) during vaso-occlusive episodes. This finding is consistent with other reports (Klug et al. 1982; Russell et al. 1984) of changes indicative of endothelial damage in the cerebral and splenic vasculature of patients with sickle cell disease. Solovey et al. (1997) examined the viability, origin, and surface phenotype of circulating endothelial cells in the steady state and during painful episodes in patients with sickle cell anemia. They found that the mean number of circulating endothelial cells is significantly higher in patients with sickle cell anemia in the steady state than in normal controls. During painful crises, the number of circulating endothelial cells increases to levels significantly higher than those in the steady state. Moreover, endothelial cells in circulation are microvascular in origin and have an activated phenotype as evidenced by the expression of four adhesion molecules: intercellular adhesion molecule 1 (ICAM-1), vascular adhesion molecule-1 (VCAM-1), E-selectin, and P-selectin. These studies suggest that the vascular endothelium is activated in patients with sickle cell anemia and that adhesion proteins on activated endothelial cells may play a role in the vasculopathy of sickle cell disease (Solovey et al. 1997).

PHASES OF THE ACUTE PAINFUL EPISODE

The literature strongly suggests that the uncomplicated sickle cell painful crisis requiring hospitalization has four distinct phases: prodrome, initial phase, established phase, and resolving phase. Table VII and Fig. 10 show the temporal relation of these phases to the severity of pain, their synonyms and their typical estimated duration. Plotting all the observations reported in the literature on a specific day of the painful crisis, whenever applicable, shows that clinical and laboratory objective signs emerge along a certain pattern that is illustrated in Fig. 10 and listed in Table VIII.

Table VII
Phases of the acute sickle cell painful crisis

Phase	Possible Synonym(s)	Duration
Prodromal	Precrisis	Up to 2 days before crisis
Initial	First Evolving Infarctive	Days 1 and 2 of the crisis
Established	Second Postinfarctive Inflammatory	Days 3–7 of crisis
Resolving	Last Healing Recovery Postcrisis	Post day 7 of crisis

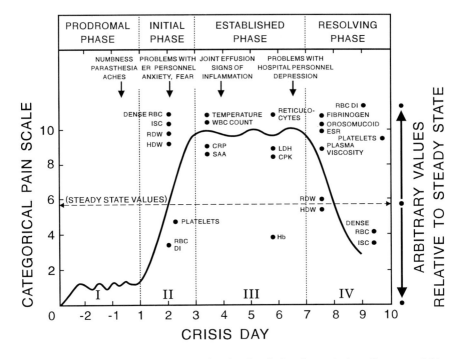

Fig. 10. A typical profile of the events that develop during the evolution of a severe sickle cell painful crisis in an adult in the absence of overt infection or other complications. Such events are usually treated in the hospital with an average stay of 9–11 days. Pain becomes most severe by day 3 of the crisis and starts decreasing by day 6 or 7. The Roman numerals refer to the phase of the crisis: I, prodromal phase; II, initial phase; III, established phase; and IV, resolving phase. Dots on the X axis indicate the time when changes became apparent and dots on the Y axis indicate the relative value of changes in comparison to the steady state indicated by the horizontal dashed line. Arrows indicate the time when certain clinical signs and symptoms may become apparent. Values shown are those reported at least twice by different investigators; values that were anecdotal, unconfirmed, or that were not reported to occur on a specific day of the crisis are not shown. Abbreviations: ISC, irreversibly sickled cells; RDW, red cell distribution width; HDW, hemoglobin distribution width; RBC DI, red cell deformability index; CRP, C-reactive protein; SAA, serum amyloid A; LDH, lactate dehydrogenase; CPK, creatinine phosphokinase; Hb, hemoglobin; ESR, erythrocyte sedimentation rate (Ballas 1995b with permission).

The prodromal phase

A premonition of painful crisis (prodromal or precrisis phase) was first mentioned by Diggs (1965), who noted that one mother could predict that her child would develop a painful crisis by noting that the "fingernails were pale." This observation was not pursued further until Murray and May (1988) used a structured questionnaire with 102 patients and reported that 58% experienced a prodromal phase of an impending painful crisis up to 24 hours before developing features typical of their usual crises (Fig. 10). Symptoms

Table VIII
Major changes in objective signs during the evolution of the sickle cell painful crisis

Prodromal Phase	Initial Phase	Established Phase	Resolving Phase
Decreasing	*Decreasing*	*Peak*	*Peak*
RBC deformability	RBC deformability	Temperature	Fibrinogen
	Platelets	WBC count	Orosomucoid
Increasing		Dense cells	ESR
Dense RBC	*Increasing*	ISC	
	Temperature	RDW	*Decreasing*
	WBC count	HDW	Temperature
	Dense cells	Reticulocytes	WBC Count
	ISC	LDH	Dense Cells
	RDW	CRP	ISC
	HDW	SAA	RDW
	ESR		HDW
	LDH	*Nadir*	CRP
	CRP	RBC deformability	
	Fibrinogen	Hb	*Increasing*
	Orosomucoid		RBC deformability
	SAA	*Increasing*	Plasma viscosity
		Fibrinogen	Platelets
		Orosomucoid	
		Plasma viscosity	
		ESR	

Note: Parameters shown are those reported at least twice by different investigators. ISC, irreversibly sickled cells; WBC, white blood cell; RDW, red cell distribution width; HDW, hemoglobin distribution width; ESR, erythrocyte sedimentation rate; LDH, lactate dehydrogenase; CRP, C-reactive protein; SAA, serum amyloid A; Hb, hemoglobin.

mentioned during the prodromal phase included numbness, aches, and paresthesia in the sites subsequently affected by pain. Akinola et al. (1992) studied 20 patients with sickle cell anemia over 16 months. Patients were visited regularly at home by a nurse practitioner and were taught to keep a diary of clinical events and to mark a visual analog scale. Twelve of 14 premonitions were followed by a typical painful crisis that required either home treatment (n = 4) or hospitalization (n = 8). Objective laboratory findings during this premonitory phase included decreased RBC deformability, increased number of both dense RBC, and irreversibly sickled cells (ISC) as compared to corresponding values in the steady state (Akinola et al. 1992).

The initial phase

The initial phase (also called first, evolving, or infarctive phase) is heralded by the onset of typical crisis pain that increases gradually in severity and reaches a peak by the second or third day of the crisis (Fig. 10). Given the paucity of objective signs during this initial phase, patients experience problems with care providers in the emergency department (Ballas 1990b). Routine laboratory data may not be atypical, which often discourages the treating physician from repeating tests. Fear, anorexia, and anxiety are usually present in this initial phase (Diggs 1965; Ballas 1990b). Major red cell changes during this phase include decreased deformability, increased dense cells, increased ISC, increased red cell distribution width (RDW), and increased red cell Hb distribution width (HDW) as compared to steady-state values (Fabry et al. 1984; Lawrence and Fabry 1986; Billet et al. 1988a, Akinola et al. 1992; Ballas and Smith 1992). The increase in dense RBC and ISC may be: (1) relative and secondary to preferential trapping of deformable discoid cells in the microvasculature, (2) absolute due to de novo formation of ISC, or (3) a combination of both (Ballas and Smith 1992). Other cellular changes in this phase include a decrease in the platelet count compared to steady state (Van der Sar 1970; Haut et al. 1973; Alkjaersig et al. 1976).

The established phase

The established phase (also called second, postinfarctive, or inflammatory phase) is characterized by the persistence of severe steady pain and typically lasts four to five days in adults (Fig. 10). Signs and symptoms of inflammation become predominant during this phase. Fever (Diggs 1965; Samuels-Reid and Scott 1985; Ballas et al. 1988), leukocytosis (Diggs 1965; Buchanan and Glader 1978; Billet et al. 1988b; Akinola et al. 1992), swelling, tenderness, and joint effusions (Schumacher 1975; Ballas et al. 1988; Serjeant 1992) are common. In addition, serum levels of acute-phase reactants such as C-reactive protein and serum amyloid A (Lawrence and Fabry 1986; Becton et al. 1989; Akinola et al. 1992) reach their peak values during this phase. Signs of hyperhemolysis including decreased Hb, increased reticulocyte count, and increased lactate dehydrogenase (LDH) may be seen. Tissue damage, especially bone marrow infarction, may be another source of increased LDH values. An increase in creatinine phosphokinase (CPK) usually indicates skeletal muscle injury. Billet et al. (1988b) reported dramatic increase in CPK values on days 5–8 of the crisis as compared to the level on days 1–3. Depression and problems with hospital care providers (Ballas 1990b), who may become suspicious of patients because of the heavy use of opioid analgesics for several days, occur toward the end of this phase and the start of the resolving phase.

The resolving phase

The resolving phase, also called last, healing, recovery, or postcrisis phase, is signalled by a gradual decrease in pain severity and may last 1–2 days (Fig. 10). Significant erythrocyte changes in this phase include a decline in the abnormalities of the initial phase with increased RBC deformability, decreased dense cells, and decreased ISC below steady-state values. Both RDW and HDW return toward steady-state values. However, rebound thrombocytosis occurs and another set of acute-phase reactants (fibrinogen and α1-acid glycoprotein or orosmomucoid) reach peak values in this phase. Plasma viscosity and erythrocyte sedimentation rate (ESR) increase above baseline values during this recovery phase. The significance of these changes will be addressed below.

Unsettled issues

The realization that the sickle cell painful crisis is a dynamic process that evolves along four phases, each of which has clinical and laboratory characteristics, raises the following issues that require further consideration both in basic research and clinical practice.

The steady state. A consensus is needed on the definition of the steady state. The prevailing definition is that it is a pain-free period following a painful episode that lasts at least one month and, according to the studies of Kenny et al. (1985), Akinola et al. (1992), and Ballas and Smith (1992), ends one to three days prior to the next crisis; i.e., it should not include the prodromal phase of a subsequent evolving painful crisis. Moreover, the painful crisis needs to be standardized as to its first day, which is generally accepted as the day a patient begins to seek treatment in a medical facility. An alternative definition should be the day on which typical crisis pain develops irrespective of whether it is treated at home (the stoic patient) or in a medical facility.

Prodromal phase. The prodromal phase of the crisis is an intriguing entity and needs further study. If such a phase could be well characterized it would offer an avenue, such as the initiation of preemptive analgesia, to abort an evolving crisis (Katz et al. 1992; McQuay 1992) to prevent the propagation of painful episodes.

The inflammatory process. The inflammatory response to vaso-occlusion secondary to sickling is poorly understood and needs further exploration. The acute sickle cell painful episode may constitute a prototype to study the complexities and intricate ramifications of the inflammatory response.

Is a resolving crisis a risk factor for the development of a new crisis? Ballas and Smith (1992) reported that 20% of recurrent crises occur within one week after the resolution of a previous painful crisis. They hypothesized that the resolving phase of the crisis involves an increased level of deformable cells that are potentially capable of adhering to endothelial cells of the microvasculature and eventually blocking the microcirculation. Moreover, elevation of the reticulocyte count during the resolving phase of the crisis could increase the number of young reticulocytes expressing the $\alpha_4\beta_1$-integrin complex (Swerlick et al. 1993). The latter could bind to activated endothelial cells via interaction between erythrocyte $\alpha_4\beta_1$ and endothelial cell vascular cell adhesion molecule-1 (VCAM-1). Besides the RBC alterations, other changes in plasma are thought to predispose to vascular occlusion in the resolving phase of the crisis, including increased plasma viscosity, fibrinogen, and platelet count, which together constitute a hypercoagulable state. Moreover, Blei et al. (1993) reported that elevated plasma levels of intercellular adhesion molecule-1 (ICAM-1) in the steady state of sickle cell disease increase further during vaso-occlusive crises. Another potential problem is reperfusion injury after a period of ischemia (Jennings et al. 1960; Engler and Covell 1987). Although the mechanism is unclear, one hypothesis is that reperfusion of ischemic tissue activates circulating leukocytes and results in new tissue damage (Breda et al. 1989; Byrne et al. 1992). Further studies are needed to monitor the development of these changes during the evolution of the sickle cell crisis in an effort to identify therapeutic approaches to prevent the propagation or relapse of painful episodes.

Clinical and laboratory features of painful episodes. The relative incidence of certain clinical findings and laboratory changes during the evolution of painful crises is not known and needs further evaluation. It is not clear what percentage of crises are associated with certain clinical and laboratory signs such as joint effusion, myonecrosis, and thrombocytopenia in the initial phase of the crisis, increased plasma viscosity, and so on. More studies are also needed to determine the incidence of clustering of certain signs and symptoms of painful episodes. For most patients, painful episodes are sometimes characterized by joint effusions, while at other times hepatic crises, for example, are most prevalent. Identification of the factors responsible for clustering of certain abnormalities may offer approaches for early preventive therapy.

Impact on treatment of pain. Finally, important questions arise: How do these interesting and dynamic features of the painful crisis relate to the bedside management of patients in pain? How many tests or studies should be performed during the evolution of the crisis to prove its existence? Should the treating physician doubt the existence of a painful episode without checking all possible parameters that could change during the painful crisis? Perhaps the most cost-effective approach to treating painful crises is to believe the patient, administer analgesics as needed to achieve pain relief, watch for side effects of analgesics, monitor Hb and reticulocyte values, and do only those tests that may alter the course of management, such as cultures to rule out coexistent infection. An alternative approach for documenting the onset of a painful crisis is to establish reliable steady-state data on each patient (the simplest and least costly would be RDW, HDW, Hb, reticulocyte and platelet counts, and one of the acute-phase reactants that changes early in the crisis such as C-reactive protein or SAA), and compare these data to values determined at the initial phase of the crisis and serially thereafter. The compilation of detailed hematological, biochemical, rheological, immunological, and biophysical profiles should perhaps be left to those researchers who are interested in elucidating the role of the multiple factors that interplay during the evolution of the battling sickle cell painful crisis.

ILLUSTRATIVE CASES

CASE 4.1

A 35-year-old African American man was diagnosed with sickle cell anemia in early childhood. His clinical course was characterized by frequent painful episodes and complicated by cholelithiasis, seizure disorder due to meperidine use, spontaneous penumothorax during one of his acute painful episodes, pneumonia, and priapism. Table IX presents his baseline hematological, biochemical, and clinical data. His painful crisis usually involved his chest, low back, extremities, and occasionally, abdomen. Between 1991 and 1995 he was hospitalized 65 times for a total of 333 days. During that same period he was treated 431 times in the emergency department for acute painful episodes and was seen 130 times in the outpatient office. He consumed about 30 tablets of oxycodone (5 mg each) with acetaminophen (325 mg each) per week as an outpatient. In the emergency department and the hospital his painful episodes were treated with parenteral hydromorphone (Dilaudid) and Vistaril. He has three siblings with sickle cell anemia, one of whom had fatal acute chest syndrome at the age of 23 years. He is divorced, has one child, and has been unemployed for several years.

CASE 4.2

A 33-year-old African American man with sickle cell anemia was diagnosed in early childhood. A previous report documented a complication of chronic leg ulcers (Ballas et al. 1995b). He is a college graduate with a B.S. degree in chemistry and is employed as an analytic chemist in a major

Table IX
Baseline hematological, biochemical, and clinical
characteristics of the patients described

	Patient 4.1	Patient 4.2
Age/sex	35/M	33/M
Diagnosis	SS	SS
α Genotype	αα/αα	αα/ααα
β^S Haplotype	Benin/CAR	Benin/CAR
Hb, g/dl	9.6	5.3
Reticulocytes, %	12.8	16.4
MCV, fl	83	100
Hb F, %	< 2	< 2
WBC, $10^3/\mu l$	14.4	9.5
Platelets, $10^3/\mu l$	554	423
Albumin, g/dl	4.2	4.4
Creatinine, mg/dl	0.9	1.3
Bilirubin T/D, mg/dl	1.8/0.4	6.5/0.9
ALP (alkaline phosphatase), IU/l	131	93
LDH (lactate dehydrogenase), IU/l	413	549
AST (aspartate aminotransferase), IU/l	32	47
ALT (alanine aminotransferase), IU/l	16	16
GGT (γ-glutamyl transpeptidase), IU/l	16	27
Annual ED visits	86	< 1
Annual admissions	13	< 1
Annual hospital days	67	< 3
Oxycodone use at home (mg/month)	1280	80

pharmaceutical company. Moreover, he is a licensed minister who volunteers his time in the prison system, visits residents of nursing homes, and assists counselors in a drug rehabilitation center. Major laboratory and clinical features of his disease are listed in Table IX. It is noteworthy that he rarely develops painful episodes that require treatment in a medical facility. He is married with one child, and has a stable and supportive family environment. Major complications of his disease include bilateral leg ulcers, cholecystectomy following an attack of acute cholecystitis with chlolelithiasis in 1985, another attack of abdominal pain and fever due to bilirubin stone in the common bile duct that was removed by cholangiopancreatography in 1990, and occasional attacks (three or four per year) of transient priapism that wake him up around 2 or 3 A.M. and last about one hour.

Comment on Cases 4.1 and 4.2

These two cases demonstrate that mild anemia in the steady state usually predisposes a patient to severe disease with frequent painful crises. The two patients described have several molecular and hematological similarities. Both are men of comparable age, are homozygous for the sickle gene, are doubly heterozygous for the Benin/CAR β haplotype, and have low Hb F level. Despite these similarities, their painful episodes differ significantly in frequency (Table IX). Paradoxically, this disparity may be due to the difference in the severity of the anemia in the steady state. Patient 4.1, with frequent painful crises, has relatively milder anemia than patient 4.2. As was mentioned above, the higher the Hb level in sickle cell anemia the higher is the blood viscosity, which in turn predisposes to vaso-occlusion. The fact that patient 4.2 had five a genes may be, in part, responsible for the severity of the anemia. The serum bilirubin, LDH, and AST levels of patient 4.2 reflect more severe hemolytic anemia in the steady state than seen in patient 4.1 (Table IX).

5

Acute Regional Pain Syndromes

There was a faith healer from Deal
Who said: "Although pain isn't real,
If I sit on a pin, and it punctures my skin
I dislike what I fancy I feel."
— Anonymous

Strictly speaking, there is but one real evil: I mean acute pain. All other
complaints are so considerably diminished by time that it is plain the grief
is owing to our passion, since the sensation of it vanishes when that is over.
— Lady Mary Wortley Montagu, 1689–1762

The acute sickle cell painful episode may involve any region of the body. Vaso-occlusion may affect certain organs and often requires special diagnostic procedures and therapeutic approaches. The clinician who assumes that painful episodes are simply transient crises may miss the diagnosis of serious pathology that, left unexplored, may be potentially fatal or associated with irreversible organ damage. This chapter will review acute painful episodes that involve specific regions of the body and present unique features that may require skillful clinical expertise coupled with appropriate diagnostic procedures and therapeutic approaches. An acute sickle cell painful episode may, as it progresses, involve all the regions reviewed below. Such involvement is usually transient and disappears with the resolution of the crisis. This chapter will also address the less common regional pain syndromes that may result in serious complications if not diagnosed.

CRANIOFACIAL PAIN SYNDROMES

HEADACHE

Headache often accompanies acute painful episodes, especially during their initial phase. Tension headache is the usual manifestation of the anxiety that accompanies the acute painful experience. The incidence and characteristics of headache in sickle cell disease have not been well studied. One review of 31 patients with sickle cell disease found that eight (26%) had headache (Hughes et al. 1940); another study of 142 patients reported 26 (18%) with headache (Patterson et al. 1950). These investigators, however, did not have reliable electrophoretic tests to diagnose sickle cell syndromes. Moreover, they did not elaborate on detailed aspects of the headache such as location, characteristics, etiology, or mechanism. Sabbagh and Keder (1996) reported headache in two patients with sickle cell disease (one with SS and the other with Hb SC) seemingly due to increased serum prolactin secondary to pituitary adenoma. This association, however, may be circumstantial since headache may be one of the symptoms of painful episodes. Moreover, serum prolactin levels may increase due to physiological/metabolic stressors (insomnia, anxiety, renal failure, hepatic disease, etc.) or certain drugs (opioids, neuroleptics, tricyclic antidepressants, etc.) that are often associated with painful crises. Recent reports on sickle cell disease have not addressed headache and its prevalence, incidence, pathophysiologic mechanism, and management.

Occasionally the acute painful episode may involve tender swelling of the scalp. In such cases patients may refer to the discomfort as headache, and innocuous touch of the scalp when combing hair or resting the head on a pillow elicits excruciating pain (allodynia) often described as "my head is blowing off." Patients sleep while sitting up to avoid any contact with the scalp that may accentuate the pain. Painful crises involved the skull in 5.5% of the patients studied by Serjeant et al. (1994). Expansion of the bone marrow of the skull leads to widening of the diploic space and thinning of the outer table (Fig. 1). The trabeculae in the diploic space may give rise to the "hair on end" appearance (Fig. 1) in less than 5% of patients with sickle cell anemia (Baker 1964).

Migraine headache and the sudden headache that accompanies cerebral hemorrhage will be addressed in Chapter 7.

FACIAL BONE INFARCTS

Although bone infarction is a common manifestation in patients with sickle cell anemia (Lutzker and Alavi 1979; Keeley and Buchanan 1982; Korent et al. 1982, 1984), facial bone infarcts are rare (Garty et al. 1983; Royal et al. 1988). Thus, only 5% of the painful crises reported by Ballas and Delengowski (1993) involved the jaw. Patients complain of pain, swelling, and tenderness over the involved area. It is important to rule out osteomyelitis of facial bones, which, untreated, may lead to central nervous system involvement with meningitis or cavernous sinus thrombosis.

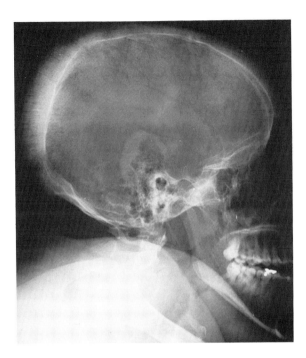

Fig. 1. The rare "hair on end" appearance and diploic thickening of the skull in a patient with sickle cell anemia.

ILLUSTRATIVE CASE 5.1

A 21-year-old African American man with sickle cell anemia was admitted to the hospital with an acute painful episode involving his right jaw, elbow, low back, and both thighs, knees, and shins. He also complained of frontal headache. He denied fever, chills, cough, nausea, vomiting, diarrhea, photophobia, or sonophobia. The pain was similar to that of his usual crises except that he was experiencing pain in the jaw for the first time. It was dull and achy and not as sharp and throbbing as the pain in the other regions, which he had rated with an intensity score of 10 on a 10-point scale. By the third hospital day the jaw pain worsened and was associated with swelling and tenderness over the right side of the face.

A limited three-phase bone scintigraphy of the right jaw, following an intravenous administration of 25 mCi of ^{99m}Tc, showed no evidence of hyperemia on the dynamic or blood pool images. Delayed images showed an area of photopenia (Fig. 2) in the region of the right mandible. This finding was consistent with an infarct and there was no increased activity to suggest osteomyelitis. Symptomatic treatment included oral hydration and parenteral hydromorphone. By the eighth hospital day the swelling and pain over the right jaw had decreased and the patient felt much better.

Fig. 2. Scintigraphy of facial bones following the intravenous injection of ^{99m}Tc shows acute infarction of the angle of the right mandible (arrow).

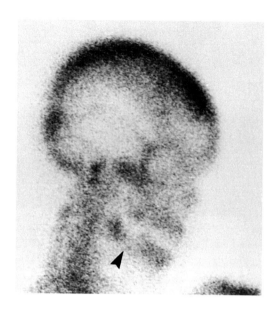

Comment on Case 5.1

Differential diagnosis of pain, swelling, and tenderness over the jaw includes bone infarction and osteomyelitis. Bone scintigraphy ruled out the latter. Bone infarction in sickle cell anemia usually involves the long axial bones. The jaw is involved in only 3% of the cases. The development of collateral blood circulation and revascularization of infarcted bones usually leads to complete resolution in two to four weeks.

OCULAR PAIN

Ocular manifestations of sickle cell disease are mainly caused by decreased blood flow in the small capillaries of the retina due to occlusion by sickle RBC. Most of these patients are asymptomatic. Retinopathy occurs more often in Hb SC disease than in sickle cell anemia and is rare prior to adolescence (Goldberg 1972; Armaly 1974; Ballas et al. 1982).

Occasional ocular pain may be due to orbital infarction or the orbital apex syndrome. Infarction of periorbital bones is rare in patients with sickle cell anemia (Garty et al. 1983) and may be associated with unilateral or bilateral periorbital hematoma or edema (Garty et al. 1984). Al-Rashid (1979) reported one patient with orbital apex syndrome secondary to sickle cell anemia. This syndrome is characterized by marked restriction of mobility of the globe associated with proptosis, lid edema, reduction of vision, and pain in the orbital region and forehead. Ocular complications of sickle cell disease also include orbital abscess formation in association with orbital infarction (Sidmen et al. 1990). Traditionally, surgical drainage of orbital abscesses has been the treatment of choice in addition to intravenous antibiotics.

LONG BONES AND JOINTS

DACTYLITIS (HAND-FOOT SYNDROME)

Hand-foot syndrome, or dactylitis, is the earliest clinical manifestation of sickle cell anemia and occurs most commonly in infants and young children between the ages of 6 months and 2 years (see Case 3.1 in Chapter 3), with a few reported cases in children up to age 7 years (Watson et al. 1963; Espinosa 1979; Stevens et al. 1981a). The clinical picture is characterized by acute, often symmetric painful swelling of the dorsa of the hands or feet. Swelling usually involves the soft tissues over the metacarpals or metatarsals and proximal phalanges of the hands and feet (Fig. 3). The cardinal signs of inflammation—tenderness, erythema, and warmth—are usually present. The edema is nonpitting. Fever up to 103°F (39.4°C) and leukocytosis may occur. Radiographs taken at the onset of soft tissue swelling usually do not show bony abnormalities. Bony changes appear after one or two weeks and include irregular areas of radiolucency, subperiosteal new bone formation, cortical thickening, and bone destruction. The episode is usually self-limited and resolves within one week, but recurrent attacks are common. Treatment is symptomatic, and if the attack persists, the clinician should consider acute osteomyelitis.

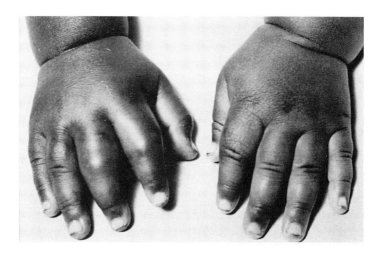

Fig. 3. Hands of a child with dactylitis (Diggs 1965 with permission).

The pathophysiologic events that lead to dactylitis seem to be due to complete necrosis of the bone marrow and of the inner third of the cortex of affected bone (Weinberg and Currarino 1972). The carpal and tarsal bones have a vascular supply similar to that of epiphyses of long bones in that each has several vessels rather than a single nutrient artery. Precipitating factors of dactylitis include environmental cold (Marsten and Shah 1964; Stevens et al. 1981a) and infections (Victor and Imperiale 1957).

Because it is often the first clinical manifestation of sickle cell anemia, dactylitis should be thoroughly explained to parents of infants diagnosed after newborn screening. Parent education should include detailed description of the problem, photographs showing the swollen hands or feet of infants with dactylitis, and the principles of management. Unprepared parents confronted with the first attack of hand-foot syndrome feel helpless and unable to relieve their infant's pain immediately, which may generate feelings of guilt and frustration.

ARTHROPATHIES

Aseptic inflammation

Pain in the joints and bone is a common component of the acute sickle cell painful episode because the sinusoidal circulation of the bone marrow provides an ideal location for sickling (Lukens 1981). Obstruction of blood flow by sickled erythrocytes causes ischemia leading to regional hypoxia and acidosis which, in turn, further increase the rate of sickling. Any joint may be directly involved during painful crises, producing painful arthritis with variable amounts of effusion. Synovial fluid is typically non-inflammatory with abundance of mononuclear cells. Reaction to juxta-articular bone infarcts or synovial ischemia and infarction seems to be the probable mechanism of sickle arthropathy. Mann and Schumacher (1995) described an unusual patient with inflammatory sickle arthropathy characterized by the presence of crystal-like arrays of polymerized sickle hemoglobin in red cells that were enfolded and phagocytized by the cells of the synovial fluid, suggesting that sickled red cells sometimes directly provoke an inflammatory response. Joint pain is usually throbbing or sharp and progressive in severity. The joints most frequently affected are the knees, followed in decreasing frequency by the shoulders, elbows, hips, wrists, and ankles (Ballas and Delengowski 1993; Serjeant et al. 1994). Joint involvement may be unilateral or symmetrical and can be associated with swelling, tenderness, erythema, and warmth. Joint swelling may occur early during the painful episode or may appear after few days. The pathophysiologic events responsible for swelling are not well known and may be related to the generation of bradykinin and other mediators of inflammation as was discussed in Chapter 4.

In most cases, needle aspiration of synovial fluid from swollen joints demonstrates evidence of mild aseptic inflammation (Kaul et al. 1996). Some providers discourage the tapping of joints because the yield for infectious agent is minimal and the risk for superinfection may be high (Kaul et al. 1996). In taking such an approach, however, providers should consider the clinical picture of each patient and carefully analyze the risk/benefit ratio of needle aspiration.

Septic arthritis

Bacterial arthritis is less common than osteomyelitis in sickle cell disease (Givner et al. 1981; Buchanan 1994). Causative organisms include *Salmonella* species, *Staphylococcus aureus*, *Streptococcus pneumoniae*, and *Escherichia coli* (Adeyokunnu and Hendrickse 1980; Syrogiannopoulos et al. 1986; Epps et al. 1991). Septic arthritis shares many clinical features with acute bone infarction secondary to vaso-occlusion. Change in the character of pain, chills and fever, and leukocytosis with a left shift in the differential should alert the physician to this possibility. Positive blood culture is a strong indicator of septic arthritis. Direct aspiration of joint fluid is essential to identify the offending organism by Gram stain and culture. Management includes symptomatic treatment with analgesics, hydration, and surgical drainage followed by a two- to six-week course of appropriate parenteral antibiotics.

ILLUSTRATIVE CASE 5.2.

A 25-year-old African American man with sickle cell anemia was admitted to the hospital with an acute painful episode involving his low back, thighs, knees, and legs. The pain was throbbing and sharp, similar to that of his usual crises, with an intensity score of 10 on a 10-point scale. In addition, he complained of a burning and tingling sensation over his legs. Physical examination revealed a temperature of 100.1°F (37.8°C), pulse of 125/minute, normal blood pressure and respiratory rate, and nonpitting swelling and tenderness of both legs. The treatment plan included hydration and 150 mg parenteral meperidine every two hours and 50 mg hydroxyzine (Vistaril) intramuscularly every four hours.

On the third hospital day he complained of pain in his left shoulder, which he had not experienced during past crises and that was somewhat different in character than the pain in his back and legs. By the seventh hospital day this new pain became excruciating, and a physical examination showed a swollen, tender, erythematous, and warm left shoulder.

Radiographs of the left shoulder revealed no abnormalities. Ultrasonography showed a large, complex fluid collection in the bursal space. Ultrasound-guided aspiration yielded 90 ml of purulent fluid. Blood cultures grew no organism. Gram stain of the aspirated fluid showed Gram-positive cocci and culture grew α-hemolytic streptococci and enterococcus, both sensitive to ampicillin. A catheter for drainage was placed in the left shoulder and intravenous antibiotics were given for three weeks. By that time the patient felt much better, was afebrile, the swelling of the left shoulder resolved, and the crisis pain and the pain in the left shoulder decreased significantly to a score of 5 on the 10-point scale. The drainage catheter was removed after it showed clear yellowish fluid. The patient was discharged 30 days after admission.

Comment on Case 5.2.

This case illustrates that a swollen tender joint of a patient with sickle cell disease could be septic. Initially, swelling and tenderness over his legs suggested that his shoulder pain was a component of his usual crisis pain. However, his lack of shoulder pain during previous painful episodes, fever, and leukocytosis with left shift were indicators of possible sepsis. Noteworthy in this case is that plain radiographs are not helpful in making the diagnosis of septic arthropathy. Aspiration of joint fluid was necessary to confirm the diagnosis. Finally, although the source of infection in this patient was not clear, one possibility points to the intramuscular injections of meperidine during the previous hospital admission, as he was discharged one week before readmission for the present illness.

Gout

The increased purine turnover of accelerated erythropoiesis in sickle cell anemia causes increased production of uric acid (Crosby 1955) in amounts proportional to the severity of the hemolysis. Catabolism of nucleic acids generates urate. In most patients, however, increased production of uric acid is balanced by increased renal excretion of urate (Diamond et al. 1975, 1979). This normal response occurs in patients with sickle cell anemia as it does in other patients (Reynolds 1983). Consequently, most patients with sickle cell disease have a normal or moderately elevated serum uric acid level. Damage to the renal tubules caused by infarction and hypoxia due to recurrent episodes of sickling, however, can reduce hyperuricosuria by the third decade of life. Impairment of this compensatory renal mechanism leads to more severe hyperuricemia, thus increasing the risk for the development of gouty arthritis (Reynolds 1983).

Reports of clinical gout are infrequent (Espinoza et al. 1974; Rothschild et al. 1980; Leff et al. 1983), but usually involve the knees, wrists, and small finger joints rather than the big toe as is typical of classical gout (Serjeant 1992). Gout that is associated with sickle cell anemia has high prevalence in women and relatively young patients (Reynolds 1983). Gout may be underdiagnosed in a disease associated with recurrent joint pain and may be mistaken for the usual acute painful episodes of sickle cell disease. Hyper-uricemia alone is not sufficient to establish the diagnosis, which requires the demonstration of uric acid crystals in joint fluid.

Avascular necrosis

Involvement of the hip and shoulder joints is the most important clinical aspect of avascular necrosis. The resultant chronic pain syndrome will be discussed in Chapter 6.

Other arthritides

Other types of arthritis that may occur in patients with sickle cell disease include rheumatoid arthritis, systemic lupus erythematosus (SLE), arthritis associated with inflammatory bowel disease, and systemic necrotizing vas-culitis (Kastanis et al. 1987; Manci et al. 1987; Marino and McDonald 1990; Serjeant 1992). Whether the coexistence of these arthritides with sickle cell disease is coincidental or has a causal relationship is unsettled at present.

LONG BONES

Bone infarction

The clinical picture of infarction of the long bones includes localized swell-ing, pain, erythema, warmth and tenderness over the affected area, and fever. Juxta-articular areas of long bones are the most frequent sites of involvement, and localized swelling may occur, especially in the anterior tibial areas. The pathophysiologic basis includes bone destruction and periosteal reaction with progressive formation of new cortical bone and narrowing of the medullary space, which become evident within two weeks after the onset of symptoms (Golding 1956; O'Hara 1967; Ennis et al. 1973; Bohrer 1987; Serjeant 1992). An inflammatory reaction triggered by localized ischemia likely causes the periosteal reaction and new bone formation. Long bone infarction thus dif-fers from the typical acute painful vaso-occlusive crisis, which is probably caused by infarction of the bone marrow. Mallouh (1987) found subperi-osteal bleeding with acute bone infarcts in children with sickle cell anemia. Needle aspiration of the serosanguinous fluid quickly decreased tenderness.

Acute osteomyelitis

Osteomyelitis of the long bones is also characterized by tenderness, swelling, and fever. Clinically, it is difficult to distinguish osteomyelitis from infarction or acute painful vaso-occlusive episode (Table I). Scanning techniques with ^{99m}Tc sulfur colloid or MRI may identify osteomyelitis. The diagnosis, however, must be confirmed by bone biopsy to identify the offending organism and its antibiotic sensitivity. Failure to confirm osteomyelitis usually suggests a diagnosis of sterile bone infarction, which is at least 50 times more common than bacterial osteomyelitis (Keeley and Buchanan 1982).

Staphylococcus aureus is the most common cause of bacterial osteomyelitis in the general population, but few reports (Sadat-Ali et al. 1985; Epps 1991) have found it to be the most common cause in patients with sickle cell disease. Several reports (Diggs 1967; Barrett-Connor 1971b; Adeyokunnu and Hendrickse 1980; Mallouh and Talab 1985; Ebong 1986; Syroginannopoulos 1986; Bennett 1990) have indicated that *Salmonella* species are the most frequently identified bacterial organisms causing osteomyelitis in sickle cell disease, particularly *S. typhimurium*. Exceptions may occur in certain geographic areas. The susceptibility to infection by *Salmonella* may reflect the ability of this organism to flourish in partially necrotic bone.

CHEST PAIN

PAIN OF CARDIAC ORIGINS

High output failure, right heart or congestive heart failure, cardiac hemosiderosis, and cardiomegaly are known to complicate sickle cell anemia in some patients. In addition, myocardial ischemia and infarction have been reported in sickle cell anemia (Martin et al. 1983). One study showed a high

Table I
Differential diagnosis of long bone infarcts

	Painful Crisis	Bone Infarct	Osteomyelitis
Pathophysiology	Bone marrow occlusion	Bone destruction	Infection
Pain and tenderness	Yes	Yes	Yes
Swelling and erythema	Yes	Yes	Yes
Fever	Yes	Yes	Yes
Leukocytosis	Yes	Yes	Yes
Bandemia	No	No	Yes
Positive blood culture	No	No	Yes/No

prevalence of mitral valve prolapse (25% of patients) in sickle cell disease (Lippman et al. 1985), but other groups did not confirm this finding (Simmons et al. 1988). The signs and symptoms of mitral valve prolapse (chest pain, dyspnea, fatigue, syncope, palpitations, etc.) are similar to those of sickle cell disease and, if there is an association between these two disorders, may demonstrate the changeable manifestations of sickle cell disease.

ACUTE CHEST SYNDROME

The full-blown clinical picture of acute chest syndrome includes chest pain, fever, leukocytosis, dyspnea, hypoxia, *new* pulmonary infiltrates on X-ray film of the chest, and decreasing hemoglobin level. Pain is pleuritic in most patients. Abdominal pain may indicate involvement of adjacent dia-phragmatic pleura. These signs and symptoms vary from mild to severe and even life threatening. The syndrome may be caused by pulmonary edema, rib or sternal infarction, pneumonia, pulmonary infarcts due to in situ sick-ling, pulmonary fat embolism, or pulmonary embolism. Acute chest syn-drome occurs in approximately 50% of hospitalized patients with sickle cell anemia (Vichinsky and Lubin 1980; Ashcroft and Serjeant 1981; Sprinkle et al. 1986). These episodes account for 15% of acute admissions and are potentially fatal (Barrett-Connor 1971a; Davies et al. 1984; Athanasou et al. 1985; Serjeant 1992). Acute chest syndrome has become the most common cause of death and the second most common cause of hospitalization in sickle cell disease and is closely associated with painful crises, especially in adults (Thomas et al. 1982; Vichinsky 1991; Gill et al. 1995; Vichinsky and Styles 1996). Acute chest syndrome is most common in sickle cell anemia followed by sickle-β^o-thalassemia, Hb SC disease, and sickle-β^+-thalassemia (Castro et al. 1994). α-Thalassemia has no effect on the incidence of acute chest syndrome. Predisposing factors include young age (highest in children aged 2 to 4 years), high steady-state Hb level, low steady-state fetal hemoglobin, and high steady-state leukocytosis (Castro et al. 1994; Vichinsky et al. 1994).

Diagnostic work-up should include X-ray of the chest, cultures of spu-tum and blood, monitoring of arterial blood gases and Hb level, ventilation and perfusion (V/Q) scans, analysis of sputum, bronchial washings, and urine for fat globules, and ruling out of thrombophlebitis in the pelvis or lower extremities. Blister cells (Fig. 4) have been described in the peripheral smear of patients with pulmonary infarcts secondary to sickle cell disease (Karayalcin et al. 1972). The treatment plan (Table II) includes antibiotic ther-apy and oxygen; exchange transfusion may be helpful in severe cases. Cau-tion should be exercised in giving opioids to the hypoxic patient. Tachypnea usually accompanies the acute chest syndrome, and depression of respiration

Fig. 4. Blister cells (arrows) in the peripheral blood of a patient with sickle cell anemia and acute chest syndrome.

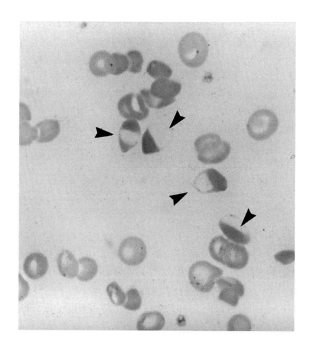

and sedation are to a point desirable therapeutic goals of opioid analgesic. The respiratory rate should be monitored; a decrease to 10 or fewer respirations per minute in a heavily sedated patient indicates that opioids should be decreased or discontinued. Heparin is usually reserved for the patient with proven pulmonary embolism. Recurrent episodes of thrombophlebitis with pulmonary embolism may justify the insertion of inferior vena caval filter, especially when it is difficult to achieve adequate anticoagulation. Repeated attacks of acute chest syndrome with pulmonary infarcts predict the onset of pulmonary hypertension, pulmonary failure with cor pulmonale, and terminal adult respiratory distress syndrome (Powars et al. 1988; Powars 1990). Moreover, the "sudden death syndrome" in adults may be related to chronic sickle cell lung disease via a sudden episode of pulmonary hypoxia.

Table II
Recommendations for the treatment
of acute chest syndrome

Oxygen
Intravenous fluids: $3L/M^2/24h$
Incentive spirometry
Antibiotics
Analgesics (parenteral opioids)
Transfusion: simple or exchange

Given the relative frequency of acute chest syndrome in sickle cell anemia and the need to monitor arterial blood gases, it is important to establish baseline blood gases and pulmonary function tests for all patients. These determinations will be of value in evaluating patients with acute onset of pulmonary signs and symptoms (Walker et al. 1979).

Pulmonary edema

Chronic anemia is usually associated with a chronic increase in cardiac output, which, in turn, may reduce the cardiovascular reserve necessary to handle volume expansion. Patients with sickle cell anemia may develop pulmonary edema during the course of routine intravenous hydration for an uncomplicated acute painful episode. Haynes and Allison (1986) reported that 10% of patients who received 50% normal saline at an intravenous rate of 200 ml per hour developed pulmonary edema. An increase in pulmonary capillary pressure and a decrease in the oncotic pressure seen with vigorous intravenous fluid administration are contributory factors to the development of pulmonary edema. Moreover, the use of opioid analgesics increases the pulmonary capillary permeability and constitutes another predisposing factor to pulmonary edema. Vigorous and aggressive hydration thus requires caution and close monitoring of patients with sickle cell anemia.

Rib and sternal infarction

The sine qua non in diagnosing acute chest syndrome is a radiograph showing new pulmonary infiltrates, which may be due to pneumonia, pulmonary infarction, fat embolism, or pulmonary embolism. In the absence of pulmonary infiltrates the most likely diagnosis is acute painful crisis involving the musculoskeletal components of the chest wall. Careful physical examination with palpation of the chest wall often identifies the painful area and reproduces the patient's symptoms. The most characteristic clinical finding in acute chest wall syndrome is tenderness over the ribs (Rucknagel et al. 1991) or the sternum (Ballas and Park 1991). This symptom is often difficult to evaluate because the patient may resist uncomfortable maneuvers. Bone infarction may be confirmed by bone scintigraphy following the intravenous injection of ^{99m}Tc-methylene diphosphonate (Fig. 5). Rib/sternal in-farction may predispose patients to typical acute chest syndrome (Rucknagel et al. 1991; Bellet et al. 1995) in a sequence of infarction, pain, inflammatory response, conscious hypoventilation due to splinting, and pleuritis. Hypoventilation may lead to atelectasis and development of the radiographic changes indicative of acute chest syndrome. Thoracic bone infarction is

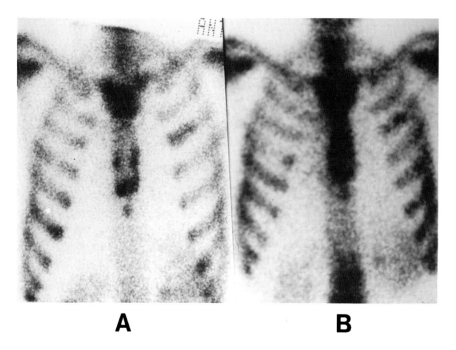

A   **B**

Fig. 5. Spot views of the chest wall taken after intravenous administration of 20 mCi of ^{99m}Tc MPD show infarction of the sternum in a patient with sickle cell anemia. **A:** Decreased activity within the body of the sternum compatible with acute pain infarction. **B:** A repeat scan two months later depicts healing of the sternal infarct and the infarction of the ribs (Ballas and Park 1991 with permission).

common and in one study was found in nearly 40% of patients hospitalized with acute painful episodes (Sadat-Ali et al. 1993). Bellet et al. (1991) reported that the use of incentive spirometry can prevent the pulmonary complications (atelectasis and infiltrates) associated with the acute chest syndrome in patients with sickle cell disease who are hospitalized with chest or back pain above the diaphragm.

Pneumonia

The relative incidence of pneumonia in patients with sickle cell disease is estimated to be 25 to 100 times greater than in the general population (Barrett-Connor 1971a, 1973; Seeler et al. 1972). The reported frequency of infection as a cause of the acute chest syndrome seems to vary with age and time. Thus, Barrett-Connor (1971a, 1973), in a retrospective study, found that bacterial pneumonia accounted for greater than 50% of episodes of pulmonary crises in children, whereas Poncz et al. (1985), in a prospective study, found bacterial pneumonia in only 12% of episodes of acute chest in children. In older children and adults an infiltrate is seldom caused by a bacterial infection (Lukens 1981). The decline in the reported frequency of infectious etiology of the acute chest syndrome may be due to the increasing use of prophylactic antibiotics and pneumococcal vaccine. However, there has been no aggressive, prospective search to elucidate the role of infection as a cause of the acute chest syndrome. A multicenter study is now in progress to determine the etiology, clinical course, and treatment of this complication of sickle cell disease (Vichinsky, personal communication).

Among the microorganisms that cause pneumonia in sickle cell disease, pyogenic bacteria *(Streptococcus, E. coli,* and *Klebsiella*) are common. Other organisms include *Mycoplasma, Chlamydia, Legionella,* and several viral agents such as influenza, cytomegalovirus (CMV), respiratory syncytial virus (RSV), parvovirus B19, adenovirus, and parainfluenza (Serjeant 1992). The ischemic lung injury resulting from infarction may increase the virulence of the bacterial and viral infections.

Pneumonia in sickle cell disease has certain distinguishing features (Bromberg 1974; Serjeant 1992). Multiple-lobe, middle-lobe, and bilateral infiltration are common. Prolonged course despite antibiotics is common and recurrences of pneumonia occur in up to two-thirds of patients. The impaired access of oxygen to inflamed and consolidated lung with consequent regional hypoxia promotes local sickling and vaso-occlusion and thus delays and complicates resolution of the infection. Mortality from lung infection in sickle cell anemia is estimated to be less than 5%.

Pulmonary thromboembolic disease

This group includes pulmonary infarction (in situ sickling), pulmonary fat embolism, and pulmonary embolism. The frequency and etiology of this noninfectious acute chest syndrome are unknown. It is possible that infectious and noninfectious complications contribute to the development of acute chest syndrome; pulmonary infarction, pulmonary fat embolism, and pulmonary emboli have been reported as causes (Johnson and Verdegen 1988; Francis and Johnson 1991). Certain extrapulmonary factors may initiate acute chest syndrome (Table III). Rib/sternal infarctions can cause splinting of the chest wall and hypoventilation as was mentioned above. Respiratory suppression secondary to opioid analgesia may lead to atelectasis and hypoxia and consequent pulmonary infection or infarction (Barrett-Connor 1971a, 1973; Palmer et al. 1983; Davies et al. 1984). This link may explain the possible association of painful crises with concomitant acute chest syndrome. Acute pulmonary edema secondary to hydration or transfusion may initiate or worsen the clinical picture (Haynes and Allison 1986). Acute chest syndrome seems

Table III
Extra-pulmonary factors that initiate
acute chest syndrome

Rib infarction
Respiratory suppression
Opioid analgesics
Acute pulmonary edema
Overhydration
Rapid transfusion
Surgery
Bronchoreactive lung disease

to be the most common complication following surgery in patients with sickle cell disease (Homi et al. 1979). Bronchoreactive lung disease may be another predisposing factor to acute chest syndrome (Handelsman and Voulalas 1991).

Pulmonary fat/bone marrow embolism in patients with SCD appears to be more common than previously thought (Vichinsky et al. 1994). The characteristic clinical picture is that of severe bone pain, usually in long bones, followed by dyspnea, hypoxia, and fever. Tissue infarction of the bone marrow within the long bones seems to generate a source of fat and necrotic tissue that has been demonstrated on autopsy. At the same time, serum levels of secretory phospholipase A_2 ($sPLA_2$), an inflammatory mediator, increase in ACS and liberate free fatty acids from membrane phospholipids of damaged tissue that are believed to cause the acute lung injury associated with fat embolism (Styles et al. 1996)

LOW BACK PAIN SYNDROME

During acute sickle cell painful episodes, pain occurs most frequently in the low back in the area of the lumbar spine (Ballas and Delengowski 1993; Serjeant et al. 1994). Causes of low back pain in sickle cell disease are listed in Table IV. Pathophysiologically, low back pain results from bone changes due to marrow hyperplasia, tissue ischemia, and infection.

MARROW HYPERPLASIA

Erythroid hyperplasia within the marrow of the vertebral bodies exerts pressure on the trabeculae that destroys the finer trabeculae and leads to radiolucency and prominence of the remaining vertical, thicker trabeculae. This process results in typical radiographic changes showing the coarse

Table IV
Differential diagnosis of acute
low back pain in sickle cell disease

Acute vaso-occlusive episode
Marrow hyperplasia
   Structural changes of lumbar spine
Tissue ischemia
   Avascular necrosis of vertebrae
Infection
   Infective spondylitis
Other causes
   Pyelonephritis
   Referred pain
      Pneumonia
      Pancreatitis
      Cholecystitis
      Bowel infarction

trabecular and striated pattern (Fig. 6) that suggests the diagnosis of sickle cell disease (Reynolds 1987). The vertebrae may be flattened with an increased width to height ratio (Diggs et al. 1937; Middlemiss and Raper 1966). Changes in shape due to compression cause concave depression of one or both end-plates. Typically the depression of the compression deformity is

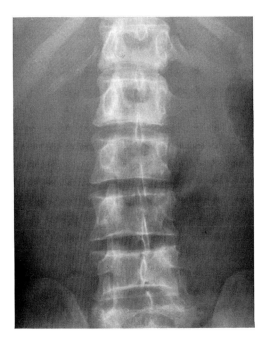

Fig. 6. Lumbar spine of a patient with sickle cell anemia showing the coarse trabecular and striated pattern produced by marrow hyperplasia.

arcuate and involves the entire end-plate (Reynolds 1987). Structural changes in the vertebral bodies due to marrow hyperplasia were found in 44% of patients with sickle cell disease in one study from Saudi Arabia (Sadat-Ali et al. 1993).

TISSUE ISCHEMIA

The vertebrae, like the rest of the skeleton, suffer from recurrent small infarcts reflected clinically by recurrent episodes of low back pain. Repeated episodes of localized sickling lead to gradual obliteration of the branches of the nutrient artery while the periosteal circulation remains intact (Fig. 7) (Bunn and Forget 1986). A "fish-mouth" or step-like depression (Fig. 8) seen in some patients is probably caused by avascular necrosis or infarction of the central portion of the vertebral body and may lead to vertebral collapse (Bohrer 1981; Reynolds 1987). Sadat-Ali et al. (1993) reported that avascular necrosis leading to collapse of the vertebral bodies occurred in 27% of their patients with sickle cell disease.

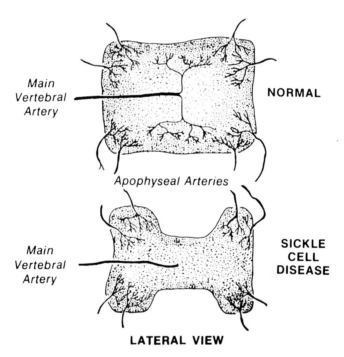

Fig. 7. The probable pathogenesis of vertebral body collapse. The central depression of the vertebral end-plates is caused by inhibition of bone growth from ischemia due to obstruction of the fine branches of the main vertebral artery by sickle cells (Bunn and Forget 1986 with permission).

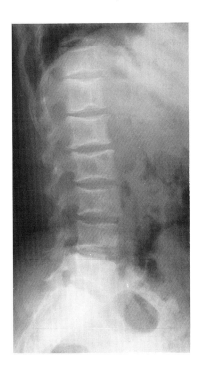

Fig. 8. "Step-like" or "fish-mouth" deformity of the lumbar vertebrae of a patient with sickle cell anemia.

INFECTION

Infective spondylitis is a serious complication of sickle cell disease. It was diagnosed in 24% of the patients reported by Sadat-Ali et al. (1993); most patients required anterolateral decompression and bone grafting. This infection is similar to osteomyelitis in etiology and management.

The pain of acute pyelonephritis is usually localized in the costovertebral angles and associated with fever and urinary signs and symptoms. Referred pain due to pancreatitis, cholecystitis, and bowel infarction will be discussed below.

ABDOMINAL PAIN

The abdomen is the second most common site of pain in sickle cell disease after musculoskeletal pain (including chest wall). The cause may be intra-abdominal pathology or pain referred from the lungs with pneumonia or from the lower ribs and the femoral heads with avascular necrosis. Specific pain syndromes due to sickle cell disease are listed in Table V and include left and right upper quadrant syndrome and acute abdomen, as will be discussed below.

Table V
Differential diagnosis of abdominal pain in
sickle cell disease

Left upper quadrant syndrome
  Splenic sequestration
  Acute pancreatitis
Right upper quadrant syndrome
  Calculous cholecystitis
  Acute viral hepatitis
  Hepatic sequestration
  Hepatic crisis
  Intrahepatic cholestasis
Other acute abdominal pain episodes
  Abdominal crisis (pseudo-acute surgical abdomen)
  Bowel infarction
  Girdle syndrome

LEFT UPPER QUADRANT SYNDROME

Acute splenic sequestration crisis

The spleen is the first organ to suffer from the destructive effects of sickle microvasculopathy that eventually lead to functional asplenia and autosplenectomy. During infancy the spleen is enlarged in about 75% of patients with sickle cell anemia. Children between the ages of 5 months and 2 years are most vulnerable to splenic sequestration that varies in severity from mild to life-threatening episodes. In its full-blown picture acute splenic sequestration is characterized by a pentad of: (1) rapid fall in hemoglobin concentration, (2) rise in reticulocyte count, (3) fall in platelet count, (4) sudden increase in spleen size associated with acute pain and tenderness in the left upper quadrant, and (5) signs and symptoms of hypovolemia (Emond et al. 1985; Solanki et al. 1986). Most reports of acute splenic sequestration involve children with sickle cell anemia under 6 years of age (Topley et al. 1981; Thomas et al. 1982). Minor episodes may resolve spontaneously but severe ones can be fatal and may be mistaken for the sudden infant death syndrome. Fibrosis occurs by the age of 8 years and the risk for splenic sequestration decreases (Powars 1976; Topley et al. 1981). Nevertheless, older children and adults with persistent splenomegaly in certain sickle cell syndromes (sickle cell anemia with two a-gene deletions, Hb SC disease, and sickle-b-thalassemia) continue to be vulnerable for acute splenic sequestration episodes. Casey et al. (1994) described a 3-year-old black girl with Hb SC disease and the signs and symptoms of acute splenic sequestration but whose spleen was not enlarged on physical examination. Abdominal ultrasonography, however, documented splenomegaly. Thus, sudden drop in hemoglobin level in young children should raise the possibility of splenic sequestration in the absence of palpable splenomegaly.

The pathophysiologic mechanisms that lead to acute splenic sequestration are not well understood. One possible mechanism is acute obstruction of the venous flow from the spleen with a resultant damming effect associated with sudden enlargement of the spleen due to pooling of red cells and platelets (Altman et al. 1951; Itzchak et al. 1978). The acidotic environment of the spleen, due to its sluggish circulation, stimulates sickling, increases viscosity, and contributes to further obstruction of blood flow. Infection can cause even more vascular engorgement in addition to the rapid acceleration of sickling. Obstruction of the venous flow may be related to abnormal rheological properties of sickle erythrocytes (Jensen and Lessin 1970). Moreover, scanning electron microscopy has demonstrated trapping of rigid sickle cells in the splenic cords of patients with sickle cell anemia (Barnhart et al. 1976).

Treatment of acute splenic sequestration consists of rapid restoration of intravascular volume and oxygen-carrying capacity. This goal is achieved by the transfusion of sickle-negative RBC at a rate of 15–20 ml/kg with careful monitoring to avoid sudden overexpansion of blood volume that may precipitate pulmonary edema. After successful treatment the spleen usually shrinks within a few days and gradually regains its baseline size.

Acute episodes of splenic sequestration tend to recur within a few months to a year after the initial sequestration crisis. Thus, splenectomy has been recommended for those patients who survive the initial severe episode (Serjeant 1992). The onset of splenic sequestration correlates with the increased risk for septicemia from *Streptococcus pneumoniae* and *Haemophilus influenzae* type b, and it is recommended that all patients with sickle cell syndromes receive pneumococcal and *H. influenzae* vaccines. As was mentioned for dactylitis, it is important to educate the family about acute splenic sequestration so the parents can be alert for early symptoms and seek immediate medical intervention.

Splenic sepsis

Beet (1949) first reported the occurrence of splenic abscess in association with sickle cell disease. Chun et al. (1980) reviewed 176 cases of splenic sepsis and found that 12% were associated with sickle cell disease. Patients affected usually are children, adolescents, or young adults. Signs and symptoms are nonspecific and include fever, abdominal pain, and tenderness in the left upper quadrant. A high index of clinical suspicion is needed to make an early diagnosis. Sonography or CT scan of the abdomen may show cyst formation or evidence of tissue breakdown in the spleen (Cavenagh et al. 1994). Management includes splenectomy and intravenous antibiotics. The organisms that most frequently cause splenic sepsis include staphylococci, streptococci, and *Salmonella* species. Functional asplenia or hyposplenia appears to be a predisposing factor to splenic sepsis.

Acute pancreatitis

Acute pancreatitis has been described in sickle cell disease (Kumar et al. 1989; Sheehan et al. 1993; Ballas et al. 1995b). The evidence that it is associated with sickle cell disease is circumstantial. Occlusion of the pancreatic duct by gallstones seems the most likely cause of acute pancreatitis. One reported case (Ballas et al. 1995b), however, showed persistent elevation of serum lipase and amylase for several months after cholecystectomy with no evidence of stones in the common bile duct or pancreatic duct. This observation suggests that acute pancreatitis may, in some cases, be secondary to in situ vaso-occlusion due to sickling.

RIGHT UPPER QUADRANT SYNDROME

The right upper quadrant syndrome (RUQ) refers to a patient with sickle cell disease who has pain in this region. Differential diagnosis of this entity includes acute sickle cell painful episode, acute cholecystitis, viral hepatitis, hepatic sequestration, hepatic crisis, and intrahepatic cholestasis.

Cholelithiasis, choledocholithiasis, and cholecystitis

At least two-thirds of adult patients with sickle cell anemia have hepatomegaly. The incidence of pigmented gallstones is about 30% in patients older than 10 years and approaches 70–75% in adults (Ballas et al. 1982; Vichinsky and Lubin 1980). About 90% of adult patients with sickle cell anemia and cholelithiasis had cholecystectomy either prophylactically or after an acute episode of calculous cholecystitis (Ballas et al. 1982). Acute cholecystitis may occur at any age and the stones are often multiple and pigmented. Less than 10% of patients with cholelithiasis develop cholecystitis (Vichinsky and Lubin 1980). The prevalence of choledocholithiasis in unselected patients with sickle cell disease is not known but seems to be less than 5% in patients with gallstones according to a survey of steady-state patients (McCall et al. 1977).

Acute cholecystitis should be treated conservatively with appropriate antibiotics and hydration until defervescence of the acute attack. Elective cholecystectomy may then be performed. Treatment of asymptomatic cholelithiasis remains controversial. Conservative measures such as restriction of fatty diet may be helpful. When gallstones are associated with chronic abdominal pain, elective cholecystectomy may be warranted. Unfortunately, only 50% of patients obtain relief of the pain following surgery (Vichinsky and Lubin 1980). Advocates of elective surgery for asymptomatic stones argue that surgical morbidity in a properly prepared sickle-cell patient is minimal whereas morbidity in an emergency cholecystectomy is high (Vichinsky and Lubin 1980). Laparoscopic cholecystectomy seems to be well tolerated by patients and associated with fewer complications than the traditional incisional surgical procedure (Ballas, unpublished observations).

Acute viral hepatitis

The clinical, laboratory, and liver findings of patients with sickle cell anemia and viral hepatitis seem to be more complicated, more prolonged, and associated with significantly higher bilirubin levels than in control groups (Barrett-Connor 1968, Serjeant 1992). Chuang et al. (1997) indicated that autoimmune liver disease and sclerosing cholangitis may occur with greater frequency in patients with sickle cell disease.

Hepatic sequestration

Acute hepatic sequestration is characterized by hepatic enlargement associated with significant fall in Hb level and no appreciable disturbance in liver function tests. Hatton et al. (1985) first described the problem in two adult patients with sickle cell anemia and associated infection. Davies and Brozovic (1989) documented hepatic sequestration with associated infection in two young children (18 months and 4 years of age), which suggests the syndrome may be present once autosplenectomy has occurred. Its most likely mechanism seems to be sequestration of sickled erythrocytes in the liver. The clinical progression is generally less acute than in splenic sequestration, and develops over a few hours to days. The liver becomes progressively enlarged and palpable and may be painful as the capsule stretches. Other signs are falling hemoglobin level and bone pain. Therapy is symptomatic and blood transfusion may be indicated if the Hb level falls below 5 g/dl. Hepatic sequestration may be easily overlooked unless the size of the liver is regularly monitored in patients with acute sickle cell crisis involving the right upper quadrant.

Hepatic crisis

Hepatic crisis is the most common liver complication in sickle cell disease (Vichinsky and Lubin 1980; Johnson et al. 1985). It may occur in 10% of patients admitted for painful crisis (Diggs 1965; Johnson et al. 1985). An attack is characterized by right upper quadrant abdominal pain, jaundice, hepatomegaly, fever, leukocytosis, dark urine, and often bone or joint pain. Serum transaminases and serum bilirubin are elevated to variable degrees. According to some reports the serum bilirubin rarely goes above 15 mg/dl (Sheehy 1977; Sheehy et al. 1980). Others, however, reported relatively mild course of hepatic crisis in children with serum bilirubin level as high as 57 mg/dl (Buchanan et al. 1977). Most of the elevated serum bilirubin (> 50%) is usually unconjugated. The clinical picture may simulate acute cholecystitis, choledocholithiasis, or viral hepatitis. Liver biopsy helps to distinguish hepatic crisis from viral hepatitis by showing sinusoidal obstruction by sickle cells, hypertrophy of Kupffer cells, and engorgement with RBC (Fig. 9). Additional findings may include hemosiderosis, occasional bile stasis, and mild centrolobular necrosis. The condition is usually transient but may last two to three weeks before complete resolution. Some authors recommended treatment with intravenous fluids and antibiotics, and elective cholecystectomy for gallstones (Vichinsky and Lubin 1980). Simple or exchange blood transfusion may be indicated (see below).

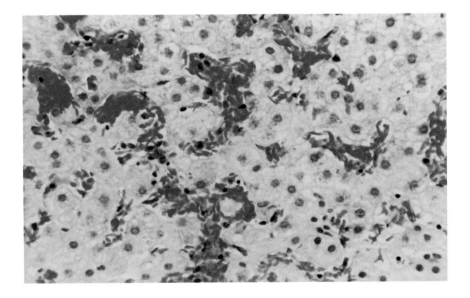

Fig. 9. Liver biopsy from a patient with sickle cell anemia and hepatic crisis showing engorgement of hepatic sinusoids with sickled erythrocytes.

Intrahepatic cholestasis

This severe form of hepatic crisis may, in rare cases, be complicated by fulminant cholestasis leading to hepatic coma and death. An attack of intra-hepatic cholestasis is characterized by sudden onset of abdominal or right upper quadrant pain, increasing jaundice (with conjugated bilirubin as high as unconjugated bilirubin), a progressively enlarging liver, light stools, and hyperbilirubinemia without urobilinogenuria. The clinical picture suggests cholestatic jaundice or choledocholithiasis but with no evidence of common duct obstruction or cholangitis. The prothrombin time (PT), partial thrombo-plastin time (PTT), lactate dehydrogenase, and liver enzymes are all el-evated. Total serum bilirubin level may be over 100 mg/dl. Liver biopsy shows similar changes to those described in hepatic crisis but in a more severe form associated with lymphocytic infiltration, paracentral necrosis, cholestasis, and dilated canaliculi containing bile plugs.

Intrahepatic cholestasis is a potentially fatal complication of sickle cell disease if not treated promptly. In early reports (Wade 1960; Sheehy et al. 1980) only one of eight patients survived. The advent of exchange transfu-sion as a therapeutic modality (Sheehy et al. 1980; Stephan et al. 1995) reversed this prognosis. In this author's opinion, patients who are suspected of having hepatic crisis should be watched carefully by monitoring their clinical status, hematological parameters, serum bilirubin, liver function, and coagulation profile. If the total serum bilirubin level increases to values greater than 50 mg/dl or the PT increases to values greater than 20 seconds, then *total* blood exchange should be performed by replacing the removed blood with washed sickle-negative RBC and fresh frozen plasma (Talacki and Ballas 1990). The procedure should be repeated until the Hb S decreases to less than 30% and the serum bilirubin and PT decrease to acceptable values.

Other acute abdominal painful episodes

An abdominal sickle cell painful crisis is characterized by severe, usu-ally generalized, abdominal pain and signs of peritoneal irritation. It may also be accompanied by fever, leukocytosis, and markedly elevated levels of lactate dehydrogenase. Clinically, a severe abdominal crisis may closely mimic an acute abdomen and may lead to an exploratory laparotomy in search for surgically correctable pathology. Patients with sickle cell disease who arrive at the emergency department with an acute abdominal crisis may be misdiagnosed with acute appendicitis or acute cholecystitis and undergo laparotomy and often "prophylactic" appendectomy and/or cholecystectomy (Ballas et al. 1995b). In the author's experience about one-third of adult patients with sickle disease give history of appendectomy. Whether the procedure was done for true acute appendicitis or misdiagnosis of abdominal crisis is unknown at present. Nevertheless, a 30% incidence of acute appendicitis is much higher than in the general population and raises questions about the authenticity of the diagnosis. Thus, acute abdominal pain in sickle cell disease should be considered a painful episode until proven otherwise.

The abdominal pain has been attributed to enlarged mesenteric and retroperitoneal lymph nodes, bone marrow hyperplasia, infarction of the vertebral bodies, hepatobiliary disease, splenic disease, or mesenteric arterial thrombosis (Leivy and Schnabel 1932; Gage and Gagner 1983). The abdominal pain seen in crisis may persist for several days, although protracted episodes lasting longer than five days are not unusual (Lukens 1981). Differentiation from other causes of acute abdominal pain may be difficult.

Pain in the trunk in association with abdominal distention has been referred to as girdle syndrome (Brozovic et al. 1987; Davies and Brozovic 1989). It is thought to result from sickling in the mesenteric blood supply. Fluid levels may be visible on radiographs of the abdomen. Mild cases are self-limiting over a two- to five-day period and are treated symptomatically with intravenous fluids because gut absorption is impaired. More severe cases have associated involvement of the liver and lungs, and in very severe cases multiorgan failure including acute chest syndrome should be considered. Such patients may have markedly distended loops of bowel and require nasogastric suction and exchange transfusion. Infarction of segments of gut can occur, so it is important to involve surgeons in the evaluation of these patients.

GENITOURINARY PAIN

PRIAPISM

Priapism (Powars and John 1996), a persistent painful penile erection, is a debilitating complication of sickle cell disease. Controlled studies are lacking, therapeutic approaches are controversial and often conflicting, and medical and surgical therapy fail in most patients. Pathophysiologic mechanisms that precipitate an attack are not well understood. The decreased rate of blood flow through the penis during normal erection allows increased oxygen extraction. As a result hypoxia promotes sickling with consequent congestion of the corpora, sludging, further impairment of venous outflow, and worsening hypoxia (Emond et al. 1980; Gradisek 1983). Venous outflow from the corpora is reduced but not completely obstructed. Most cases of priapism (about 75%) occur between midnight and 6 A.M. and after normal sexual intercourse (Seeler 1973a; Baron and Leiter 1978; Emond et al. 1980).

Acidosis resulting from dehydration and hypoventilation during sleep may be a precipitating factor.

Two distinct patterns of priapism are bicorporal and tricorporal. A magnetic resonance (MR) scan of the penis can differentiate the two patterns. Bicorporal priapism involves both corpora cavernosa and is more common in children. It is characterized by short, repetitive, reversible painful episodes referred to as "stuttering priapism," with detumescence occurring within a few hours after the onset of erection. This pattern has good prognosis and is associated with normal sexual function. The reported prevalence of stuttering priapism varies widely from about 2% of men with sickle cell disease in a retrospective study by Sharpsteen et al. (1993) to between 40% and 60% of men with sickle cell disease according to other investigators (Emond et al. 1980; Serjeant 1985). Tricorporal priapism involves both corpora cavernosa and the corpus spongiosum and is more common in older patients. It is characterized by painful erection that may last up to several days or weeks and may be followed by complete or partial impotence. Its reported prevalence also varies widely between 6.5% (Sharpsteen et al. 1993) and 38% (Emond et al. 1980) of men with sickle cell disease. Sharpsteen et al. (1993) reported that sickle cell-related organ failure such as stroke, chronic lung disease, chronic renal failure, and chronic leg ulcers were observed more frequently in men who had tricorporal priapism. In their study death occurred in nine adult patients (25% of men with priapism) within five years of the first episode of priapism. They concluded that priapism in adult males is a marker of severe disease and identifies patients who are at risk for other sickle cell-related organ failure syndromes.

Management of priapism is highly controversial. Major goals of treatment include pain relief and prevention of impotence. Precipitating factors should be sought and corrected if possible. These include infection of the prostate or bladder, recent trauma, medications with autonomic side effects, and alcohol ingestion (Galloway and Harwood-Nuss 1988). Initial treatment in the emergency department should include vigorous hydration and opioid analgesics. Catheterization of the urinary bladder may be indicated to promote emptying. The administration of benzodiazepines or pseudoephedrine HCl may be helpful in some patients. Hypertransfusion or exchange transfusion to permit the entry of normal RBC to the engorged area and enhance oxygenation is an acceptable approach to persistent priapism (Seeler 1973a; Baron and Leiter 1978; Talacki and Ballas 1990). Siegel et al. (1993), however, reported significant neurological complications (headache, seizures, and obtundation requiring ventilatory support) in patients with priapism who had exchange transfusion. Patients responding to transfusion therapy usually experience detumescence within 24 to 48 hours. Many authors believe medical treatment should be instituted prior to surgery (Gradisek 1983). Recent studies suggest that if detumescence has not begun within 24 hours following the completion of a transfusion, significant response is unlikely and a shunt operation should be considered. However, no evidence supports surgical intervention as the initial mode of therapy (Baron and Leiter 1978; Gradisek 1983). Surgical procedures vary from simple needle aspiration with irrigation to various shunt procedures between the cavernosa and spongiosum (Gradisek 1983). Without intervention, severe priapism results in impotence in more than 80% of patients. The combination of transfusions and surgery can decrease this to 25-50%. Patients who become impotent may benefit from psychological counseling and the insertion of prosthetic penile implants.

PELVIC CRISES

In the author's experience some patients with sickle cell disease may complain of acute painful episodes involving the low abdomen, inguinal areas, the genitalia, and the inner aspect of both thighs. The pain is described as similar to that of the usual painful episodes and is associated with tenderness in the involved areas. This constellation of signs and symptoms suggests pelvic pain due to vaso-occlusive episodes. The incidence, prevalence, and mechanism of this type of painful episode needs further documentation and study.

INFECTION

Urinary tract infection and pyelonephritis cause pain by themselves and, moreover, may precipitate acute sickle cell painful episodes. In addition, pyelonephritis is usually associated with fever, leukocytosis, and back pain that may be mistaken for acute painful episodes. It is advisable to order urinalysis, and urine and blood cultures in all patients with back pain, especially with fever.

MUSCLE PAIN

Although bone and joint infarction has been well documented during the acute painful crises of sickle cell disease, muscle involvement has not been well described and documented. Dorwart and Gabuzda (1985) noted symmetric myositis and fasciitis six times in 36 consecutive painful crises in two patients during two years of observation. Muscle biopsies showed muscle and facial necrosis. Despite the finding of necrosis by biopsy, levels of serum creatinine phosphokinase never exceeded 500 IU/l (normal level is less than 10 IU/l), and serum aldolase was repeatedly normal. The necrotizing myositis and fasciitis were self-limited and recurrent. They occurred suddenly during prolonged sickle cell crises, had the same monotonous appearance each time, and involved the deltoids and thigh muscles symmetrically. The condition was painful and disabling while acute and had no satisfactory explanation.

Valeriano-Marcet and Kerr (1991) described four patients with sickle cell painful episodes, symmetric proximal muscle pain, and swelling as prominent features of their attacks. Muscle biopsies showed acute myonecrosis with a minimal inflammatory reaction and myofibrosis with abundant collagen deposition. Chronic sequelae consisted of muscle induration, atrophy, and contractures. It is not clear, however, whether these changes are due to ischemic myopathy secondary to vaso-occlusion or to repeated intramuscular injections of opioid analgesics. Nevertheless, ischemic myopathy in sickle cell disease seems to be underdiagnosed or not well recognized because its manifestations overlap with those of painful crises and because providers tend to lump all the complaints of patients with sickle cell disease as "just another crisis."

6

Chronic Pain Syndromes

Pain, whose unchecked and familiar speed
Is howling, and keen shrieks day after day.
— Percy Bysshe Shelley, 1792–1822

LEG ULCERS

PREVALENCE AND INCIDENCE

Leg ulceration is a common complication of sickle cell anemia (Diggs and Ching 1934; Serjeant 1974). Although it occurred in the first four cases of sickle cell disease reported in the English literature, it was not recognized as a specific complication until 1940 when Cummer and La Rocco (1940) suggested a causal relationship. The incidence and prevalence of skin ulceration shows great variation in reported series. In the West Indies, of the patients with sickle cell disease, 65% between the ages of 15 and 19 years and 75% of those over 30 years had active leg ulcers (Serjeant 1974). Similarly, a 75% incidence was reported in the United States earlier in this century (Wolfort and Kirzak 1967; Serjeant 1974; Alleyne et al. 1977). Recent representative data from a large cooperative study in the United States found active leg ulcers at entry in 2.5% of 2075 patients aged 10 years or older and in none of 1700 patients less than 10 years old (Koshy et al. 1989). The prevalence rate of leg ulcers elsewhere in the world varies from almost none in Saudi Arabia (Perrine et al. 1978; Al-Momen 1991) to 4% in London (Brozovic and Anionwu 1984) and 10% in Africa (Akinyanju and Akinsete 1979; Konotey-Ahulu 1979; Adedeji 1988; Durosinmi et al. 1991).

PREDISPOSING FACTORS

Table I summarizes predisposing factors. Among sickle cell syndromes, sickle cell anemia is most often associated with leg ulceration, which is are rarely seen in patients with Hb SC disease or sickle-β^+-thalassemia (Koshy

121

Table I
Factors that increase the risk of leg ulcers in sickle cell disease

Factor	Risk
Type of sickle cell syndrome	Hb SS > Sickle-β^0-thal > Sickle-β^+-thal > Hb SC
Gender	Males > females
Age	Incidence increases with age
Total Hb level	High incidence in patients with very low Hb level
Hb F level	Negative correlation of incidence with Hb F level
α Genotype	Hb SS with four α genes > Hb S with two α genes
β Haplotypes	High incidence in patients with CAR haplotype
Antithrombin III	Deficiency increases risk
HLA type	Greater with HLA-B35 and HLA-CW4 types
Geography	Jamaica > USA > London > Saudi Arabia

et al. 1989). Data on leg ulcers from the cooperative study of the clinical course of sickle cell disease (Koshy et al. 1989) identified five risk factors: leg ulcers were more common in males than in females and in older patients, and less common in patients with α-gene deletion, high total Hb level; and high levels of Hb F. Powars et al. (1990a,b) reported that leg ulcers were more common in patients with sickle cell anemia who were also carriers of the CAR β-haplotype. Cacciola et al. (1989) found antithrombin III deficiency in patients with sickle-β-thalassemia and chronic leg ulcers; treatment with antithrombin III concentrate produced a favorable outcome. Other factors reported to increase the risk of leg ulcers include tissue type HLA-B35 and HLA-CW4 (Ofosu et al. 1987).

PATHOPHYSIOLOGY

Ulceration of the skin in sickle cell anemia seems to be the result of multiple factors. Leg ulcers may appear spontaneously, or following infection or trauma. Trauma, even minor, to an area of compromised blood supply may initiate the ulcer. Diggs (1973) indicated that an ulcer may start as an insect bite, pimple, skin abrasion that becomes infected, a bruise, or as a hemorrhagic infarct that first appears as a tender nodule. Wrinkling, roughening, and hyperpigmentation of the skin usually occur over the site where the ulcer will appear. It progresses to a nodular swelling associated with pain, tenderness, and pruritus, and eventually skin ulceration. Extravasation of plasma into interstitial fluid follows trauma and results in localized edema that compresses tissue around the injury. Consequently, blood flow through the capillaries decreases and arterial pressure increases. The precapillary arterioles expand, arterial blood is shunted away from the traumatized area, and tissue ischemia and damage worsen. The aging process causes vessels to lose their anastomotic network and become end-arteries, resulting in further obstruction and necrosis (Serjeant 1974). Other reported factors that may enhance blood stasis and skin necrosis include reduced red cell deformability (Ballas 1991), adherence of sickle RBC to the endothelium (Hebbel et al. 1980a,b), increased blood viscosity (Phillips et al. 1991), the presence of circulating immune complexes (Morgan and Venner 1981), or activated blood coagulation (Cacciola et al. 1989). Secondary infection of the ulcer with undermining of the edges delays healing and causes progressive extension of skin ulceration. Surprisingly, venous insufficiency is not known to be a cause of leg ulcers in sickle cell disease (Billet et al. 1991).

CLINICAL FEATURES

The most common site for the appearance of leg ulcers is the distal third of the leg, especially on the inner area, just above the ankles and over the medial melleoli (Fig. 1). No site of the skin, however, is spared from possible involvement, and ulcers have been reported over the dorsum of the foot, elbows, and thighs. Leg ulcers may be single or multiple, and an estimated one-third occur bilaterally (Serjeant 1974; Koshy et al. 1989; Ankra-Badu 1992). They vary in size from a few millimeters in diameter to huge ulcers that may circle around the leg. They may be shallow, superficial erosions of the dermis or very deep craters with tendons visible at their base. They are usually discrete, sharply marginated, round, oval, and punched out in appearance. They may be covered with a dry, serous, or seropurulent crust. Leg ulcers tend to be indolent, and heal slowly over months to years.

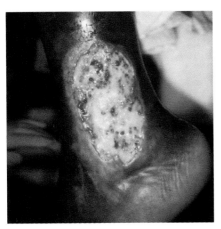 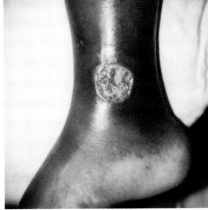

Fig. 1. Leg ulcers in a patient with sickle cell anemia.

Direct involvement of the periosteum is unusual but periosteal reaction may occur in 60% of cases (Serjeant 1974). Scars of healed ulcers are thin, atrophic, smooth, glossy, and surrounded by a pigmented areola. Healed ulcers often recur within a few months.

Leg ulcers, especially when large, cause the affected patient considerable grief. The ulcers are painful, tender, unsightly, and often associated with foul smell. Patients tend to avoid social interactions for fear of embarrassment. The pain associated with leg ulcers may be severe, excruciating, penetrating, sharp, and stinging. In many patients, opioid analgesics are needed to achieve some pain relief (see Chapter 10).

MANAGEMENT

Treatment of leg ulcers requires significant patience on the part of providers and patients. Careful and regular nursing care coupled with patient education and counseling is of paramount importance. Small ulcers may heal in few weeks, but complete healing can take several months to years. Table II summarizes various methods of treatment reviewed by Phillips et al. (1994).

Table II
Summary of methods used to treat leg ulcers

Local Measures	Agents that Promote Tissue Granulation
Bed rest, elevation of legs	Benzoyl peroxide
Wet to dry dressings	Dextranomer (Debrisan)
Hydrotherapy (whirlpool therapy)	Gelatin sponge (Gelfoam)
Disinfecting Agents	*Other Modalities*
Soaps	Unna boots
Acetic acid (1.01%)	Blood transfusion/exchange
Hexachlorphene (PHisoHex)	transfusion
Hydrogen peroxide	Topical hyperbaric oxygen
Povidone-iodine (Betadine)	Oral zinc sulfate
Silver sulfadiazine (Silvadene)	Erythropoietin
Sodium hypochlorite (Dakin's Solution)	RGD peptide matrix
Aluminum acetate (Burow's Solution)	Recombinant human granulocyte-
Topical antibiotics	macrophage colony stimulating
Debridement	factor (rh GM-CSF)
Surgical	Collagen matrix dressings
Medical (enzymes)	Lyophilized type-1 collagen
Collagenase (Santyl, Biozyme C)	Antithrombin III
Fibrinolysin and desoxyribonuclease	Electrical stimulation
(Elase)	Skin grafting
Trypsin (Granulderm)	*Circ Aid Legging*
Sutilans (Travase)	
Hydrocolloid dressings (DuoDERM)	

Treatment should start with good local care that includes rest, elevation of the affected leg, and wound care with wet to dry dressing soaked in a disinfecting agent (Table II), and whirlpool therapy. Infected ulcers may be treated with topical or systemic antibiotics. Large ulcers associated with abundant necrotic tissue may require debridement either surgically (in severe cases) or medically. Several agents are available to achieve rapid debridement (Table II) and are well tolerated with painful ulcers. Patients should be informed that debridement will cause the ulcer to enlarge at first as dead tissue is removed. Agents that promote tissue granulation should be used after the removal of devitalized tissue by debridement. Oral zinc therapy (600 mg per day) may be beneficial in some patients (Serjeant 1992). Leg ulcers that persist beyond six months present a challenge to the treating physician and the patient.

Failure to respond to the measures mentioned above may justify trying the other modalities listed in Table II, although no controlled trials have examined these modalities. The benefit/risk ratio for each patient should be carefully analyzed. Uncontrolled trials, mostly anecdotal, reported healing of sickle leg ulcers with transfusion (Chernoff et al. 1954; Talacki and Ballas 1990), erythropoietin in combination with hydroxyurea (Al-Momen 1991), arginine butyrate (Sher and Olivieri 1994), hyperbaric oxygen (Heng 1983; Ravina et al. 1983; Heng et al. 1984), arginine-glycine-aspartic acid (RGD) synthetic peptide matrix (Wethers et al. 1994), recombinant human granulocyte-macrophage colony stimulating factor (rhGM-CSF; Pieters et al. 1995), collagen matrix dressing (Reindorf et al. 1989), lyophilized Type-1 collagen (Mian et al. 1991), antithrombin III (Cacciola et al. 1989), and electrical stimulation (Ballas et al. 1995b). The induction of Hb F production by hydroxyurea or other agents seems to be promising. Hydroxyurea reportedly improves leg ulcers in patients with myeloproliferative disorders (Nguyen and Margolis 1993). Although controlled studies have not been reported to support the role of Hb F induction in the management of leg ulcers, further analysis of the data in a multicenter trial of hydroxyurea (see Chapter 12) may provide further information into the role of hydroxyurea in treating recalcitrant leg ulcers (Charache et al. 1995).

Finally, if all else fails, skin grafting may be considered. Some studies report a degree of success (Heckler et al. 1977; Spence 1985; Khouri and Upton 1991) and others a high rate of failure (Koshy et al. 1989). To be successful skin grafting should be done on clean, debrided ulcers, and should be preceded and followed by transfusion or exchange transfusion to keep the percentage of Hb S low (< 30%) to break the cycle of sickling, vaso-occlusion, and tissue necrosis and to promote healing.

Because leg ulcers may recur after minimal trauma, the use of Circ Aid leggings as a preventive measure may be advisable (Ballas et al. 1995b). These nonelastic (special Velcro) lower-extremity orthoses with ankle straps are custom-made and may be worn during the day and at work.

AVASCULAR NECROSIS

AVASCULAR NECROSIS OF THE FEMORAL HEAD

Avascular necrosis (also referred to as aseptic necrosis, osteonecrosis, or ischemic necrosis) of the epiphyses is an important complication of sickle cell disease. It is second only to the spleen as the most commonly observed sickle-cell-induced organ failure (Powars 1990). Acute diaphyseal infarction of long bones is less common in adults than in children. Avascular necrosis of the epiphyses, however, becomes more common, recurrent, and chronic in adults with sickle cell disease and may cause considerable morbidity because of persistent pain and limitation of movement. The hip joint seems to be the most common site of avascular necrosis and is the subject of several studies and reports. Involvement of the shoulder is less common, and the knees and other large joints are rarely involved (Bohrer 1987).

Predisposing factors

Risk factors for avascular necrosis of the femoral head include genotype, age, frequency of painful episodes, hemoglobin/hematocrit level, α-gene deletion, mean corpuscular volume, and serum aspartate aminotransferase (AST) (Milner et al. 1991). Early studies (Smith and Conley 1954; Hill et al. 1975) suggested that avascular necrosis of the femoral head was more common in Hb SC disease but this finding was probably due to patient selection because patients with Hb SC disease lived longer and were more likely to be affected with age. In the natural history study in the United States where 2590 patients over 5 years of age at entry were followed prospectively for an average of 5.6 years, patients with hemoglobin SS genotype and α-thalassemia (and possibly those with S-β°-thalassemia) were at higher risk for avascular necrosis of the femoral head compared to other genotypes. Age, frequency of painful episodes, Hb level, and α-gene deletion showed positive correlation with avascular necrosis. In Hb SC disease and sickle-β+-thalassemia, however, avascular necrosis seems to be associated with lower incidence of painful crises. Patients with sickle cell anemia and α-gene deletion have a higher incidence of avascular necrosis (Ballas et al. 1989b; Milner et al. 1991) because their relatively high hematocrit increases blood viscosity and, thus, enhances microvasculopathy in the aforementioned anatomic sites. The mean corpuscular volume and serum aspartate aminotransferase were negatively correlated with avascular necrosis. The significance and pathophysiology of this finding are not well understood at present.

Prevalence and incidence

Sickle cell anemia is the most common cause of avascular necrosis of the hip in children (Hernigou et al. 1991; Serjeant 1992). The overall prevalence of avascular necrosis in sickle cell syndromes is about 10% and patients with homozygous sickle cell anemia and concomitant α-thalassemia are at particular risk with a prevalence greater than 20% (Ballas et al. 1989b; Milner et al. 1991; Ware et al. 1991; Serjeant 1992). The risk of developing avascular necrosis increases with age, and almost 50% of patients with sickle cell anemia develop avascular necrosis by age 35.

The prevalence and incidence of avascular necrosis of the femoral head in sickle cell syndromes was determined by a prospective study of 2590 patients who were followed for an average of 5.6 years (Milner et al. 1991). At entry 9.8% of patients had avascular necrosis of one or both femoral heads. Prevalence was highest among patients with sickle-β°-thalassemia (13.1%) followed by sickle cell anemia (5.8%). None of the patients with sickle-β+-thalassemia younger than 25 years had avascular necrosis on entry. Follow-up data showed significant differences in age-adjusted incidence rates; the highest rate occurred in patients with sickle cell anemia and concomitant α-thalassemia (4.46 per 100 patient years) (Table III).

Table III
Incidence of avascular necrosis of the femoral head per 100 patient-years

Age at diagnosis (years)	Hemoglobin Genotype					All Genotypes
	SS	SS, α-Thal	Sβ°	SC	Sβ+	
5–9	2.51	1.31	2.78	0.00	0.00	1.77
10–14	1.05	4.69	5.25	0.87	1.70	2.21
5–14	1.41	3.64	4.29	0.66	1.53	2.09
15–24	2.58	3.45	1.90	2.11	1.11	2.83
25–34	3.44	6.35	4.40	1.89	2.54	3.50
35–44	0.02	4.41	8.03	5.15	11.47	3.57
≥45	2.36	9.45	0.00	2.59	30.02	4.51
35– ≥45	0.98	6.34	6.66	4.13	13.83	3.85
Crude rate	2.31	4.47	3.65	2.02	3.04	2.88
Age-adjusted rate	2.35	4.46	3.63	1.91	3.27	—

Source: Milner et al. 1991, with permission.

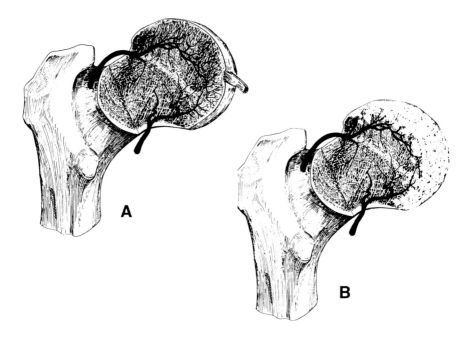

Fig. 2. A: Arterial blood supply to the head of the femur; **B:** necrosis due to occlusion of capillaries by sickled cells at distal portion where hypoxia is maximal and collateral circulation inadequate (Diggs 1965 with permission).

Pathophysiology

The femoral head is the most common site of necrosis owing to the poor anastomotic network and the stress of weight bearing. Sherman (1959) described local damage to extremely small vessels in association with disintegration of the hip in sickle cell disease. Diggs (1965) noted that occlusion of vessels is more likely to occur in the portion that is farthest from the arterial blood supply, as is the case in the vessels supplying the head of the femur (Fig. 2). Thus, avascular necrosis of the hip results from severe ischemia of the medullary bone. Occlusion of the osseous circulation leads to necrosis and to an increase in intramedullary pressure that causes further vascular compromise (Ficat 1985; Mankin 1992). Without treatment, this sequence of pathologic events may lead to total collapse of the femoral head.

Clinical features

Avascular necrosis of the hip causes chronic severe pain and morbidity in patients with sickle cell disease. The pain is generally worse on walking and relieved by rest and may be accompanied by a moderate limitation of motion and a limp when the patient bears weight on the affected extremity.

Continued weight bearing on a softened femoral head results in collapse and damage to the articular surface. The clinical picture varies considerably. Some patients are asymptomatic, others may have minimal pain despite gross destruction of the femoral head, and still others may have severe pain (Diggs 1967; Chung and Ralston 1969; Lee et al. 1981; Sebes and Kraus 1983; Iwegbu and Fleming 1985). Most patients need a cane to assist with ambulation; some may need a brace, crutches, or reconstructive surgery.

In their prospective study, Milner et al. (1991) found that about 47% of the patients who developed avascular necrosis had no pain or limitation of motion at the time of diagnosis. About 21% of these patients, however, reported symptoms of pain or had limitation of motion in the affected joint at a later date.

Fig. 3 shows examples of the radiological picture of avascular necrosis in sickle cell disease. Ficat et al. (1983) proposed a four-stage radiographic classification as summarized in Table IV. Knowing the stage of the disease is important in choosing the most appropriate therapeutic approach (see below). At the time of diagnosis of avascular necrosis 47.4% of the patients showed stage II disease, 29.6% showed stage III, and 23% showed stage IV (Milner et al. 1991).

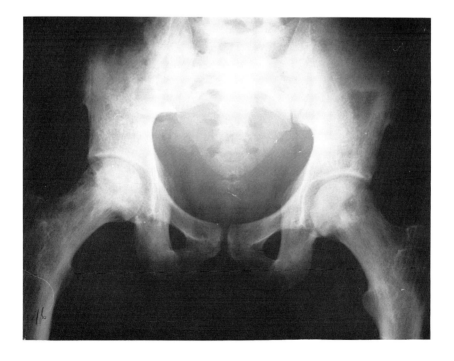

Fig. 3. Avascular necrosis of the femoral head in sickle cell disease.

Table IV
Radiological classification of avascular necrosis

Stage I	Normal plain radiograph, abnormal MRI
Stage II	Sclerosis, radiolucent areas, and lytic areas on radiography
Stage III	Subepiphyseal radiolucency, flattening of femoral head, and widening of the joint space
Stage IV	Sclerosis and/or fragmentation of the epiphysis, collapse of the femoral head, and narrowing of the joint space

Treatment

Treatment of symptomatic avascular necrosis of the femoral head in patients with sickle cell disease can be medical or surgical. Medical treatment includes analgesia, reduction of weight bearing on the affected joint, and physical therapy. Severe pain may entail the use of opioid analgesics, especially in patients with history of recurrent acute painful episodes and tolerance to nonopioid analgesics (see Chapter 9). Bed rest is recommended, especially if the femoral head is severely involved. Reduction or elimination of weight bearing may allow a weakened epiphysis to heal without collapse. The use of a cane or a walker may be useful in reducing weight bearing in mild cases. Total immobility with braces or crutches could have an adverse psychological effect on children, adolescents, or young adults. Education and counseling is of paramount importance in these situations. Physiotherapy helps maintain muscle tone and rebuild muscle mass. Transfusion therapy does not seem to play an important role with this complication of sickle cell disease.

Advanced forms of avascular necrosis require total bone replacement. Results of hip arthroplasty in sickle cell disease are not as encouraging as results of arthroplasty performed for an arthritic hip (Saito et al. 1989). Placement of an internal prosthesis may be difficult due to the presence of hard sclerotic bone in sickle cell disease. Other problems associated with hip arthroplasty in sickle cell disease include an increased incidence of infarction (Hanker and Amstutz 1988; Clarke et al. 1989), a failure rate of about 50%, and a high morbidity due to loosening of both cemented and uncemented prostheses (Clarke et al. 1989). Recent techniques of arthroplasty may improve the life expectancy of hip prostheses.

Other reported surgical techniques for the treatment of avascular necrosis of the femoral head include the injection of acrylic cement (Herrigou et al. 1993) and core decompression (Styles and Vichinsky 1996). The latter is recommended in early stages (I or II) of avascular necrosis. Controlled trials are needed to verify the value of these new surgical techniques.

AVASCULAR NECROSIS OF OTHER JOINTS

Although avascular necrosis tends to be most severe and disabling in the hip area, it is a generalized disorder in that the femoral and humeral heads and the vertebral bodies may be affected. Avascular necrosis of the vertebral column was discussed in Chapter 5. The limited terminal arterial blood supply and the paucity of collateral circulation make these three areas especially vulnerable to sickling, vaso-occlusion, and subsequent bone damage.

Sickle cell disease is a frequent cause of avascular necrosis of the humeral head, especially in children and young adults. The prevalence and incidence of avascular necrosis of the humeral head in sickle cell disease was determined by a prospective study of 2524 patients who were followed for an average of 5.6 years (Milner et al. 1993). At entry, 5.6% had radiographic evidence of avascular necrosis in one or both shoulders. The results showed little difference in age-adjusted prevalence among genotypes but striking differences in age-specific rates. No sickle-β^+-thalassemia patients younger than 25 years of age had avascular necrosis on entry. The highest age-adjusted incidence rate was found in sickle cell anemia patients with concomitant α-thalassemia (4.85 per 100 patient-years), followed by sickle-β^o-thalassemia (4.8 per 100 patient-years), sickle-β^+-thalassemia (2.61 per 100 patient-years), sickle cell anemia without α-thalassemia (2.54 per 100 patient-years), and Hb SC disease (1.66 per 100 patient-years). Only about 21% of patients reported pain or had limited range of movement at the time of diagnosis.

CHRONIC OSTEOMYELITIS

Chronic osteomyelitis is a continuous infectious process of bone. Acute osteomyelitis may evolve into a chronic bone infection with typical radiographic changes (David et al. 1987). In sickle cell anemia, chronic osteomyelitis is rare and may follow acute osteomyelitis associated with the insertion of a hip or shoulder prosthesis. Inappropriate management can result in significant bone destruction and necrosis with persistent foci of inflammation. Those sites may continue to reinfect the area with a progressive bony response characterized by sequestration and involucrum formation. With healing the shaft will demonstrate increased bone density (David et al. 1987). Chronic osteomyelitis in sickle cell anemia is difficult to treat; prolonged antibiotic therapy may suppress the infection but rarely eradicates it. Persistent infection is one cause for the recurrence of acute sickle cell painful episodes.

INTRACTABLE PAINFUL EPISODES

A few patients with sickle cell disease have intractable painful episodes and take opioid or nonopioid analgesics on a chronic basis. They have no evidence of precipitating cause such as infection, dehydration, or ischemia. Many of these patients are often referred to as "problem" patients or "difficult" patients, and their management is a challenge to the treating physician, as will be discussed in Chapters 10 and 13.

CHRONIC ARTHROPATHY SECONDARY TO IRON DEPOSITION

Arthropathy is a common and disabling complication of idiopathic hemochromatosis (Adams and Speechley 1996). Multiply transfused patients with sickle cell disease, especially adults, suffer from hemosiderosis due to iron deposition in the reticuloendothelial system. With progressive iron accumulation, tissue damage may occur, including a chronic form of arthropathy. This sequence of events, however, has not been proven by well-designed studies.

7

Other Pain Syndromes

But pain is perfect misery, the worst of evils, and,
excessive, overturns all patience.
    —John Milton, *Paradise Lost*, 1608–1674

Pain is God's megaphone to arouse a deaf world.
    —Clive S. Lewis, 1898–1963

HEADACHE

Patients with sickle cell disease often complain of headache, one of the most common pain syndromes that afflicts the population at large. There are three major types of headache that occur in association with sickle cell disease and deserve special mention. Their recognition has important implications for diagnosis, pathophysiology, and management. These three types are: (1) acute painful episode involving the head, (2) headache secondary to the involvement of the central nervous system, and (3) migraine headache.

Type I was discussed in Chapter 5. The onset of severe headache associated with changes in mental status suggests complications involving the central nervous system. Changes in mental status include disorientation, confusion, and lethargy. Fever and stiffness of the neck warrant tests for meningitis, which occurs predominantly in infants and young children (Barrett-Connor 1971b) and is usually caused by *Streptococcus pneumoniae*. Thus, management of headache in infants and young children with fever and alterations in mental status should include examination of the cerebrospinal fluid and the administration of appropriate antibiotic therapy.

In adult patients with sickle cell disease, the onset of a new, severe, and persistent headache raises the possibility of cerebral hemorrhage, especially if the pain worsens and is associated with changes in the mental status. Computed tomography or magnetic resonance imaging of the head clarifies the diagnosis (Fig. 1).

Neurologic complications (including infarction, hemorrhage, seizure disorder, infection, sensorineural hearing loss, and spinal cord infarction) occur

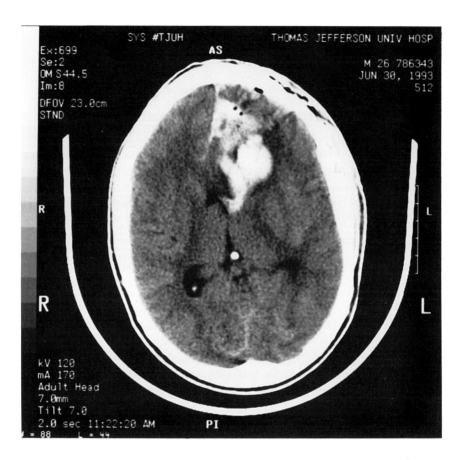

Fig. 1. Intracerebral hemorrhage in a patient with sickle cell anemia (Ballas et al. 1995b with permission).

in 25% of patients with sickle cell disease and are most common in sickle cell anemia. Cerebral infarction is more frequent in children, whereas intra-cerebral hemorrhage is more prevalent in adults (Powars et al. 1978; Powars 1976, 1990; Lubin and Vichinsky 1991). Microaneurysms involving fragile, dilated vessels, which develop as compensatory collateral circulation around areas of infarction, seem to be responsible for hemorrhage in adults. Unlike other vascular beds, large vessels rather than microvessels seem to be the site of occlusion with consequent infarction. About two-thirds of children with cerebral infarction (who are not transfused) may develop further ischemic events within three years (Powars 1976; Powars et al. 1978).

For a child with cerebral infarction secondary to vaso-occlusion, exchange transfusion or hypertransfusion is the appropriate therapy to maintain an Hb S level below 30%. Red cell transfusions are usually provided for a minimum of five years, after which the continuation of transfusion therapy is individualized. It is not known whether chronic transfusion therapy is indicated for adults with cerebral infarction secondary to vaso-occlusion. Similarly, the appropriate management of an adult patient with cerebral hemorrhage is unknown. A thorough search for aneurysms and consideration of surgical intervention is recommended (Ballas et al. 1995b).

MIGRAINE HEADACHE

Migraine headache has been described in patients with sickle cell disease (Ballas et al. 1995b), but the type, prevalence, and incidence rates in this patient population are not known. Migraine headache in patients with sickle cell disease may be mistaken for a manifestation of the acute painful episodes. The association of migraine with sickle cell disease raises several questions. Sickle cell disease is a vaso-occlusive disease whereas migraine is due to vasodilation and its treatment includes the use of vasoconstricting agents (Saper et al. 1993). Whether one disease precipitates or exacerbates the other is not known. The stress of a migraine attack may precipitate an acute sickle cell painful episode or vice versa. In the author's experience patients who suffer from both diseases often, but not always, indicate that the sickle cell painful episode precipitates an attack of migraine headache. The treatment of migraine in patients with sickle cell disease should not include vasoconstrictive agents, such as sumatriptan, because these drugs may precipitate or worsen acute painful vaso-occlusive episodes. The use of antidepressants in this combination may be useful (Ballas et al. 1995b).

NEUROPATHIC PAIN

Neuropathic pain describes a group of disorders believed to be caused by functional abnormalities of the central nervous system (Fields 1987). The common mechanism shared by these disorders presumably involves aberrant somatosensory processing in the central or peripheral nervous system. Accordingly, a pathophysiologic classification divides these disorders into central and peripheral neuropathic pain. As will be discussed below, both these types of pain are rarely reported in association with sickle cell disease. This paucity of reports may represent an authentic low incidence or inability of care providers to differentiate neuropathic pain from the pain associated with the acute vaso-occlusive episodes typical of sickle cell disease.

CENTRAL NEUROPATHIC PAIN

Central pain, according to the International Association for the Study of Pain (IASP), is caused by a lesion or dysfunction in the central nervous system (Merskey 1986). Given that sickle cell disease involves the CNS, we would expect that central neuropathic pain might occur in this disease. As was mentioned above, and except for acute headaches that may accompany cerebral hemorrhage or infection, central pain is virtually not reported in sickle cell disease.

Most reported neurological complications of sickle cell syndromes involve the CNS and include cerebral infarction (Powars et al. 1978; Frempong 1991), intracranial hemorrhage (Powars 1976; Powars et al. 1978, Frempong 1991; Balkaran et al. 1992), cognitive dysfunction (Swift et al. 1989; Adams 1994), hearing loss (Todd et al. 1973), and a few cases of spinal cord infarction (Rothman and Nelson 1980). The most common and the most striking neurological complication of sickle cell anemia is stroke due to cerebral infarction. The observed frequency varies from 6% to as high as 34% (Sarnaik and Lusher 1982). If untreated, cerebral infarction may recur in two-thirds of affected patients. Central poststroke pain has an estimated incidence of 1–2% of all stroke patients (Boivie 1994). Reports of central poststroke pain in sickle cell disease are absent from the literature. In fact, children who develop strokes due to sickle cell anemia and who are treated with chronic transfusion or exchange transfusion experience significant decrease (or even total absence) of painful episodes compared to their peers without stroke and without chronic transfusion. The reasons why poststroke pain is not described in sickle cell disease are unknown. One possibility pertains to the location of the infarct, which usually involves the cerebrum and rarely involves the brain stem, the thalamus, or the spinal cord.

Other types of central pain such as painful epileptic seizure, multiple sclerosis, Parkinson's disease, and syringomyelia have not been described in association with sickle cell syndromes.

PERIPHERAL NEUROPATHIC PAIN

The rarity of peripheral nerve infarction in sickle cell disease may be due to unusual anatomical and pathophysiological characteristics of the microvascular network that supplies peripheral nerves (Shields et al. 1991). Peripheral nerves receive their blood supply from the arteriae nervorum, derived from main adjacent arteries and composed of numerous interconnecting nutrient vessels (Sunderland 1978). At the nerve, the nutrient arteries divide and subdivide several times into ascending, descending, penetrating, secondary, and tertiary branches to form an extensive plexus of anastomotic microvascular network, within and around the nerve, that supplies blood to the epi-, peri-, and endoneurium (Sunderland 1945, 1978). This rich and complex interconnecting network of nutrient vessels may protect peripheral nerves from infarction because of its ability to maintain adequate blood circulation even if the patency of a primary nutrient vessel is compromised. Moreover, such a network can shunt blood to compensate for focal zones of aberrant perfusion (Durward 1948; Sunderland 1978; Bell and Weddell 1984a,b).

The microvascular capillary network of peripheral nerves has another feature that protects the nerves from ischemia due to vaso-occlusion. Accurate measurements have shown that the capillaries of peripheral nerves in animals are approximately twice as large in diameter (8–9 vs. 3–4 mm) as those of muscle and other tissues (Bell and Weddell 1984a,b). Lipowsky and Sheikh (1987) used intravital microscopy to measure the size of nailfold capillary loops but found no difference between controls and patients with sickle cell anemia. Nailfold capillaries, however, may not be representative of capillaries in muscle and other organs (Lipowsky and Sheikh 1987).

The size of capillaries of nerves may explain why peripheral nerves are protected from vaso-occlusion by sickled cells and the consequent ischemia. Resistance to blood flow in a vessel varies inversely as the fourth power of the radius of the vessel ($R = K/r^4$, where R = resistance to blood flow, K = constant, and r = vessel radius). Thus, small conglomerates of stiff sickled cells would be less likely to impede blood flow in a nerve where the demand for oxygen is relatively low than in muscles where oxygen demand is high.

Mental nerve neuropathy

Peripheral neuropathy has been reported in a few patients with sickle cell disease (Konotey-Ahulu 1972; Kirson and Tomaro 1979; Adams 1994). Lesions of the mental nerve associated with numbness of the chin have been most often described and are believed to result from bone compression due to mandibular bone infarction (Table I).

Peripheral neuropathy with lead poisoning. Lead poisoning in children is characteristically manifested by encephalopathy, whereas peripheral neuropathy is relatively rare (Seto and Freeman 1964; Barltrop 1971). The reverse is true in adults with plumbism. However, some reports indicate that peripheral neuropathy is the most common mode of presentation when lead poisoning occurs in children with sickle cell anemia. Of 15 children with lead poisoning and peripheral neuropathy, six had sickle cell anemia or Hb SC disease (Anku and Harris 1974; Erenberg et al. 1974). The symptomatology of lead neuropathy in sickle cell anemia includes the classically described drop foot and peripheral muscle weakness.

Table I
Types of peripheral neuropathy reported in patients with sickle cell disease

Mental nerve neuropathy

Periphral neuropathy with lead poisoning

Multiple cranial neuropathies, trigeminal neuralgia, and vascular headaches

Acute proximal median mononeuropathy

Sodium cyanate–induced neuropathy

Entrapment neuropathy
  Carpal tunnel syndrome
  Tarsal tunnel syndrome
  Brachial plexopathy

Neurogenic pain (? sympathetically maintained pain)

Acute demyelinating polyneuropathy (Guillain-Barré syndrome)

Multiple cranial neuropathies, trigeminal neuralgia, and vascular headaches. Asher (1980) reported the case of a 29-year-old woman with sickle cell disease complicated by avascular necrosis of both femoral heads and by chronic renal failure necessitating hemodialysis. Prior to renal transplantation her sickle cell disease was quiescent with no painful episodes. She was maintained on periodic transfusion to keep her sickle hemoglobin about 40%. Following renal transplantation her sickle cell disease worsened and she experienced painful episodes and developed simultaneous trigeminal and facial neuropathies, trigeminal neuralgia following the resolution of the trigeminal sensory neuropathy, and vascular headaches. She probably experienced more frequent painful crises because the transplanted kidney produced erythropoietin that led to increasing levels of sickle hemoglobin, as has been report in similar cases (Spector et al. 1978). Carbamazepine nearly completely relieved the signs and symptoms of trigeminal neuralgia.

Acute proximal median mononeuropathy. Shields et al. (1991) described a 26-year-old woman with sickle cell anemia who developed features of an acute ischemic median mononeuropathy during an acute painful crisis. Symptoms included numbness in the right thumb, index, and middle fingers, and weakness of the right hand. She also complained of intense localized pain in mid-humerus. Neurological examination showed loss of superficial sensation in the right median nerve distribution and weakness of median-innervated muscles. Electrodiagnostic studies documented conduction block of the proximal median nerve at the level of the mid-humerus with a mild degree of axonal loss. Together, the clinical and electrophysiological features suggested an ischemic mechanism from the sickling process. She was treated symptomatically and within a few weeks the sensory and motor deficits of the right hand improved significantly.

Sodium cyanate-induced neuropathy. Sodium cyanate was tried as a therapeutic agent in sickle cell disease in the 1970s (Harkness and Roth 1975). Although animal studies and short-term clinical trials showed little evidence of toxicity, three patients with sickle cell disease who were maintained on long-term sodium cyanate therapy developed severe debilitating peripheral neuropathy (Charache et al. 1974; Peterson et al. 1974; Harkness and Roth 1975). They all experienced marked weight loss. Each had muscle weakness of upper and lower extremities; distal muscles were more severely affected than proximal. All three patients had gait disturbance with drop foot and depressed deep tendon reflexes in the ankles. Two patients had noted paresthesias in the hands and feet, one for six weeks and the other for four or five months before the onset of overt weakness. Nerve conduction velocity measurements indicated a diffuse abnormality of both sensory and motor nerves. Sural nerve biopsies in two of the patients revealed a decreased number of myelinated fibers in both, segmental demyelination in one, and linear rows of myelin ovoids in the other. In one patient the predominant abnormality was segmental demyelination and remyelination; while the other patient had histological features typical of axonal degeneration (Ohnisi et al. 1975). After discontinuing cyanate therapy, all three patients gradually improved and regained nearly normal function within nine to 12 months, with improvement in nerve conduction.

Further evidence that sodium cyanate was responsible for the neuropathy came from physical examination and nerve conduction studies of 25 other patients who received this treatment. Subclinical neuropathy was found in 14 of these patients (Peterson et al. 1974). The association of peripheral neuropathy with cyanate resulted in the termination of the therapeutic trial of this compound.

Entrapment neuropathy. Ballas and Reyes (1997) described other types of peripheral neuropathy in sickle cell disease including entrapment neuropathy, neurogenic pain, and Guillain-Barré syndrome (Table I). Carpal tunnel syndrome was observed in eight patients during acute sickle cell painful episodes. In six patients it was bilateral and one patient also had bilateral tarsal tunnel syndrome. Signs and symptoms of carpal tunnel syndrome included burning pain, numbness, tingling sensation, swelling over the thenar area, and positive Tinel and Phalen's signs. A ninth patient had right brachial plexopathy during an acute painful episode. EMG confirmed the diagnosis of entrapment neuropathy. In eight patients the signs and symptoms of entrapment neuropathy resolved with the resolution of the sickle cell painful crisis. In the ninth patient the signs and symptoms of carpal tunnel syndrome resolved within two months after the diagnosis. The pathophysiologic events that lead to entrapment neuropathy during acute painful episodes seem to be straightforward. Sickle cell painful episodes are often associated with edema secondary to inflammation, which in turn generates pressure on adjacent nerves, such as the median nerve, and leads to the signs and symptoms associated with entrapment.

Neurogenic pain. Ballas and Reyes (1997) described three patients with sickle cell disease who developed neurogenic pain that seems to show some features of sympathetically maintained pain during acute painful episodes (numbness, tingling sensation, swelling, decreased sensory sensation, and trophic changes). The signs and symptoms of this type of neuropathy seem to be the result of neurogenic inflammation caused by the release of various neuropeptides from unmyelinated nociceptive nerve endings (Schwartzman 1992; Hernanz et al. 1993). These compounds include substance P, neurokinin A and B, vasoactive intestinal peptide, and calcitonin gene-related peptide. These neuropeptides cause, among other problems, vasodilatation, increased vascular permeability, and relaxation of smooth muscles; the pain and swelling generated spread locally and distally via the sympathetic system. Involvement of the sympathetic system is thought to result from an abnormal reflex arc related to internuncial neurons (Schwartzman and McLellan 1987; Rosen 1989; Jänig 1992). Thus, afferent pain information reaches the spinal cord and is, in turn, relayed to the sympathetic ganglia via the internuncial neurons in the spinal cord. This process initiates efferent symptoms of autonomic arousal mediated by norepinephrine and associated with vascular spasm, ischemia, and further inflammation.

Acute demyelinating polyneuropathy. Ballas and Reyes (1997) also described a patient with sickle cell anemia and a variant of acute demyelinating polyneuropathy (or Guillain-Barré syndrome) known as the C. Miller-Fisher variant (Ropper 1992). The association between the diseases, however, seems to be incidental rather than causal.

FIBROMYALGIA AND MYOFASCIAL PAIN

This syndrome differs from the myonecrosis and myofibrosis described in Chapter 5. Fibromyalgia and myofascial pain are the most commonly used terms to describe a common chronic pain syndrome involving muscles, ligaments, and fasciae. This syndrome is also known by many other names such as nonarticular rheumatism, muscular rheumatism, fibrositis, and psychogenic rheumatism.

Fibromyalgia pain can be persistent, severe, and disabling and afflicts females about five times more commonly than males. The characteristic patient is a woman aged 20–45 years who has diffuse chronic pain. Physical examination reveals no abnormalities except for scattered tender points that are painful on palpation. Pain often arises from mild to moderate trauma or muscle overuse and if not properly treated can persist for prolonged periods. Traditionally, the pain is subdivided into localized and diffuse fibromyalgia. IASP defines diffuse myofascial pain syndrome as aching musculoskeletal pain associated with discrete predictable tender points and stiffness (Merskey 1986). Localized myofascial pain syndrome involves one muscle or a group of adjacent muscles. These tender areas are commonly known as trigger points. Simple techniques directed at stretching trigger points in combination with antidepressant medications are the mainstay of therapy (Travell 1976; Travell and Simmons 1983, 1991).

Fibromyalgia has not been reported in association with sickle cell disease. Again, its occurrence may be mistaken for sickle cell pain. Those patients with intractable chronic crisis pain described in Chapter 6 may suffer from chronic fibromyalgia with superimposed acute painful episodes. Such a possible combination needs further explanation and study.

AIDS AND SICKLE CELL DISEASE

AIDS may occur concomitantly in patients with sickle cell disease (Steiner and Ballas 1996). AIDS is associated with several pain syndromes (O'Neill and Sherrard 1993), but types of pain syndromes that may arise when sickle cell disease and AIDS coexist are not known and, to date, have not been reported.

8

Munchausen Sickle Cell Painful Episodes

He was so absorbed in his never-ceasing pain that it had almost become a habit with him.
— Alexandre Dumas, "The Black Tulip," 1802–1870

Patients with sickle cell disease often suffer from severe recurrent episodes of acute pain that require treatment with parenteral opioid analgesics. Some patients may wander from hospital to hospital in search of adequate treatment that offers pain relief. In urban areas such actions may easily be misconstrued as drug-seeking behavior. A provider may be confounded by an African American patient who complains of pain, demands opioid analgesics, and has a history of hospital shopping but who shows no objective signs of painful crisis. Some providers who have no experience or interest in sickle cell disease may conclude that such patients are malingerers demonstrating drug-seeking behavior or Munchausen sickle cell painful crisis. This chapter will elucidate what is known about Munchausen sickle pain and demonstrate that it is manifested by patients who do not have sickle cell disease.

The term "Munchausen syndrome" was coined by Asher (1951) for Baron Hieronymus Karl Friedrich von Munchausen, a storyteller of alleged heroic deeds in the German calvary. Persons with this syndrome suffer from factitious disorders and feign physical or psychological symptoms so as to assume the sick role (American Psychiatric Association 1994). The fourth edition of the *Diagnostic and Statistical Manual of Mental Disorders* (DSM-IV) of the American Psychiatric Association (1994) lists three criteria for the diagnosis of factitious disorders: (1) a sine qua non feature pertains to the intentional production of physical or psychological signs or symptoms; (2) the major motivation for the factitious behavior is to assume the sick role; and (3) the absence of external incentives for the behavior. Factitious disorders differ from malingering (Table I). Malingering is characterized by the intentional production of false or grossly exaggerated physical or

Table I
Differences between factitious disorders and malingering

Production of Signs and Symptoms is . . .	Factitious Disorders	Malingering
Intentional	Yes	Yes
False	No	Yes
Unconscious	Yes	No
To obtain external incentives	No	Yes
To assume the sick role	Yes	No
Due to lying	Yes	Yes

psychological symptoms, motivated by external incentives such as avoiding military duty or work, obtaining drugs, evading criminal prosecution, or obtaining financial compensation. In factitious disorders the production of symptoms is presumed to be unconscious, and external incentives are absent. Evidence of an intrapsychic need to maintain the sick role suggests factitious disorders.

Malingering in patients with sickle cell disease is the exception rather than the rule, and probably occurs in less than 1% of patient encounters. It may be suspected in patients who, soon after hospital admission, request letters to exempt them from court appearance because they are sick and then request discharge from the hospital soon after the date of the court appearance passes. There are, however, anecdotes of patients with sickle cell disease who died soon after discharge from medical facilities and who had received little or no treatment because they were suspected of malingering or drug-seeking behavior. Thus, it is advisable to believe patients and take their complaints seriously (Payne 1989b; Ballas 1990b). By doing so, the provider would be offering benefit to more than 99% of patients at a risk of being fooled by an occasional patient. A nonjudgmental approach of belief in treating patients with sickle cell disease would thus be overwhelmingly in favor of benefit.

There are three types of factitious disorders: (1) those with physical symptoms, (2) those with psychological symptoms, and (3) atypical (American Psychiatric Association 1994). Munchausen syndrome is an example of a factitious disorder with predominantly physical signs and symptoms. An essential feature is a tendency for the patient to give a fabricated but plausible history and seek out care by wandering from hospital to hospital.

Munchausen syndrome has two subtypes (Nadelson 1979): prototypical and nonprototypical. Patients with the first type are usually unemployed men who drift from hospital to hospital. Both men and women who demonstrate the nonprototypical syndrome often simulate illness and stay in one place for months or years. The patients with Munchausen sickle cell painful crisis seem to fit the nonprototypical pattern.

To date, the literature includes seven reports of patients with Munchausen sickle cell painful episodes. Two patients who fabricated the signs and symptoms of sickle cell anemia on numerous occasions but who had normal hemoglobin electrophoresis were described by Lindenbaum (1974), who first used the terms hemoglobin Munchausen to designate this condition. A third case described a young man with hemolytic anemia and painful episodes ascribed to "sickle" but with normal hemoglobin electrophoresis (Fisher 1974). A fourth example of Munchausen sickle cell painful crisis occurred in a patient who repeatedly fabricated the signs and symptoms of acute painful episodes but who had sickle cell trait plus severe iron deficiency anemia that required blood transfusion (Ballas 1992). The fifth, sixth, and seventh examples (Ballas 1996c) were young persons who feigned the symptoms of painful crises and who had diabetes with hypertension, seizure disorder, and asthma, respectively.

Table II lists the characteristics of the seven reported patients with Munchausen sickle cell crises. All were young adults who demonstrated

Table II
Characteristics of reported patients with Munchausen sickle cell painful crisis

Age (Y)/ Sex	Feigned Diagnosis	Coexistent Disease*	Exposure to Patients with SCD	Reference
31/M	Hb SC	IDDM hypertension	Yes; friends	Ballas 1996c
28/F	SS	Seizure disorder	Yes; cousin	Ballas 1996c
21/M	SS	Asthma bone infarcts	Yes; significant other	Ballas 1996c
22/F	SS	Severe IDA (Hb AS)	Yes; nephew and cousin	Ballas 1992
28/F	SS	IDA, UTI (Hb AC)	Yes; she is a nurses' aide	Lindenbaum 1974
22/F	Hb SC	PID	Probably yes; other patients	Lindenbaum 1974
20/M	"Sickle"	Hemolytic	Probably yes; other patients	Fisher 1974

Abbreviations: Hb SC, hemoglobin SC disease; SS, sickle cell anemia; Hb AS, sickle cell trait; Hb AC, hemoglobin C trait; IDDM, insulin-dependent diabetes mellitus; IDA, iron deficiency anemia; UTI, urinary tract infection; PID, pelvic inflammatory disease.
*All seven patients demonstrated pathological lying (pseudologia fantastica).

pathological lying (pseudologia fantastica). It is interesting that most of the patients had other authentic disease processes but they elected to change their diagnosis to painful episodes and feign the appropriate syndromes so as to make their history plausible and obtain the desired treatment. This situation differs from the classical description of Munchausen syndrome in which the patients are basically disease free and feign symptoms to obtain treatment. Perhaps the exposure to relatives, friends, or other patients with sickle cell disease (Table II) was a factor in adopting and internalizing the diagnosis of sickle cell disease. Ballas (1996c) suggested referring to this type of factitious acute sickle cell painful episode as secondary Munchausen syndrome in contradistinction to the primary type with no underlying disease process.

The motives for Munchausen syndrome are complex and in any specific patient may never be clearly defined (Asher 1951). The primary motive in patients with factitious sickle cell crises most likely includes the desire to be the center of attention. Other motives such as the desire to obtain free room and board (O'Shea et al. 1984) and opioid analgesics are unlikely secondary incentives. It is also conceivable that some patients were truly convinced that they had sickle cell disease because they were misinformed repeatedly by previous physicians who might have diagnosed them without the benefit of hemoglobin electrophoresis. Persons with sickle cell trait are known to develop symptoms when they misunderstand the diagnosis or misinterpret the information given in counseling.

Patients who show signs and symptoms of sickle cell disease should be properly tested to confirm the diagnosis. This confirmation becomes particularly important prior to major interventions such as surgery and prior to the repeated use of opioid analgesics. Moreover, knowing the exact type of sickle cell syndrome is important in the follow-up of patients because certain complications occur more frequently in one type of sickle cell syndrome than others (Chapter 2). Knowing the exact diagnosis is also important in educating and counseling affected patients and their families, in prenatal diagnosis, and in newborn screening.

Part III

Pharmacologic Therapy
of Sickle Cell Pain

9

Pharmacology of Analgesics and Adjuvants

Among the remedies which pleased God to give man
to relieve his suffering, none is so efficacious as opioids.
— Anonymous physician, 1600

Grief for a while is blind, and so was mine.
I wish no living thing to suffer pain.
— Percy Bysshe Shelley, 1792–1822

PHARMACODYNAMICS AND PHARMACOKINETICS OF ANALGESIC DRUGS

This section is *not* meant to be a comprehensive review of the pharmacodynamics and pharmacokinetics of analgesic drugs. That vast subject is beyond the scope of this book. This brief section will explain commonly used words that describe the properties of analgesic agents, for example, bioavailability, half-life, and steady state. The significance of these terms may be more evident in the sections of this chapter discussing analgesics and adjuvants to analgesics, and in Chapter 10, and may provide the basis for the rational use of analgesic agents.

PHARMACODYNAMICS

Definition

Pharmacology is a science that studies drugs. Pharmacodynamics is a branch of pharmacology that studies the mechanism of action of drugs and their biochemical and physiological effects (Ross 1996b). Most drugs exert their effect via interactions with tissue receptors to which they are bound and, hence, trigger a series of biochemical and physiological cellular events that culminate in a response that is characteristic of the drug in question

149

(Ross 1996b). This sequence of events can be schematically illustrated as follows:

Drug + receptor → drug/receptor complex → response

Drug receptor. A drug receptor, usually a protein, is a macromolecular component of the organism (Ross 1996b). Drugs that act via this mechanism bind to extracellular receptors that transduce the information into the cell by various mechanisms. The four major classes of receptors are: (1) receptors with enzymatic activity, (2) receptors coupled to G proteins (guanine nucleotide binding proteins), (3) ion channel receptors, and (4) transcription factors (DiPalma 1990; Ross 1996b).

Receptor protein kinases constitute the majority of receptors with enzymatic activity. When stimulated, receptors with tyrosine-specific protein kinase activity, for example, activate this enzyme to enhance the transport of nutrients and ions across the cell membrane. Insulin receptors function by this mechanism to increase glucose transport into insulin-dependent tissues such as muscle and adipose tissues. Other receptors that are tyrosine protein kinases include those for epidermal growth factors, platelet-derived growth factor, and some lymphokines.

Receptors coupled to G proteins (guanine nucleotide binding proteins) exert their effect either by opening an ion channel or by inhibiting/stimulating specific enzymes. Examples of G protein-coupled receptors include those for opioid analgesics, biogenic amines, eicosanoids, and several peptide hormones. The sequence of events is as follows:

Drug (first messenger) + receptor → drug/receptor complex

Drug/receptor complex + G protein + GTP → activated G protein

Activated G protein → regulates the activity of specific effectors

Activated effectors → generate second messenger

Second messenger → enzyme stimulation → efflux or influx of ions and
  nutrients

Activated ion channel receptors enhance the influx of extracellular ions into the cell. Examples of these receptors include the nicotine cholinergic receptor, the GABA receptor for γ-aminobutyric acid, and receptors for glutamate, aspartate, and glycine. The GABA receptor is an ionophore for chloride ions, and its activation selectively opens a channel for Cl^- and causes the influx of extracellular Cl^- into the cell.

Receptors that function as transcription factors are soluble DNA-binding proteins that regulate the transcription of specific genes. They include receptors for steroid hormones, thyroid hormones, vitamin D, and the retinoids and differ from other receptors in that they are associated with the nucleus of the cell and penetrate into target cells when activated.

PHARMACOKINETICS

Definition

Pharmacokinetics is a branch of pharmacology that studies the factors affecting drug movement in the body. A certain drug must be present in adequate concentration at its site of action to produce its specific effect. The degree to which a certain drug reaches its site of action or the fraction of the dose that reaches the systemic circulation following administration by any route is referred to as its bioavailability. Opioid analgesics have low bioavailability. The higher the bioavailability the better the chances that the drug in question will exert its specific effect at a given dose. The relationship between the concentration of a certain drug in plasma and its characteristic effect is, therefore, much more important than its dose and effect. Understanding basic pharmacokinetic principles and applying them to patient care will lead to rational drug therapy where the amount of analgesic drug delivered to the target tissue can be controlled safely (DiPalma et al. 1990; Ross 1996a).

The major factors that affect the concentration of a drug in the systemic circulation (or its pharmacokinetics) include absorption, distribution, biotransformation, and elimination.

Absorption

Absorption refers to movement across various cellular membranes and pertains to various transport mechanisms involved not only in absorption from the gastrointestinal tract, but also in the distribution and elimination of drugs. Transmembranal transport mechanisms include filtration, simple diffusion, facilitated diffusion, active transport, and endocytosis. Filtration and simple diffusion are dominant factors in most drug absorption, distribution, and elimination (DiPalma et al. 1990; Ross 1996a).

The most common method by which ionic components with low molecular weight enter cells is via filtration through membrane channels. Filtration refers to the transport of drug molecules that fit through membrane pores consequent to the flow of water through the pores due to osmotic differences across the membrane. The extent of filtration varies from cell type to cell type because of differences in the pore size.

Simple diffusion is another mechanism by which substances cross membranes without the active participation of components in the membranes. Lipid-soluble compounds use this method to enter cells at a rate proportional to the concentration gradient across the membrane and the lipid/water partition coefficient of the drug. Lipophilic opioid analgesics, such as meperidine and fentanyl, employ this method to enter cells.

Carrier-mediated transport provides selectivity to the uptake process and is used to describe both active transport and facilitated diffusion. Active transport is responsible for the movement of a number of organic acids and bases across membranes of renal tubules and hepatic cells. In contrast to active transport, facilitated diffusion does not require energy and so cannot prevail against a concentration gradient. Glucose transport into erythrocytes is a good example.

Endocytosis is responsible for the transport of large molecules such as proteins and colloids. Although endothelial cells employ this transport mechanism extensively, its importance in drug action is uncertain.

Drug absorption from the gastrointestinal tract occurs primarily via passive processes: filtration and simple diffusion. Factors that affect absorption from the gastrointestinal tract include the surface area for absorption, blood flow to and the concentration of the drugs at the site of absorption, and the physical state of the drug. The absorption of nonionized and lipophilic forms of drugs is favored in the gastrointestinal tract because such components employ passive processes to cross cellular membranes.

Drug absorption from intramuscular and subcutaneous routes occurs by simple diffusion across the gradient from the drug pool to plasma. The solubility of the injected drug in the interstitial fluid and the size of the capillary network at the site of injection affect its rate of absorption. The intravenous route of drug administration circumvents the problems encountered with other procedures and more quickly achieves the desired plasma concentration.

Distribution

After absorption or injection into the blood stream, a drug is usually distributed into intersticial and cellular fluids. Several physiological factors and physiochemical properties of the drug play a major role in the pattern of distribution including solubility, volume of distribution, and protein-drug binding.

Lipid-soluble or lipophilic drugs that permeate membranes efficiently are not limited in their distribution and tend to accumulate in body fat. Other drugs may accumulate in muscle or liver. A drug that is sequestered in a certain tissue may function as a reservoir that prolongs its action in the same tissue or at a different site through the circulation.

The volume of distribution refers to the extent of dilution of a drug within the body at a time of maximum distribution. Together with drug clearance (see below) it plays a role in determining the amount of the drug that will reach the target tissues.

Drug distribution may also be limited by drug binding to plasma proteins, especially albumin for acidic drugs and α1-acid glycoprotein for basic drugs. Because only the free (unbound) fraction of drug can cross biologic membranes, binding to plasma proteins limits a drug's concentration in tissues and thus decreases the apparent volume of distribution of the drug. Plasma protein binding will also reduce glomerular filtration of the drug because this process is highly dependent on the free drug fraction.

Biotransformation

After it enters the blood stream and is distributed to tissues, a drug is subject to specific metabolic pathways referred to as biotransformation reactions. These culminate in the production of inactive metabolites that are readily excreted from the body. In some cases, however, intermediary metabolites with biological activity or toxic properties may be generated during the progression of the transformation reactions. First-pass elimination, functionalization reactions, and conjugation reactions are major processes involved in biotransformation (DiPalma et al. 1990; Mather et al. 1996; Ross 1996a).

The first-pass effect is commonly considered to involve the biotransformation of a drug during its first passage through the portal circulation of the liver. Drugs that are administered orally enter the portal circulation and can be biotransformed by the liver prior to reaching the systemic circulation. Therefore, drugs with a high first-pass effect are biotransformed quickly, which reduces the oral bioavailability and the systemic blood concentrations of the compounds. Administration by the intravenous, intramuscular, and sublingual routes allows the drug to attain concentrations in the systemic circulation and to be distributed throughout the body prior to hepatic metabolism. Drugs administered by inhalation are not subjected to a significant first-pass effect unless the respiratory tissue is a major site for the drug's biotransformation. The bioavailability of drugs administered rectally is sensitive to the position of the preparation in the rectum (Mather et al. 1996). Correct placement in the middle part of the rectum leads to absorption mainly via the inferior and middle rectal veins into the systemic system and thus avoids the hepatic first-pass effect. Placement too high in the rectum results in greater absorption into the portal system via the superior rectal veins.

Biotransformation reactions involving the oxidation, reduction, or hydrolysis of a drug are classified as phase I (or nonsynthetic) functionalization reactions; these chemical reactions may result in either the activation or inactivation of a pharmacologic agent. Oxidations are the most numerous of these many types of reactions. Phase II (or synthetic) reactions, which almost always result in the formation of an inactive product, involve conjugation of the drug (or its derivative) with an amino acid, carbohydrate, acetate, or sulfate. The conjugated form(s) of the drug or its derivatives may be more easily excreted than the parent compound.

Prodrugs are an example of agents that are activated via phase I biotransformation. Prodrugs are pharmacologically inactive compounds that, after administration, are converted to an active drug. Inactive sulindac, for example, is reduced to sulindac sulfide, an active nonsteroidal anti-inflammatory drug, and codeine, a prodrug, is demethylated to morphine.

Elimination

Drugs are eliminated from the body either unchanged or as breakdown metabolites generated by the biotransformation reactions. Water-soluble compounds are more efficiently eliminated by excretory organs than are lipid-soluble drugs. Elimination of the latter group of compounds is dependent on their metabolism to more water-soluble metabolites.

Elimination of drugs occurs primarily through the kidney and the hepatobiliary system. The kidney is the most important organ for elimination of drugs and their metabolites. Elimination is achieved via glomerular filtration, active tubular secretions, and passive tubular reabsorption. Metabolites of drugs produced in the liver are excreted into the intestine through the biliary system. Some metabolites may be excreted in the feces and often may be reabsorbed and repeatedly cycled through the hepatobiliary circulation.

Factors that contribute to the rate of drug elimination include clearance and half-life (DiPalma et al. 1990; Mather et al. 1996; Ross 1996a). Clearance is equal to the product of blood flow to that organ and its extraction ratio, which is defined as the difference in drug concentration between blood entering and leaving the organ, divided by the entering concentration. Total body clearance is defined as the rate of removal of a drug from the body and is the sum of the individual clearance rates of the kidney, liver, lung, and other organs. It is an expression of the total volume of distribution cleared from the drug per unit time.

The elimination half-life (T½) defines the time required for the blood concentration of a certain drug to decrease by 50% of the original value. It is a measure of the rapidity with which the blood concentration of a drug changes. It is inversely related to clearance and directly related to the volume of distribution. Thus, a drug with a short T½ will be subject to rapid clearance and vice versa. Mathematically, clearance = K x Vd/T½, where K = constant (0.693), Vd = volume of distribution, and T½ = half-life.

Steady state

Steady state refers to a constant or stable drug concentration that occurs when drug elimination equals availability. This important concept must be considered to achieve a rational regimen for long-term drug administration. To achieve acceptable pain relief, for example, it is important to maintain steady-state concentration of a drug within a known therapeutic range. The steady state will be achieved if the rate of drug elimination equals the rate of drug administration assuming complete bioavailability.

Drug-drug interaction

Patients with sickle cell pain often receive a combination of various drugs including opioid analgesics, NSAIDs, adjuvant analgesics, and antibiotics. Such drugs may interact and the response elicited may be equal to, greater than, or less than the sum of the effects of the individual compounds. Synergism, potentiation, additive effect, and antagonism are some of the common terms that describe the pattern of drug-drug interaction.

Synergism refers to a situation in which two drugs act at the same site or on the same biologic unit (cell, tissue, or organ) and the combined effect of the two drugs exceeds the sum of their individual effects. For example, both acetaminophen and codeine have analgesic activity, but the combination has greater analgesic activity than that of either drug used alone. *Potentiation* is similar to synergism, but the term is usually reserved for cases in which two drugs act differently and one has a less significant effect alone. For example, adjuvant analgesics potentiate the analgesic effect of opioids. An *additive effect* occurs when the combined effect of two drugs acting by the same mechanism is equal to that expected by simple addition (DiPalma et al. 1990).

Antagonism is the interference of one drug with the action of another. *Pharmacologic antagonism* is the interaction that occurs through receptor-mediated events; for example, naloxone blocks the effects of hydromorphone at μ and κ receptor sites. *Dispositional antagonism* is an alteration in the absorption, distribution, biotransformation, or excretion of a compound so that less compound can reach the active site; for example, chronic administration of phenobarbital enhances the metabolism of many drugs through the hepatic drug microsomal metabolizing system and reduces their effects. *Functional,* or *physiologic, antagonism* occurs when two compounds produce opposite effects on the same system; for example, histamine-induced bronchoconstriction is antagonized by epinephrine, a bronchodilator. *Chemical antagonism* results from a chemical interaction between compounds that neutralizes their effects; for example, deferoxamine chelates with iron to reduce its concentration throughout the body (DiPalma et al. 1990) and thus reduces the harmful effects of iron overload in hypertransfused patients with sickle cell disease.

NONOPIOID ANALGESICS

Nonopioid analgesics comprise a heterogeneous group of compounds that differ in chemical composition and structure but share pharmacological and therapeutic properties. They include acetaminophen, dipyrone, NSAIDs, local anesthetics, capsaicin, and tramadol. The "analgesic ladder" approach of the World Health Organization (1990) emphasizes the potential value of the nonopioid and adjuvant analgesics in the management of cancer pain. These agents themselves have become important in the management of acute and chronic pain of mild to moderate severity. They are also useful in treating severe pain when combined with opioids to provide an additive analgesic effect (World Health Organization 1990). Table I lists the common nonopioid analgesics. It includes local anesthetics and capsaicin, which others may consider as adjuvants. Nonopioid analgesics, by definition, are chemically different than opioids and their primary clinical use is to provide analgesia. Local anesthetics, capsaicin, and tramadol fit this definition. Corticosteroids, however, are adjuvants because their usual primary clinical indication is to provide anti-inflammatory effect and, secondarily, analgesia.

Nonopioid analgesics have several advantages over opioids (Table II) and the following general advantages: (1) they are useful in treating mild to moderate pain; (2) they are widely available and some do not require a

Table I
Classification of nonopioid analgesics

Acetaminophen (Tylenol, Paracetamal)
Dipyrone (Metamizol, Novalgin)
Nonsteroidal anti-inflammatory drugs
Local anesthetics
  Oral agents
    Mexiletine (Mexitil)
    Tocainide (Tonocard)
  Topical Agents
    EMLA
Topical analgesics
  Capsaicin (Zostrix)
  Other preparations
Tramadol (Ultram)

Table II
Differences between nonsteroidal anti-inflammatory
drugs and opioid analgesics

	NSAIDS	Opioids
Ceiling effect	Yes	No
Addiction potential	No	Yes
Tolerance	No	Yes
Physical dependence	No	Yes
Sedation, confusion	Rare	Common
Mechanism of action	Mostly peripheral	Mostly central
Systemic side effects	More common	Less common
"Street value"	None	High

prescription or access to medical staff; (3) additive analgesia can be obtained when they are combined with opioids or adjuvants; (4) they can be administered by patient or family for feasible home management of pain; (5) some of these medications are inexpensive; and (6) they do not produce tolerance or physical/psychological dependence. Their disadvantages include a ceiling effect and greater likelihood of adverse systemic effects than with use of opioids (Ferrer-Brechner and Ganz 1984; Beaver 1988). The ceiling effect refers to a dose above which there is no additional analgesic effect although duration of the effect may be increased. The anti-inflammatory effect of NSAids has no ceiling.

ACETAMINOPHEN (TYLENOL, PARACETAMOL)

Unlike the NSAids, acetaminophen is nonacidic, has no significant anti-inflammatory effect (Skjelbred et al. 1984), is less expensive, and has fewer side effects. Its major advantages include analgesia and antipyresis that seem to result from a central mechanism (Piletta et al. 1991). Gastrointestinal toxicity is rare, and it does not impair platelet function (Drug Facts and Comparison 1997). Acetaminophen has been implicated in papillary necrosis of the kidney (Kincaid-Smith 1986; Whelton and Hamilton 1991). The recommended adult oral or rectal dose should not exceed 6000 mg per day in four to six divided doses (Wallenstien 1975; Sunshine and Olson 1989). Doses that exceed the recommended maximum can cause hepatic toxicity. Patients with concomitant liver disease can develop severe hepatotoxicity even when the drug is taken according to therapeutic recommendations (Seeff et al. 1986). Acute overdosage can produce hepatic necrosis, and death can occur after the ingestion of a single dose of 25 g or more (Insel 1996). As patients with sickle cell disease may have concurrent liver disease, the total daily dosage of this analgesic should be monitored. Acetaminophen has no cross-reactivity in patients with NSAID hypersensitivity. In children the oral dose of acetaminophen is limited to 10–15 mg/kg three or four times a day. When administered rectally in children, the dose may need to be as high as 35–45 mg/kg to achieve therapeutic plasma concentration (Houck et al. 1995; Montgomery et al. 1995). The metabolism of acetaminophen in infants is different than that in adults (Miller et al. 1976; Rumack and Peterson 1978). Infants preferentially conjugate acetaminophen to the sulfate metabolite rather than the glucuronide metabolite. With age, children gradually excrete more of the acetaminophen as the glucuronide metabolite, and by the age of 12 years the glucuronide to sulfate ratio approaches adult values. This developmental change in the metabolism of this drug correlates with a dramatic increase in liver toxicity after acetaminophen overdose in children over 12 years of age versus younger children (Rumack and Peterson 1978).

DIPYRONE (METAMIZOL, NOVALGIN)

Dipyrone has analgesic, antipyretic, and antispasmodic effects. It is a phenylpyrazole sodium salt prodrug. After ingestion it is hydrolyzed to biologically active metabolites that are believed to inhibit prostaglandin synthesis (Levy 1986; Roth 1986). It was removed from the market in the United States and other countries because of its association with agranulocytosis. Nevertheless, it continues to be used in many other countries (Levy 1988). Dipyrone may be given orally, intramuscularly, or intravenously. The average analgesic dose is 500–1000 mg orally or 50–200 mg parenterally, and the maximum allowable daily dose is 3000 mg orally or 800 mg parenterally in three to four divided doses.

NONSTEROIDAL ANTI-INFLAMMATORY DRUGS (NSAIDS)

Classification

Table III lists the major classes of NSAIDs, their doses, and shelf lives (Ferrante 1993a). They are weakly acidic compounds with ionization constants ranging from 3 to 5 (Brooks and Day 1991). Acetylsalicylic acid (aspirin), ibuprofen (Advil), naproxen (Alleve), and ketoprofen (Orudis) are available over the counter. NSAIDs differ in potency with respect to their analgesic, antipyretic, and anti-inflammatory effects (Rooks et al. 1982, 1985). Ketorolac, for example, has anti-inflammatory activity at doses higher than those eliciting analgesia (Rooks et al. 1982, 1985).

Table III
Clinical pharmacology of the various nonsteroidal anti-inflammatory drugs

Drug	Average Analgesic Dose (mg, p.o.)	Dose Interval (hours)	Maximal Daily Dose (mg)	Half-life (T½, h)
Salicylates				
Acetysalicylic acid (aspirin)	500–1000	4–6	6000	4–15
Nonacetylated salicylates				
Salicyl salicylate (Disalcid)	1500	2–4	5000	4–15
Diflunisal (Dolobid)	1000	8–12	1500	7–15
Choline magnesium trisalicylate (Trilisate)	1500	6–12	4000	4–15
Pyrazoles				
Phenylbutazone (Butazolidine)	100	6	400	40–80
Proprionic acid derivatives				
Ibuprophen (Motrin, Advil)	200–400	4–6	3200	2
Naproxen (Naprosyn, Anaprox)	500	6–8	1500	13
Fenoprofen (Nalfon)	200	4–6	3200	2
Ketoprofen (Orudis)	75	8	225	2
Suprofen (Suprol)	200	4–6	1200	2
Flurbiprofen (Ansaid)	50–100	6–12	300	3–4
Acetic acid derivatives				
Idomethacin (Indocin)	25	8–12	100	3–11
Ketorolac (Toradol)	10	4–6	40	3–11
	30 i.m.	6	150	3–8
Sulindac (Clinoril)	200	12	400	16
Tolmetin (Tolectin)	400	6–8	1600	1–2
Diclofenac (Voltaren)	50–100	6–12	200	2
Etodolac (Lodine)	800	8–12	1200	7.3
Nabumetone (Relafen)	500	24	2000	22.5–30
Anthranilic acid derivatives				
Mefenamic acid (Ponstel)	500	6	1500	2–4
Mecolfenamate (Meclomen)	100	6	400	2–3
Oxicams				
Piroxicam (Feldene)	20	24	20	30–86

Clinical pharmacology

All the NSAIDs are available orally and are rapidly absorbed from the gastrointestinal tract after ingestion (Brooks and Day 1991). Almost all are metabolized in the liver and their inactive metabolites are excreted in the urine (Brooks and Day 1991). Three of the NSAIDs—salicyl salicylate, nabumetone, and sulindac—are inactive prodrugs and must be converted to active metabolites by the liver (Simon and Mills 1980). Most NSAIDs are highly bound (> 95%) to albumin after entry into the bloodstream (Brooks and Day 1991). The free fraction of the drug is usually increased in patients with hypoalbuminemia. Sulindac is thought to have less renal toxicity because it does not seem to affect the renal synthesis of prostaglandins as much as do other NSAIDs, and thus is preferred in patients with renal disease or threatened renal perfusion, such as those who are hypotensive or hypovolemic (Ciabettoni et al. 1984, 1987). Other investigators, however, failed to demonstrate an advantage for sulindac in these situations (Roberts et al. 1985; Quintero et al. 1986).

The NSAIDs act primarily at the level of nociceptors where pain impulses originate and thus are often described as peripherally acting compounds. They decrease the sensitivity of peripheral nociceptors to noxious stimuli, i.e., they desensitize them. A central mechanism for the NSAIDs has been recently proposed (Taiwo and Levine 1988; Malmberg and Yaksh 1993). Their antipyretic effect is thought to be central by involving the hypothalamus. NSAIDs exert their analgesic effect by inhibiting the biosynthesis of prostaglandins (Vane 1971), which reduces tissue levels and thus decreases or abolishes their action in the sensitization of nociceptors. NSAIDs decrease the synthesis of prostaglandins by inhibiting the enzyme cyclooxygenase (COX) (Fig. 1), which catalyses the conversion of arachidonic acid to cyclic endoperoxides, the precursors of prostanoids including the prostaglandins (Moncada and Vane 1979). Two isoforms are COX-1, which is constitutionally expressed in many tissues, and COX-2, which is induced by the cytokines IL-1 and TNF-α, which are secreted by activated host-defense cells such as macrophages following tissue damage (Wu 1996). Most currently available NSAIDs are nonselective and block both COX-1 and COX-2, although etodolac (Lodine) and nabumetone (Relafen) seem to have more selectivity for COX-2 than do other NSAIDs. Search for a selective COX-2 inhibitor has recently identified one compound, in an animal model, that may offer a safer alternative to NSAIDs for pain relief (Anderson et al. 1996).

Arachidonic acid can also be metabolized to an array of eicosanoids (Fig. 1) that have an important role in the inflammatory response (Bray 1986). NSAIDs do not typically inhibit the lipooxygenase but may actually enhance its activity by blocking the syntheses of prostanoids and shunting arachidonic acid to the eicosanoid pathway (Fig. 1). This mechanism explains the origin of allergic reactions and asthma with the use of NSAIDs (Izzo et al. 1991). Diclofenac, indomethecin, and meclofenamic acid inhibit both the lipooxygenase and the cyclooxygenase enzymes and thus decrease the synthesis of leukotrienes and prostaglandins (Seigel et al. 1979; Kitchen et al 1985; Boctor et al. 1986; Conroy et al. 1991). Table IV lists the routes of administration for NSAIDs.

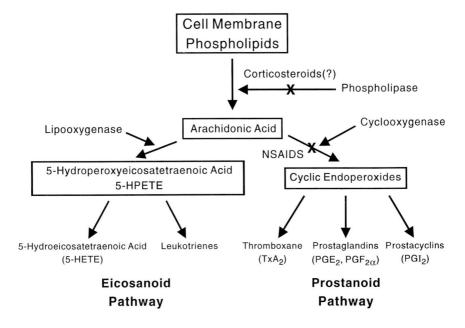

Fig. 1. Metabolism of arachidonic acid via the cyclooxygenase and lipooxygenase pathways (adapted from Ferrante 1993a with permission).

Indications for use

Most NSAIDs have Food and Drug Administration (FDA) approval for use in rheumatoid arthritis, degenerative joint disease, acute gout, ankylosing spondylitis, bursitis, tendonitis, pain, and dysmenorrhea. They are indicated alone for the treatment of pain of varying severity or in combination with opioids or adjuvants. Patients may differ in their relative response to NSAIDs, so an alternative NSAID should be considered for a patient who does not respond to a particular drug.

Table IV
Routes of administration of nonsteroidal anti-inflammatory drugs

Route	Drugs
Oral	All NSAIDS
Controlled-release form	Indomethacin, naproxen, diclofenac
Parenteral (both i.m. and i.v.)	Ketorolac, ketoprofen*, lysine acetylsalicylate*
Rectal	Indomethacin

*Not available in the United States.

Adverse effects

NSAIDs have two sets of potential adverse effects. The first is toxic and can be caused by all NSAIDs but may vary in severity among different patients and different NSAIDs. The second set of adverse effects is idiosyncratic and may be observed with some NSAIDs but not others in certain patients.

Toxic reactions. Toxic effects of NSAIDs limit their role in the treatment of pain in general and in sickle cell patients in particular. Toxicity of NSAIDs results primarily from their effect on the metabolic cascade of arachidonic acid (Fig. 1) and especially from their inhibition of the biosynthesis of prostaglandins in all organs. The three major toxic effects associated with NSAIDs are gastropathy, nephropathy, and hemostatic defects. These toxicities should not be minimized because 10–15% of patients with sickle cell disease have hepatic or renal damage due to hemoglobinopathy (Achord 1994; Falk and Jeanette 1994).

Gastropathy. Gastrointestinal toxicity occurs with decreased local tissue levels of prostaglandins, which contribute to cytoprotection of the gastric mucosa. Consequently, administration of NSAIDs results in increased gastric acid secretion, decreased mucin production and mucosal resistance, reduced bicarbonate secretion, reduced blood flow, and a decrease in sphincter tone (Roth and Bennett 1987; Semble and Wu 1987). The most serious toxic effect of NSAIDs on the gastrointestinal tract is gastric ulceration with hemorrhage, which may be severe in some patients. The risk of hemorrhage is further increased by concomitant platelet dysfunction caused by NSAIDs (see below). Symptoms of NSAID gastropathy include bloating, dyspepsia, nausea, vomiting, abdominal pain, constipation or diarrhea, anorexia, and bleeding. Risk factors for the development of NSAID gastropathy include history of gastric bleeding, history of peptic ulcer disease, smoking, alcohol consumption, old age, and high doses of NSAIDs.

A variety of approaches have been attempted to reduce the risk of bleeding caused by NSAIDs and to improve their gastrointestinal tolerance. These approaches include the use of histamine H_2 antagonists to reduce the incidence of duodenal ulcers (Delhotal-Landes et al. 1988; Langmen 1989), omeprazole (Prilosec) to reduce the incidence of gastric ulcers (Walan et al. 1989), and misoprostol (Cytotec) to inhibit both gastric and duodenal ulceration (Graham et al. 1988; Roth et al. 1989, 1988; Agrawal et al. 1991). The use of these agents for prophylaxis against NSAIDs-associated gastropathy is complex and controversial (Hawkey 1990; Soll 1990).

Nephropathy. In the kidney, prostaglandins act as vasodilators to maintain renal blood flow (Dunn 1977). Inhibition of prostaglandin synthesis may lead to a decrease of renal blood flow and glomerular filtration that results in increased serum creatinine level and sodium and water retention with edema or volume overload (Clive and Stoff 1984; Patrono and Dunn 1987). In the presence of hepatic cirrhosis, congestive heart failure, and volume depletion, NSAIDs can cause fluid retention, hyperkalemia, and impaired responsiveness to diuretics (Clive and Stoff 1984; Patrono and Dunn 1987). Risk factors for NSAID-induced acute renal failure include congestive heart failure, chronic renal failure, and intravascular renal depletion (Payne 1989a,b). Patients with sickle cell disease are at risk for developing dehydration due to an inability to concentrate their urine (hyposthenuria). Thus, hepatic and renal functions should be monitored when using these analgesics for prolonged periods.

Hemostatic defects. NSAIDs reduce platelet aggregation because they inhibit the biosynthesis of prostaglandins and thromboxane A_2 (Fig. 1). Aspirin inhibition of platelet cyclooxygenase is irreversible whereas the inhibition by the other NSAIDs is reversible (Ali and McDonald 1978; Burch et al. 1978). Thus, aspirin leads to platelet dysfunction with prolonged bleeding time for the entire life span of the platelet (6–10 days), whereas the other NSAIDs cause platelet dysfunction for five half-lives, the time required to eliminate all drugs from the body. Longer-acting NSAIDs, such as piroxicam (Feldene), pose a relative disadvantage in patients at risk for bleeding (Table III).

Idiosyncratic side effects. These effects, summarized in Table V, are not related to inhibition of the biosynthesis of prostaglandins (O'Brien and Bagby 1985). Although these reactions are rare, they can be serious in some patients (see case 9.1 below).

Recently, necrotizing fasciitis, a potentially fatal soft tissue infection involving the fat and fascia, has been associated with the administration on NSAIDs (Smith and Berk 1991; Pillans and O'Conner 1995). Those implicated in causing this complication include: oral diclofenac, piroxicam, and diflunisal; rectal indomethacin and flurbiprofen; and intramuscular diclofenac. The frequency, risk factors, and mechanism of this complication of NSAIDs are unknown and controversial.

Drug interactions

Patients with sickle cell disease are likely to have multiple organ dysfunction and may be taking other medications that may potentially interact with NSAIDs. The interested reader may wish to consult reviews on this subject (Tonkin and Wing 1988; Brooks and Day 1991). Suffice it to say that NSAIDs can increase the effect of oral anticoagulants, phenytoin, oral hypoglycemic

Table V
Idiosyncratic (nonprostaglandin-mediated) reactions
caused by nonsteroidal anti-inflammatory drugs

Reaction	Manifestations	Major Implicated Agents
Bone marrow toxicity	Aplastic anemia Agranulocytosis Red cell aphasia	Phenylbutazone
CNS symptoms	Headaches, dizziness, lightheadedness, mood alterations, blurred vision	Indomethacin
Aseptic meningitis	Headache, stiff neck, fever, photophobia	Ibuprofen, sulindac, tolmetin
Dermatologic reactions	Minor rashes to exfoliative dermatitis or toxic epidermal necrolysis	Most NSAIDs
Asymptomatic transaminasemia	Elevated lab values with no clinical signs and symptoms	Most NSAIDs
Hepatitis	Variable mechanisms	Sulindac, phenylbutazone, diclofenac
Bilateral pulmonary infiltrates	Dyspnea, nonproductive cough	Naproxen
Exacerbation of bronchospasm	Triad of asthma, nasal polyposis, and aspirin hypersensitivity (Samter's syndrome)	Aspirin, other NSAIDs
Necrotizing fasciitis	Soft tissue infection	Diclofenac, piroxicam, diflunisal, indomethacin, flurbiprofen

Source: Adapted from Ferrante 1993a, with permission.

agents, valproate, digoxin, and aminoglycosides. NSAIDs potentiate the effect of these drugs in two ways: their high affinity to proteins conveys the ability to displace these drugs from albumin; and they inhibit their metabolism. Metoclopramide, antacids, probencid, barbiturates, and caffeine, however, can enhance the effect of NSAIDs by increasing their absorption, decreasing their renal clearance, or reducing their metabolism.

Cost of NSAIDs

The cost of NSAIDs varies considerably among different preparations (Table VI). The price of generic and brand preparations also differs.

LOCAL ANESTHETICS

Oral local anesthetics

Oral local anesthetics are widely used to manage neuropathic pain (Woolf and Wiesenfeld-Hall 1985; Chabal et al. 1989). Mexiletine (Mexitil) and tocainide (Tonocard) are the two most commonly used. Mexiletine is the safest oral local anesthetic and has been used to manage both lancinating and continuous pain (Portenoy 1993). To date the literature includes no reports of the treatment of sickle pain with oral local anesthetics, perhaps because neuropathic pain is rare in sickle cell disease.

Table VI
Cost of nonsteroidal anti-inflammatory drugs for 30 days of therapy for an adult patient

Brand Name	Generic Name	Adult Dosage*		Quantity	Brand Cost ($)	Generic Cost ($)
Anaprox	Naproxen sodium	275 mg	b.i.d.	60	53.13	43.97
Ansaid	Flurbiprofen	50 mg	q.i.d.	120	108.95	89.25
Ascriptin	Aspirin	975 mg	q.i.d.	360	21.89	10.20
Cataflam	Diclofenac potassium	50 mg	t.i.d.	90	143.48	NA
Clinoril	Sulindac	200 mg	b.i.d.	60	81.48	66.27
Daypro	Oxaprozin	1200 mg	q.d.	60	82.63	NA
Disalcid	Salsalate	750 mg	q.i.d.	120	76.50	38.21
Dolobid	Diflunisal	500 mg	b.i.d.	60	80.93	64.55
Feldene	Piroxicam	20 mg	q.d.	30	86.27	65.18
Indocin	Indomethacin	25 mg	t.i.d.	90	56.33	20.13
Lodine	Etodolac	400 mg	b.i.d.	60	92.25	NA
Meclomen	Meclofenamate	100 mg	t.i.d.	90	BNA	57.23
Motrin	Ibuprofen	600 mg	t.i.d.	90	25.68	18.60
Nalfon	Fenoprofen	300 mg	q.i.d.	120	50.51	41.35
Naprelan	Naproxen, controlled release	750 mg	q.d.	60	71.73	NA
Naprosyn	Naproxen	250 mg	b.i.d.	60	52.51	45.74
Orudis	Ketoprofen	50 mg	q.i.d.	120	126.81	112.89
Oruvail	Ketoprofen	200 mg	q.d.	30	82.02	NA
Relafen	Nabumetone	1000 mg	q.d.	60	70.66	NA
Voltaren	Diclofenac	75 mg	b.i.d.	60	83.96	69.66
Voltaren-XR	Diclofenac sodium, controlled release	100 mg	q.d.	30	76.38	NA

Source: Reprinted with permission of the Pennsylvania Medical Society 1997.
Note: Cost = average wholesale price for May 1997 plus $4 dispensing fee, in U.S. dollars; NA = generic not available; BNA = brand no longer available.
*Dosage and duration may have to be adjusted for disease severity, age, and/or comorbid conditions.

Topical local anesthetics: EMLA

EMLA is an oil-in-water emulsion system in which the oil phase consists of a eutectic mixture of the base forms of 2.5% lidocaine and 2.5%
prilocaine in the ratio of 1:1. It is marketed as EMLA cream and EMLA
patch. The FDA has approved the former for marketing in the United States.
It is used widely in infants and children. This topical anesthetic provides
effective anesthesia of the skin in connection with venipuncture, lumbar
puncture, postherpetic neuralgia, debridement of infected leg ulcers, painful
ulcers, and routine immunization in children (Hallen et al. 1985; Joyce et al.
1990; Kapelushni et al. 1990; Lycka 1992; Koren 1993). In Europe EMLA
is not approved for infants less than 3 months; in the United States the
minimum age for administration is 1 month and for infants who are receiving methemoglobin-inducing agents the minimum is 12 months because of
concerns regarding a greater susceptibility to methemoglobinemia in these
situations. This age restriction was challenged by one French study (Gourrier
et al. 1996) in which EMLA cream was used on 500 neonates, 69% of
whom were premature, over two years with no evidence of toxicity due to
methemoglobin. The authors, however, cautioned not to give EMLA to neonates less than 30 weeks of gestational age, in cases of serious sepsis, and in
combination with drugs known to increase methemoglobin formation. Side
effects of EMLA include minor blanching, followed by reactive erythema
and edema, and rare occurrence of methemoglobinemia in infants less than
3 months old (Lee and Forrester 1992; Koren 1993). EMLA has not been
used to date in the management of sickle cell disease, although it may have
beneficial effect in leg ulcers.

TOPICAL ANALGESICS

Capsaicin

Capsaicin is a topical cream derived from the active ingredient in hot
red peppers and exerts its analgesic effect by depleting substance P and
CGRP in primary afferent neurons that mediate the transmission of noxious
stimuli (Jessel and Dodd 1989; Dubner 1991). Topical administration of
capsaicin may reduce central transmission of information about a noxious
stimulus. Patients with postherpetic neuralgia and with postmastectomy pain
seem to benefit from this medication (Watson et al. 1988, 1989). Again,
capsaicin has not been reported in the management of sickle cell pain.

Other preparations

Active ingredients in topical analgesics, other than capsaicin, include methylsalicylate, menthol, camphor, eucalyptus oil, turpentine oil, methylnicotinate, and mustard oil (Drug Facts and Comparisons 1997). Methylsalicylate, which occurs naturally as oil of wintergreen, is available in a variety of concentrations (8–55%) and is the most widely used by patients with arthritis. These preparations are marketed as gels, creams, ointments, liquids, sprays, lotions, and liniments. Their efficacy in the management of sickle cell pain is anecdotal and not well documented. Topical analgesics should not be applied to irritated skin or leg ulcers and should not be used concomitantly with heating pads.

TRAMADOL (ULTRAM)

Tramadol is a synthetic centrally acting analgesic not chemically related to opiates that acts as a weak agonist at opioid receptors with preferential affinity for the μ receptor. Moreover, it inhibits neuronal uptake of both serotonin and norepinephrine and stimulates the release of serotonin. Thus, functionally, it has properties of an opioid and an antidepressant. Unlike conventional opioids, tramadol has not been associated with clinically significant respiratory depression or addiction potential (Lee et al. 1993; Budd 1994; Abel 1995). The latter salutary effect, however, has recently been challenged. It seems to be as effective as acetaminophen with 30 mg codeine (Tylenol #3) with the added advantage of tricyclic antidepressant-like effect. Tramadol may be used by the oral or parenteral route and it is available in slow-release form. Only the oral form is approved for marketing in the United States. The role of tramadol in the management of sickle cell pain remains to be determined.

OPIOID ANALGESICS

INTRODUCTION

Definitions

The word opioid is a generic term that refers to all analgesic compounds that possess morphine-like properties whether they are naturally occurring or synthetic, endogenous or exogenous. The term opiate refers to naturally occurring alkaloids, such as morphine and codeine, derived from opium. The word opium is derived from the Greek word meaning "juice." Opium is

the dried, powdered mixture of 20 alkaloids obtained from the unripe capsules of poppy seeds (Ferrante 1993b; Reisine and Pasternak 1996).

Opioids vs. narcotics

The word narcotic is derived from the Greek word *narkoun*, to benumb,
and *narki*, meaning numbness or stupor. As a noun narcotic means: (1) any
drug that induces stupor, (2) a person addicted to narcotics, or (3) anything
that causes stupor. In common usage the word narcotic connotes addiction,
drug-seeking behavior, and association with abused substances. It is advisable not to use this term in a pharmacological context.

Schedules of controlled substances

Opioid analgesics are drugs that come under the jurisdiction of the Controlled Substance Act. These drugs are divided into five schedules as listed
below (Code of federal regulation 1996).

Schedule I substances. These drugs have no accepted medical use in
the United States and have a high potential for abuse. Some examples are
heroin, marijuana, LSD, tetrahydrocannabinols, benzylmorphine, dihydro-
morphine, and others.

Schedule II substances. The drugs in this schedule have a high abuse
potential with severe liability for psychic or physical dependence and include certain narcotics, stimulants, and depressants. Some examples are opium,
morphine, codeine, diphenoxylate, hydromorphone (Dilaudid), methadone
(Dolophine), meperidine (Demerol), oxycodone (Percodan, Percocet),
oxymorphone (Numorphan), levorphanol, fentanyl, and others. Schedule II
non-narcotics include amphetamine (Dexedrine) and methamphetamine
(Desoxyn), phenmetrazine (Preludin), methylphenidate (Ritalin), amobar-
bital, pentobarbital, secobarbital, etorphine hydrochloride, phencyclidine, and
glutethimide (Doriden).

Schedule III substances. The drugs in this schedule have less potential
for abuse than those in Schedules I and II, and include compounds containing limited quantities of certain narcotic drugs, such as paregoric, and non-
narcotic drugs such as derivatives of barbituric acid (except those listed in
another schedule), methyprylon (Noludar), chlorhexadol, nalorphine,
benzphetamine, chlorphentermine, clortermine, mazindol, phendimetrazine,
and anabolic steroids.

Schedule IV substances. The drugs in this schedule have less potential
for abuse than those listed in Schedule III and include barbital, phenobar-

bital, methyphenobarbital, chloralbetaine (BetaChlor), chloralhydrate, ethchlorvynol (Placidyl), ethinamate (Valmid), mephorbamate (Equanil, Miltown), paraldehyde, methohexital, fenfluramine, diethylpropion, phentermine, chlordiazepoxide (Librium), diazepam (Valium), oxazepam (Serax), clorazepate (Tranxene), flurazepam (dalmane), clonazepam (Clonopin), prazepam (Verstran), lorazepam (Ativan), mebutamate, and dextropropoxyphene (Darvon).

Schedule V substances. The drugs in this schedule have less potential for abuse potential than those listed in Schedule IV and consist of preparations containing limited quantities of certain narcotic drugs generally used for antitussive and antidiarrheal purposes. Schedule V controlled substances or any controlled substance that is not a prescription item under the Federal Food, Drug, and Cosmetic Act, may be distributed without a prescription order at retail provided that such distribution is made only by a pharmacist and not by a nonpharmacist employee even if under the direct supervision of a pharmacist. However, after the pharmacist has fulfilled professional and legal responsibilities, a nonpharmacist may complete actual cash or credit transactions or delivery.

CLASSIFICATION

According to efficacy

Opioid analgesics are classified in several ways (Foley 1982, 1985; Jaffe and Martin 1990; Wall and Melzack 1994; Drugs Fact and Comparisons 1997). One classification divides them arbitrarily into weak and strong groups according to their potency and efficacy (Table VII). Weak opioids are available in combination with nonopioid analgesics such as acetaminophen or aspirin (Table VIII). Although such combinations provide additive antipyretic and anti-inflammatory effects, they limit the amount that can be administered because a daily maximum of 6000 mg of acetaminophen, an amount contained in about 18 tablets of Percocet, is recommended to avoid hepatotoxicity.

According to receptor interaction

A physiologic classification of opioids divides them according to structure and interaction with receptors (Table IX), i.e., agonists, partial agonists, and mixed agonists/antagonists. Thus, these drugs act centrally, at the level of the dorsal horn, midbrain, and thalamus where opioid receptors abound.

Table VII
Classification of opioid analgesics according to efficacy

"Weak" opioids used orally for mild to moderate pain
Codeine
Dihydrocodeine and hydrocodone
Oxycodone (Percocet, Percodan, Roxicodone, Roxicet, Tylox)
Propoxyphene HCl (Darvon)
Propoxyphene napsylate (Darvon-N)
Pentazocine (Talwin)
"Strong" opioids used parenterally for severe pain
Morphine sulfate
Hydromorphone (Dilaudid)
Oxymorphone (Numorphan)
Levorphanol (Levo-Dromoran)
Meperidine (Demerol, Pethidine)
Methadone (Dolophine)
Fentanyl
Nalbuphine (Nubain)
Butorphanol (Stadol)
Buprenorphine (Buprenex)

CLINICAL PHARMACOLOGY

Mechanism of action

The mechanism of action of opioid analgesics is best defined by their activity at specific receptors (Vaught et al. 1982). Opioids block slow but not fast transmission of pain and raise the pain threshold by acting as ligands that bind to stereo-specific and saturable receptors in the central nervous system and other tissues (Beckett and Casey 1954; Snyder 1984; Fields 1987). Receptors mediate two major functions: chemical recognition and physiologic action. Recognition is highly specific so that only L-isomers of opioids exert analgesic activity (Leysen et al. 1983). The binding affinity or strength with which a drug binds to its receptor varies considerably among opioids (Kosterlitz 1975). Fentanyl, for example, has a higher binding affinity than morphine (Leysen et al. 1983). The binding affinities of opioids seem to correlate well with their analgesic potencies (Martin et al. 1976). Physiologically, by binding to receptors, opioids initiate a series of biochemical events including activation of G-proteins, inhibition of adenylate cyclase activity, and extrusion of postassium ions that result in hyperpolarization of cell membranes (Herz and Teschemacher 1971; Snyder 1977; Simon and Hiller 1978), which delays or prevents the transmission of painful stimuli. The endogenous opioids, endorphins, enkephalins, and dynorphins also exert their action by binding to these receptors.

There are four major types of opioid receptors (Table X): μ, κ, δ, and σ (Gilbert and Martin 1976; Martin et al. 1976; Pasternak and Wood 1986; Pasternak 1988) and two subtypes receptors termed μ_1 and μ_2 (Pasternak et al. 1980; Wood et al. 1982; Nishimura et al. 1984). Opioids interact with various receptor subtypes as shown in Table XI. Adverse effects depend on the degree of binding to receptors. To date, no known opioid analgesic selectively activates μ_1 receptors without concomitant activation of the μ_2 receptors. Such a drug would be ideal to produce analgesia without sedation. Opioid analgesics that bind more to μ_2 receptors, which mediate sedation, and less to μ_1 receptors, which mediate analgesia, may produce excessive sedation without adequate analgesia, i.e., a sleepy patient who complains of

Table VIII
Representative opioid analgesic combinations

Codeine combinations	*Ocycodone combinations*
Empirin compounds	Percodan
Aspirin (325 mg)	Oxycodone 4.5 mg
+ codeine phosphate:	Oxycodone terephthalate 0.38 mg
#3 30 mg codeine	Aspirin 325 mg
#4 60 mg codeine	Percocet, Roxicet
Tylenol with codeine	Oxycodone 5 mg
Acetaminophen (300 mg)	Acetaminophen 325 mg
+ codeine phosphate:	Tylox
#3 30 mg codeine	Oxycodone 5 mg
#4 60 mg codeine	Acetaminophen 500 mg
Fiorinal with codeine	*Propoxyphene combinations*
Aspirin 325 mg	Darvon with ASA
Caffeine 40 mg	Propoxyphene HCl 65 mg
Butalbital 50 mg	Aspirin 325 mg
Codeine 30 mg	Darvocet-N 50 (or -N 100)
Fioricet with codeine	Propoxyphene napsylate 50 (or 100) mg
Acetaminophen 325 mg	Acetaminophen 325 (or 650) mg
Caffeine 40 mg	Darvon compound (or Darvon compound-65)
Butalbital 50 mg	Propoxyphene HCl 32 (or 65) mg
Codeine 30 mg	APC (aspirin, phenacetin, and caffeine)
Hydrocodone combinations	*Pentazocine combinations*
Vicodin	Talwin compound
Hydrocodone bitartrate 5 mg	Pentazocine HCl 12.5 mg
Acetaminophen 500 mg	Aspirin 325 mg
Lortab 2.5, 5.0 or 7.5/500	Talacen
Hydrocodone 2.5, 5, or 7.5 mg	Pentazocine HCl 25 mg
Acetaminophen 500 mg	Acetaminophen 650 mg
Tussionex ER suspension	Talwin-Nx
Hydrocodone 10 mg	Pentazocine HCl 50 mg
Chlorpheniramine 8 mg	Naloxone 0.5 mg

Table IX
Classification of opioids
according to chemical structure and function

Agonists
  Naturally occurring (opium alkaloids)
    Codeine
    Morphine
  Semisynthetic opioids
    Hydrocodone (Hycodan, Vicodin, Lortab, Tussionex)
    Oxycodone (Percocet, Percodan, Roxicet, Roxicodone, Tylox)
    Hydromorphone (Dilaudid)
    Oxymorphone (Numorphan)
  Synthetic opioids
    Morphinans
      Levorphanol (Levo-Dromoran)
    Phenylpiperidines
      Meperidine (Demerol, Pethidine)
      Alfentanil
      Fentanyl
      Sufentanil
    Diphenylheptanes
      Methadone (Dolophine)
      Propoxyphene HCl (Darvon, Darvocet, Wygesic)
      Propoxyphene Napsylate (Darvon N)
Partial agonists
  Buprenorphine (Buprenex)
  Dezocine (Dalgan)
Mixed agonists-antagonists
  Pentazocine (Talwin)
  Nalbuphine (Nubain)
  Butorphanol (Stadol)

---

severe pain whenever awakened. This situation may create logistical problems in managing painful sickle crises as will be discussed in Chapter 10.

Table XII lists the parmacokinetic profiles of opioids. Understanding their characteristics permits rational use. Morphine, the prototype of opioid agonists, acts primarily at μ and δ receptors and to a lesser extent at κ receptors (Table XII) (Jaffe and Martin 1990). Opioid agonists do not have a "ceiling effect;" as the dose is increased on a logarithmic scale the increment in analgesia seems to be linear to the point of unconsciousness. Before loss of consciousness, however, undesirable side effects such as excessive sedation, mental clouding, and respiratory depression limit the maximum useful dose.

Opioid agonist-antagonists and partial agonists have agonist activity at some receptors and antagonist activity at others (Zola and McLeod 1983; Jaffe and Martin 1990; Hoskin and Hanks 1991; Wall and Melzack 1994;

Table X
Classification of opioid receptors and their effects

Receptor Type	Mediated Effects
μ_1	Supraspinal analgesia, miosis, nausea, vomiting, constipation, urine retention, pruritus, fever, euphoria
μ_2	No analgesia, apnea, sedation, respiratory depression, bradycardia, decreased gastrointestional motility
κ	Spinal analgesia, sedation, miosis, diuresis, respiratory depression
δ	Spinal analgesia, apnea, nausea, vomiting, pruritus
σ	No analgesia, dysphoria, psychotomimetic effects, tachypnea, tachycardia, mydriasis, vasomotor stimulation

Sources: Adapted from Ferrante 1993b and Benedetti and Butler 1990, with permission.

Table XI
Interactions of opioids with various receptor types

Opioid	Receptor Type			
	μ	κ	δ	σ
Agonists				
Morphine	3+	1+	2+	–
Meperidine	2+	–	2+	–
Hydromorphone	3+	–	2+	–
Oxymorphone				
Levorphanol				
Methadone	3+	–	2+	–
Fentanyl	4+	–	1+	–
Partial agonist				
Buprenorphine	Partial agonist	–	–	–
Dezocine	Partial agonist	–	+1	–
Agonist-antagonists				
Pentazocine	Antagonist	3+	?	2+
Nalbuphine	Antagonist	3+	–	1+
Butorphanol	Antagonist	2+	–	2+
Antagonists				
Naloxone	Antagonist	Antagonist	Antagonist	Antagonist
Naltrexone	Antagonist	Antagonist	Antagonist	Antagonist
Nalmefene	Antagonist	Antagonist	Antagonist	Antagonist

Sources: Adapted from Ferrante 1993b and Benedetti and Butler 1990, with permission.
Notes: Pluses (+) indicate an agonist effect: the higher the number the stronger the binding affinity to the receptor. Minuses (–) indicate no known or reported effect.

Table XII
Pharmacokinetic profiles of commonly used opioid
analgesics based on intramuscular administration

Drug	Onset (min)	Peak (h)	Duration (h)	Half-life (T½, h)
Agonists				
Morphine	15–20	0.5–1.0	3–7	1.5–2.0
Hydromorphone	15–30	0.5–1.0	3–4	2.0–3.0
Meperidine	10–15	0.5–1.0	2–3	3.0–4.0
Levorphanol	30–60	0.5–1.0	4–6	12–16
Alfentanil	Immediate	ND	ND	1–2*
Fentanyl	7–8	ND	1–2	1.5–6.0
Sufentanil	1.3–3	ND	ND	2.5
Methadone	30–60	0.5–1.0	4–6	15–30
Codeine	15–30	1.0–1.5	4–6	3.0
Oxycodone (p.o.)	15–30	1.0	3–5	ND
Propoxyphene (p.o.)	30–60	2–2.5	4–6	6–12
Oxymorphone	5–10	0.5–1.0	3–6	ND
Partial agonists				
Buprenorphine	15	0.5–1.0	6	2.2–3.5
Dezocine	15–30	0.5–2.5	2–4	2–4*
Mixed agonist-antagonists				
Pentazocine	15–20	0.5–1.0	4–6	2–3
Nalbuphine	<15	0.5–1.0	3–6	5
Butorphanol	10–15	0.5–1.0	3–4	2.5–4

Note: ND = no data available.
*Data based on i.v. administration.

Drugs Facts and Comparisons 1997). The two types of opioid agonists-antagonists are: (1) nalorphine-type mixed agonist-antagonists, which are antagonists at the μ receptor and agonists at other receptors, e.g., pentazocine; and (2) morphine-type partial agonists, which have limited agonist activity at the μ receptor, e.g., buprenorphine. Unlike opioid agonists, these agents have a ceiling effect that may limit their use in achieving pain relief.

Equianalgesic dosing equivalents

Opioid analgesics differ in potency due to their specific physiochemical and pharmacokinetic properties, but all opioids can be made equivalent or equianalgesic by adjusting for the differences in these properties by changing the dose or the route of administration. Table XIII shows an equianalgesic conversion scheme. Conversion from one opioid to another or from one route to another is extremely important in clinical practice (Foley 1985; Twycross and McQuay 1989). Nevertheless, equianalgesic conversion tables are guidelines and not indisputable dogma. Careful monitoring of the dosage to achieve pain relief without serious side effects supersedes conversion tables.

The high oral/parenteral ratio for morphine is due to its significant first-pass metabolism, which decreases its oral bioavailability to an average of 38% with a range from 15% to 64% (Routledge and Shand 1979; Sawe et al. 1981). For acute short-term use, the oral to parenteral potency ratio for morphine is six. For chronic administration this ratio decreases to two or three (Houde et al. 1975; Twycross 1975; Sawe et al. 1981; Kaiko 1986).

The parenteral routes of administration are thought to be equipotent in conversion tables by assuming equivalent bioavailability among intravenous, intramuscular, and subcutaneous administration. However, many patients with sickle cell disease and their care providers question this assumption. The subcutaneous to intravenous potency ratio in patients receiving hydromorphone was 1:1.5 or 1:2, which indicates that the subcutaneous dose must be higher than the intravenous dose to achieve the same level of analgesia (Urquhart et al. 1988; Moulin et al. 1991).

Table XIII
Equianalgesic dosing equivalents of opioids

Drug	Potency i.m./p.o.	Equianalgesic Doses[*] i.m. (mg)	p.o. (mg)
Agonists			
Morphine	6	10	60
Hydromorphone	5	1.5	7.5
Meperidine	4	75	300
Levorphanol	2	2	4
Alfentanil	NA	ND	NA
Fentanyl	NA	0.1	NA
Sufentanil	NA	0.02	NA
Methadone	2	10	20
Codeine	1.5	130	200
Oxycodone (p.o.)	NA	NA	30
Propoxyphene (p.o.)	NA	NA	130
Oxymorphone	NA	1	10[†]
Partial agonist			
Buprenorphine	NA	10	NA
Dezocine	NA	10	NA
Mixed agonist-antagonists			
Pentazocine	3	60	180
Nalbuphine	NA	10	NA
Butorphanol	NA	2	NA

Note: ND = no data available; NA = not applicable.
[*]Based on acute short-term use. Chronic administration may alter pharmacokinetics and decrease the oral:parenteral dose ratio. The morpohine oral:parenteral ratio decreases to 2:3 upon chronic dosing.
[†]Rectal administration.

Route of administration

Analgesic drugs may be given orally, intravenously, intramuscularly, subcutaneously, transdermally, or transmuscosally. Other routes, such as rectal, epidural, intrathecal, or intraventricular, are rarely used for the treatment of sickle cell pain. Not all drugs can be given by all routes. Meperidine, for example, may be given orally, intramuscularly, or intravenously, but not subcutaneously or transdermally. Oxycodone is not available for parenteral administration. Table XIV lists the approved routes of administration of the major opioid analgesics available in the Unites States (Drug Facts and Comparisons 1997).

Method of administration

Analgesic drugs may be administered by continuous intravenous drip, on a fixed schedule with rescue doses, as needed, or by PCA. The advantages and disadvantages of each method are addressed in Chapter 10.

Table XIV
Routes of administration of analgesics

Drug	Route of Administration
Morphine	p.o., i.m., i.v., s.c., r.t.m., epidural, intrathecal, i.c.v.
Hydromorphone	p.o., i.m., i.v., s.c., r.t.m.
Meperidine	p.o., i.m., i.v.
Levorphanol	p.o., i.m., i.v., s.c.
Alfentanil	i.v.
Fentanyl	i.m., i.v., t.d., o.t.m.
Sufentanil	i.v.
Methadone	p.o., i.m.
Codeine	p.o., i.m., i.v., s.c.
Oxycodone	p.o.
Propoxyphene	p.o.
Oxymorphone	i.m., i.v., s.c., r.t.m.
Pentazocine	p.o., i.m., i.v., s.c.
Nalbuphine	i.m., i.v., s.c.
Butorphanol	i.m., i.v., s.c., i.n.
Buprenorphine	i.m., i.v., s.c., s.l.g.*

Note: p.o., oral; i.m., intramuscular; i.v., intravenous; s.c., subcutaneous; r.t.m., rectal transmuscosal; i.c.v., intracerebroventricular; t.d., transdermal; o.t.m., oral transmucosal; i.n., intranasal; s.l.g., sublingual.
*The sublingual form of buprenorphine is not available in the United States. Morphine, oxycodone, codeine, and hydromorphone are available in controlled-release form. Slow-release codeine and hydromorphone are not yet available in the United States as of this writing. Sustained-release morphine is commercially available in 20-, 50-, and 100-mg oral doses.

Indications

Opioid analgesics are the major and primary pharmacologic therapy for moderate to severe pain irrespective of its etiology. In an effort to encourage appropriate management of pain, especially cancer pain, the Agency for Health Care Policy and Research (AHCPR) developed a clinical practice guideline (Jacox et al. 1994) through a rigorous scientific process. This monograph presents standards for the assessment of cancer pain. Opioids are recommended as the major class of analgesics for control of moderate to severe pain because of their effectiveness, ease of titration, and favorable risk/benefit ratio. Unfortunately, this document never mentioned sickle cell pain and thus, unintentionally, gave the impression that sickle pain need not be treated as aggressively as cancer pain. Although these guidelines targeted cancer pain, many providers are applying them for selected patients with nonmalignant pain.

Adverse effects

Side effects of opioid agonists are listed in Table XV (Jaffe and Martin 1990; Wall and Melzack 1994; Drug Facts and Comparisons 1997). Some side effects such as relief of anxiety, euphoria, and sedation are desirable in managing acute sickle pain. Neurologic side effects include euphoria, drowsiness, mental confusion, and apathy. Nausea and vomiting ensue from direct stimulation of medullary emetic chemoreceptors. Pulmonary effects include diminished tidal volume followed by depressed responses of the respiratory center to carbon dioxide. Cardiovascular effects include depressed

Table XV
Comparative analgesic effect and side effects of opioid agonists

Drug	Anal-gesia	Resp. Depr.	Seda-tion	Eupho-ria	Eme-sis	Anti-tussive	Consti-pation
Morphine	2+	2+	2+	3+	2+	3+	2+
Hydromorphone	2+	2+	1+	3+	1+	3+	1+
Meperidine	2+	2+	1+	4+	NA	1+	1+
Levorphanol	2+	2+	2+	NA	1+	2+	2+
Fentanyl	2+	1+	NA	NA	NA	NA	NA
Sufentanil	NA	NA	NA	NA	NA	NA	NA
Methadone	2+	2+	1+	NA	1+	2+	2+
Codeine	1+	1+	1+	1+	1+	3+	1+
Oxycodone	2+	2+	2+	3+	2+	3+	2+
Propoxyphane	1+	1+	1+	1+	1+	NA	NA

Note: Resp. Depr. = respiratory depression; NA = information not available responsiveness of α-adrenergic receptors causing peripheral vasodilation, reduced peripheral resistance, and inhibited baroceptors, which may result in orthostatic hypotension. Gastrointestinal effects include inhibition of peristalsis, which may cause constipation, and spasm of the sphincter of Oddi. Urinary tract manifestations are primarily urinary retention due to enhanced bladder sphincter tone.

Opioids have abuse potential; psychological dependence or addiction, physical tolerance, and physical dependence may develop upon repeated use. Chapters 10 and 13 define these terms and discuss their impact on therapy. Other complications include skin rash, itching, and central nervous system hyperirritability, with toxic doses manifesting in multifocal myoclonus and seizures. Meperidine is most notorious for the last complication; repetitive dosing results in accumulation of the active metabolite normeperidine, which produces hyperirritability, including seizures. Seizures are not unique to meperidine, but can occur with toxic doses of most narcotic analgesics (Foley 1982; Eisele et al. 1991).

Some opioid agonist-antagonists have only recently been used in sickle cell disease, so extensive clinical experience is lacking. These agents have less potential for abuse, tolerance, physical dependence, and addiction than do opioid agonists, yet some risk is associated with the chronic use of pentazocine (Zola and McLeod 1983). Their disadvantages include a ceiling effect, the precipitation of withdrawal in patients using narcotic agonists, and psychomimetic side effects such as delusions, depersonalization, dysphoria, hallucinations, vivid daydreams, nightmares, and panic. These agents should not be used in conjunction with opioid agonists or morphine-type agonist-antagonists. Partial agonists of the morphine type have one major advantage over nalorphine-type agents—the lack of psychomimetic side effects. Further studies are needed to determine the optimal role of these agents in treating sickle cell pain.

DRUG INTERACTIONS

The coadministration of clomipramine, tricyclic antidepressants, and amitriptyline may increase the plasma concentration of morphine because these agents increase its biovailability and half-life (Ventafridda et al. 1990). In contrast, the coadministration of phenobarbital and phenytoin decreases the plasma concentration of meperidine due to the enhanced metabolic rate of meperidine. Similarly, the coadministration of rifampin and phenytoin decreases the plasma concentration of meperidine.

Coadministration of adjuvants with opioid analgesics requires skillful selection and monitoring, especially when a centrally acting drug is used.

The sedative effects of an opioid may accentuate that of other agents such as antidepressants, neuroleptics, and anxiolytics. Drugs with anticholinergic effects may worsen the constipation caused by opioids. The use of meperidine in conjunction with monoamine oxidase inhibitors may cause a severe adverse reaction characterized by excitation, hyperpyrexia, convulsions, and death (Inturrisi and Umans 1986). The coadministration of neuroleptics with meperidine may cause an array of neuromuscular disorders including akathisia, dystonia, tardive dyskinesia, and neuroleptic malignant syndrome (Munetz and Cornes 1983).

Generally, the effects of morphine may be antagonized by acidifying agents and potentiated by alkalinizing agents. The concomitant use of anticholinergics with opioids, including morphine, may result in an increased risk of severe constipation and urinary retention.

CNS depressants, such as other opioids, alcohol, anesthetics, antihistamines, barbiturates, beta-blockers, chloral hydrate, glutethimide, hypnotics, monoamine oxidase (MAO) inhibitors, phenothiazines, pyrazolidone, sedatives, skeletal muscle relaxants, and tricyclic antidepressants may enhance the depressant effects of morphine. Concurrent use may result in potentiation of CNS depression and death may occur. If used concurrently with CNS depressants, dosage adjustment may be required.

Amphetamines potentiate the analgesic effect of opioids. Opioids may increase the anticoagulant activity of warfarin and other anticoagulants.

COST

The cost of opioids depends on their type (e.g., codeine is less expensive than meperidine), manufacturer (generic vs. brand), geographical area, and dispensing institution. Table XVI summarizes the current cost of the major opioid analgesics.

OPIOID ANTAGONISTS

Opioid antagonists displace agonists from receptors. Naloxone (Narcan), naltrexone (Trexan/Revia), and nalmefene (Revex) are pure antagonists of μ, κ, δ, and σ receptors. These agents are of value in reversing the sedation and respiratory depression caused by opioid analgesics as will be discussed in Chapter 10.

Naloxone is the prototype of opioid antagonists. It is available as a solution for parenteral use, preferably intravenous. Nausea and vomiting are major side effects related to the dose and speed of injection (Longnecker et al. 1973; Kripke et al. 1976). Administration of naloxone activates the

Table XVI

Cost comparison of opioid analgesics for approximately two weeks of therapy for an adult patient

Brand Name	Generic Name	Adult Dosage*	Quantity	Brand Cost ($)	Generic Cost ($)
B&O Supprettes	Opium/belladonna	15A (30 mg) or 16A (60 mg) q.d.–b.i.d. (max 4 doses/24h)	28 / 28	82.75 / 88.58	NA / 76.38
Codeine	Codeine sulfate or phosphate	30 mg q4–6h p.r.n.	84	53.51	40.98
Demerol	Meperidine	50 mg q3–4h p.r.n. / 100 mg q3–4h p.r.n.	112 / 112	89.41 / 116.47	65.03 / 102.24
Dilaudid	Hydromorphone	2 q4–6h p.r.n. / 4 mg q4–6h p.r.n.	84 / 84	39.36 / 61.72	32.75 / 49.70
Dolophine	Methadone	5 mg q3–4h p.r.n. / 10 mg q3–4h p.r.n.	112 / 112	14.01 / 20.26	13.50 / 19.59
Duragesic	Fentanyl, transdermal patch	25 µg/h q72h / 50 µg/h q72h / 75 µg/h q72h	5 / 5 / 5	57.94 / 84.87 / 127.52	NA / NA / NA
Levo-Dromoran	Levorphanol/tartrate	2 mg q4–6h p.r.n.	84	55.78	51.31
Mepergan/Fortis	50 mg merperidine/ 25 mg promethazine	1 cap q3–4h p.r.n.	112	73.94	NA
MS Contin	Morphine sulfate, extended release	30 mg q12h / 60 mg q12h	28 / 28	52.09 / 97.83	44.76 / 83.53

Drug	Form	Dosage	Quantity	Cost	Generic
Kadian		20 mg q.d.	14	19.27	NA
		50 mg q.d.	14	14.23	NA
		100 mg q.d.	14	70.15	NA
MSIR or RMS	Morphine sulfate, immediate release	10 mg q4h p.r.n.	84 supp	122.65	122.67
		15 mg q4h p.r.n.	84 tabs	20.08	23.88
	supp: 10 mg (RMS)	30 mg q4h p.r.n.	84 tabs	31.17	38.25
	conc: 20 mg/1 ml	30 mg q4h p.r.n.	126 ml conc	79.82	74.84
			1260 ml soln	110.17	71.29
	soln: 10 mg/5 ml	30 mg q4h p.r.n.			
Numorphan	Oxymorphone suppositories	5 mg q4–6h p.r.n.	84	430.72	NA
Oxycontin	Oxycodone, extended release	10 mg q12h	28	37.60	NA
		20 mg q12h	28	68.32	NA
		40 mg q12h	28	118.06	NA
OxyIR[a] Roxicodone[b]	Oxycodone, immediate release	5 mg q6h p.r.n.	56	19.11[a] 27.79[b]	NA NA
Percocet	5 mg Oxycodone/ 325 mg APAP	1 tab q6h p.r.n.	56	43.14	18.35
Percodan	4.5 mg Oxycodone/ 325 mg ASA	1 tab q6h p.r.n.	56	44.49	17.29
Tylox	5 mg Oxycodone/ 325 mg APAP	1 cap q6h p.r.n.	56	46.95	32.55

Source: Reprinted with permission of the Pennsylvania Medical Society 1997.

Note: Cost = average wholesale price for May 1997 plus $4 dispensing fee, in U.S. dollars. NA, generic not available; supp, suppository; tabs, tablets; conc, concentrate; soln, solution.

*Dosage may have to be adjusted for disease severity, age, and/or comorbid conditions.

sympathetic nervous system to produce tachycardia, cardiac arrhythmia, hypertension, and pulmonary edema (Martin et al. 1973; Michaelis et al. 1974; Tanaka 1974; Flacke and Flacke 1977).

Naltrexone (Trexan) is available in oral form and can produce sustained opioid antagonism for up to 24 hours (Martin et al. 1973). It has been used in the treatment of opioid addiction and is available in 50-mg tablets.

Nalmefene (Revex) is a long-acting opioid antagonist available as a solution for parenteral use (i.m., i.v., or s.c.). It provides protection against renarcotization and sustains reversal of opioid drug effects, including respiratory depression, sedation, and hypotension. It may also be used in the emergency department to manage known or suspected opioid overdose (Cheskin et al. 1995).

Opioid antagonism begins within two minutes after i.v. injection of nalmefene and reaches a peak within five minutes. The drug is slowly metabolized in the liver by glucuronidation to form an inactive metabolite. The half-life of nalmefene is about 11 hours, much longer than naloxone's half-life of one to two hours.

CHARACTERISTICS OF SPECIFIC OPIOIDS

Agonists

Codeine. This opiate, similar to morphine, is a naturally occurring alkaloid. It is a prodrug and is metabolized in the liver to morphine and norcodeine and excreted in the kidneys, mostly in inactive forms. About 10% of a dose of codeine is demethylated to morphine. Codeine itself has low affinity to opioid receptors so the fraction that is converted to morphine may be responsible for its analgesic effect (Misra 1978; Kitahata et al. 1982).

Codeine is the most commonly used oral opioid analgesic for the treatment of mild to moderate pain. A dose of 30 mg of oral codeine is equivalent to 650 mg of aspirin, and the combination of 30 mg codeine and 650 mg aspirin yields an analgesic effect that is comparable to 60 mg codeine (Beaver 1984).

Codeine is an excellent, dose-dependent antitussive (Sevelius et al. 1971). It is often included in medication for its antitussive effect or is combined with acetaminophen or aspirin (Table VIII) for the relief of mild to moderate pain (Cooper and Beaver 1976). The usual dose is 30–120 mg of codeine combined with 300–975 mg of acetaminophen or aspirin every four to six hours.

Hydrocodone and dihydrocodeine. In the United States, these analogs of codeine are available only in combination with acetaminophen (Vicodin, Lortab, Dihydrocodeine Plus, Synalgos-DC) or aspirin (Hycodan, Tussionex).

Oxycodone. Oxycodone is a synthetic derivative of morphine and has a similar profile. It is available for oral but not parenteral administration. It is metabolized in the liver into noroxycodone (Weinstein and Gaylord 1979; Poyhia et al. 1991). Like codeine, oxycodone is usually admixed with nonopioid analgesics in commercial preparation for the management of mild to moderate pain. Dose escalation is limited in the combination form because of a potential toxicity from the acetaminophen or aspirin component. It is also available as a single entity and doses can be increased to achieve pain relief (Kalso and Vainio 1990). A controlled-release preparation of this drug (Oxycontin) recently entered the U.S. market after receiving FDA approval. A transdermal form is under development (Tien 1991). As with some other opioids, oxycodone has strong abuse potential (Maruta et al. 1979).

Propoxyphene. Propoxyphene is structurally similar to methadone but is a weak analgesic and is only available in oral preparations. Unlike other opioid analgesics, the dextrorotatory form (dextropropoxyphene) has the analgesic effect (Jaffe and Martin 1985). It was originally considered a nonopioid analgesic and was prescribed widely in the 1960s and 1970s. In 1978, 31 million prescriptions were written for propoxyphene in the United States alone (Mather and Denson 1992). Addiction, physical dependence, and tolerance were reported so it was reclassified as a weak opioid analgesic. Moreover, its analgesic efficacy is less than that of aspirin and only slightly better than placebo (Smith 1971). In humans, propoxyphene is N-demethylated to norpropoxyphene, which has a long half-life and is associated with excitatory effects including tremulousness and seizures (Giacomini et al. 1980; Inturrisi et al. 1982). These effects, however, are rarely associated with the doses usually administered for mild to moderate pain. Propoxyphene is not commonly used to treat sickle pain.

Morphine. Morphine is a strong μ-opioid agonist that was introduced into clinical use about 200 years ago. It is a naturally occurring alkaloid derived from the opium poppy, which is still the major source as its biochemical synthesis is difficult. It is hydrophilic and thus is rapidly distributed to tissues and organs and is probably sequestered in nonfat tissues such as skeletal muscles (Stanski et al. 1978; Murphy and Hugg 1981). It may be administered by any route (Table XIV) and is available in immediate-release, controlled-release, and sustained-release oral formulations (Maccarone et al. 1994). Controlled-release morphine has dosing intervals of 8–12 hours, and for several years has been commercially available in 30-, 60-, and 100-mg oral doses. A novel formulation of sustained-release morphine with a dosing interval of 24 hours has recently become commercially available in 20-, 50-, and 100-mg doses. It contains morphine as polymer-coated sustained-release pellets in a capsule for oral ingestion. Because they have a pH-dependent profile, the pellets do not release significant amounts of morphine until they have entered the small intestine.

Morphine undergoes glucuronidation at the 3 and 6 positions to yield morphine-3-glucuronide (M3G) and morphine-6-glucuronide (M6G) (Sawe et al. 1983; Paul et al. 1989). M3G is the major metabolite and has negligible affinity for opioid receptors. M3G produces hyperalgesia in rats when administered by the intrathecal and intraventricular routes and may act as an opioid antagonist (Smith et al. 1990). Human studies to evaluate the pharmacodynamics of M3G have not been performed. M6G, unlike M3G, binds to opioid receptors (Paul et al. 1989) and produces potent opioid effects in animals (Pasternak et al. 1987; Paul et al. 1989) and humans (Osborne et al. 1986; Paul et al. 1989; Hanna et al. 1990). In patients with renal insufficiency who receive morphine, M6G accumulates in the plasma and cerebrospinal fluid (Osborne et al. 1986; Portenoy et al. 1991, 1992). It has been associated with toxicity in patients with impaired renal function (Osborne et al. 1986; Hagen et al. 1991) and it may contribute to morphine analgesia even in patients with normal renal function (Portenoy et al. 1992). These data, although preliminary and needing further investigation, suggest caution when administering morphine to patients with renal failure due to the potential accumulation of M6G.

Morphine is highly histaminergic (Benedetti and Butler 1990) and is often associated with pruritus that may be severe in some cases. Consequently, it is not a popular drug among patients with sickle cell disease, as will be discussed in Chapter 10.

Hydromorphone. This morphine congener is five to seven times more potent than morphine. It is more soluble and is available in a concentrated dosage form of 10 mg/ml. It has been widely used by subcutaneous infusion in patient-controlled analgesia. Contrary to previous belief, the bioavailability of hydromorphone by continuous subcutaneous infusion is about 80% of the intravenous route (Moulin et al. 1991). An extended-release form of hydromorphone is available in countries other than the United States. Hydromorphone is not contraindicated in renal failure.

Oxymorphone. Oxymorphone is a lipophilic congener of morphine. When administered parenterally it is approximately 10 times more potent than morphine (Eddy and Lee 1959; Beaver et al. 1977; Sinatra and Harrison 1989). It is available in rectal formulation, which is about one-tenth as potent as intramuscular administration but as potent as parenteral morphine (Beaver and Feise 1977). It has a short half-life (1.2 to 2 hours) and is less likely to produce histamine release than is morphine (Hermens et al. 1985; Sinatra et al. 1988). Its major disadvantage is its high cost (Table XVI).

Levorphanol. Another morphine congener with a long half-life (12–16 hours), levorphanol is useful in patients who cannot tolerate morphine, hydromorphone, or methadone (Dixon et al. 1983; Portenoy et al. 1986). The combination of long half-life with a shorter duration of analgesia (4–6 hours) may predispose to drug accumulation following the initiation of therapy or dose escalation. In this regard it is similar to methadone.

Meperidine. This synthetic opioid is a member of the phenylpiperidine series of µ-opioid agonists. It is more lipophilic than morphine and produces faster onset and shorter duration of analgesia (2–3 hours) after parenteral administration (Lasagna and Beecher 1954; Marks and Sacher 1973). Problems with meperidine center around one of its major metabolites normeperidine. Approximately 90% of a certain dose of meperidine undergoes N-demethylation in the liver to produce normeperidine (Burns et al. 1979; Mather and Gourlay 1984), which has a half-life four to five times that of meperidine (18 vs. 3.5 hours), is twice as potent a convulsant and half as potent an analgesic as its parent compound (Armstrong and Bersten 1986). Accumulation of normeperidine after repetitive dosing of meperidine can result in central nervous system excitability characterized by subtle mood changes, anxiety, tremor, multifocal myoclonus, and seizures (Szeto et al. 1977; Eisendrath et al. 1987). Although old age and renal disease predispose patients to accumulation of normeperidine, toxicity is sometimes noted in young patients with normal renal function (Szeto et al. 1977; Kaiko et al. 1983). In patients with sickle cell disease the incidence of seizures related to the use of meperidine varies between 1% and 12% (Tobin 1989; Nadvi et al. 1995). Oral meperidine has only 25% of the analgesic effectiveness but produces just as much normeperidine. Naloxone does not reverse meperidine-induced seizures but, to the contrary, may precipitate seizures by blocking the depressant action of meperidine and facilitating the manifestation of the convulsant activity of normeperidine (Umans and Inturrisi 1982).

Factors associated with the occurrences of seizures in patients taking meperidine are: (1) doses greater than 100 mg every two hours around the clock for prolonged time; (2) alkaline urine (decreased excretion of normeperidine); (3) coadministration of phenobarbital and other enzyme-inducing drugs (increased production of normeperidine due to increased metabolism); (4) coadministration of phenothiazines (lowers seizure threshold); and (5) a history of seizures. Patients with impaired renal function are particularly at risk. Given that acute pain due to sickle cell disease typically lasts five to seven days (Shapiro 1993), use of meperidine should be limited to no more than 48 hours and daily doses should be less than 1200 mg per day unless the history indicates that the patient in question usually tolerated larger doses for a longer time.

High doses of morphine and methadone also have caused seizures

(Benedetti and Butler 1990). The incidence of such seizures in adult patients with sickle cell disease is not known, perhaps because these drugs have not been widely used for a long time, as is the case with meperidine.

Hepatic cirrhosis may cause decreased plasma clearance of normeperidine (Pond et al. 1981). Patients with hepatic cirrhosis may be relatively protected from normeperidine toxicity because of impaired hepatic function, but repetitive dosing may remove this protection (Pone et al. 1981).

Desirable properties of meperidine include the euphoria it produces (Table XV) and its association with a lower incidence of pruritus compared to morphine due to its reduced effect on histamine release (Hermens et al. 1985; Sinatra et al. 1988; Benedetti and Butler 1990). Unlike other opioids, meperidine has modest atropine-like properties so it causes mydriasis rather than miosis and rarely causes bradycardia but may cause tachycardia (Ferrante 1993b). When given in large doses, however, meperidine results in reduced myocardial contractibility, reduced stroke volume, and elevated filling pressure (Strauer 1972; Freye 1974).

Meperidine has mild antispasmodic properties. It causes less biliary spasm than does morphine after equianalgesic dosing (Radney et al. 1980). Meperidine causes less smooth muscle spasm than do other μ-opioid agonists, so it is ideal for treating patients with renal colic.

Although the role of meperidine in the management of chronic cancer pain is limited and its use in acute pain regimens is questioned, it is the most commonly used opioid analgesic in the management of hospitalized patients with sickle pain, as will be discussed in Chapter 10.

Fentanyl. This congener of meperidine is a member of the phenylpiperidine series (Table IX). Fentanyl is extremely lipophilic and is approximately 100 times more potent than morphine as an analgesic (De Castro et al. 1979; Jaffe and Martin 1990). It has been used parenterally and intrathecally to manage obstetric and postoperative pain (Holley and Van Steenis 1988; Gourlay et al. 1990). The development of transdermal (Miser et al. 1989; Calis et al. 1992) and transmucosal (Stanley et al. 1989; Fine et al. 1991) preparations have expanded its clinical utility to the management of chronic pain.

Methadone. Methadone is a synthetic μ-opioid agonist. Its long plasma half-life ranges from 13 to more than 100 hours with an average of about 24 hours. Similar to levorphanol, the discrepancy between long plasma half-life and duration of analgesia (4–8 hours) may predispose to drug accumulation following the initiation of therapy or dose escalation (Szeto et al. 1977; Eisendrath et al. 1987). Methadone is an excellent analgesic that is useful in treating chronic pain (Hansen et al. 1982; Ventafridda 1986) provided the prescriber knows its pharmacology and has experience in its use. Careful monitoring of patients coupled with stepwise dose escalation or reduction decrease the risk of delayed toxicity from methadone accumulation. Oral and parenteral preparations of methadone are available. Subcutaneous injections are reported to cause local skin toxicity and are not recommended (Inturrisi and Umans 1986).

Partial agonists

Buprenorphine. This semisynthetic opioid partial agonist binds to μ, κ, and δ receptors. It is highly lipophilic with a high affinity for opioid receptors and a subsequent slow dissociation from the receptor site, which may explain its relatively prolonged duration of analgesic effect (6–8 hours) and lack of severe abstinence effects when the drug is abruptly withdrawn (Heel et al. 1979; Bullingham et al. 1980). The high affinity of buprenorphine to opioid receptors decreases the efficacy of concomitantly administered opioid antagonists (Gal 1989). If respiratory depression occurs with this compound, large doses of naloxone may be necessary to reverse it, and central nervous system stimulants may be indicated.

Like other mixed agonists-antagonists, buprenorphine has a ceiling effect both for respiratory depression and analgesia (McQuay et al. 1979; Sekar and Mimpriss 1987). In the United States it is available only in parenteral preparation; sublingual preparations are available in other countries (Houde 1979). The pharmacokinetics of buprenorphine are unchanged in renal failure (Bullingham et al. 1982). To date buprenorphine plays a minor role in the management of sickle pain.

Agonists-antagonists

Pentazocine, nalbuphine, and butorphanol. These drugs play a minor role in the management of sickle pain. Their pharmacology is characterized by a ceiling effect for analgesia and the ability to precipitate withdrawal in patients who are physically dependent on opioid analgesics. All these drugs are available in parenteral preparations. Only pentazocine is available in oral preparations in the United States. These oral formulations combine pentazocine with naloxone or a nonopioid analgesic. Pentazocine is contraindicated in patients with cardiac dysfunction due to potential for increased blood pressure and tachycardia (Lee et al. 1976; Schmucker et al. 1980). Although abuse potential is low, pentazocine can cause physical dependence and addiction. Nalbuphine can also be used to reverse certain physiologic effects of μ agonists such as pruritus and sedation, while still maintaining analgesia (Latasch et al. 1984; Moldenhauer et al. 1985). Butorphanol is now available in intranasal preparation, which is effective for postoperative pain.

ADJUVANTS TO ANALGESICS

By definition, an adjuvant is a substance administered in conjunction with a prescription drug to enhance the effect of the principal ingredient. The usual primary indication for an adjuvant is to treat symptoms other than pain. Nevertheless, as a secondary effect adjuvants confer analgesia in some painful conditions. Although both NSAIDs and opioids control pain when used appropriately, they may induce the production of new symptoms or exacerbate preexisting symptoms such as pruritus, nausea, and sedation (Foley 1985). The combination of an adjuvant with a primary analgesic drug can potentiate the affect of the main analgesic and, often, ameliorate some of its undesirable side effects. The combination of severe sickle cell pain with anxiety, depression, pruritus, and other symptoms constitutes an indication for the use of adjuvants in the management of the various sickle cell pain syndromes. An adjuvant may be combined with the primary analgesic in any of the steps of the analgesic ladder.

To be used in the management of sickle cell pain, an adjuvant drug should meet at least one of the following criteria: (1) increase the analgesic effect of opioids (adjuvant analgesic); (2) reduce the toxicity associated with the use of the main analgesic drug (e.g., nausea or pruritus); and (3) improve other symptoms associated with sickle cell painful episodes, such as anxiety. To achieve their maximal desired effect, adjuvants are often given with the main drug at the initiation of treatment and before the side effects of the primary analgesic drug manifest.

The use of adjuvant drugs in the management of sickle cell pain entails the understanding of certain issues that are associated with this approach to therapy. First, no controlled studies have determined the efficacy of adjuvant analgesics in sickle cell pain; most of the evidence is anecdotal. Second, adjuvant drugs are often used for accepted but unapproved indications. The parenteral use of diphenhydramine (Benadryl), for example, is an accepted practice in treating sickle cell pain although it is not approved by the FDA for this purpose (Ballas 1995a). Third, both the provider and the patient must understand that the use of adjuvants is empirical and they must know the side effects of the adjuvant in question. Moreover, the provider must know the primary indications of the adjuvant, its pharmacokinetics, potential for serious side effects, its interactions with other drugs, and dosing guidelines for pain. Fourth, as is the case with opioid analgesics, there is great variability in response to adjuvants among patients and in the same patient over time. The experience of a certain patient with an adjuvant does not predict the outcome of a therapeutic trial in other patients or in the same patient at a different time. Accordingly, adjuvant drugs are often used on a trial and error basis.

Table XVII
Adjuvant drugs used in the treatment
of sickle cell pain

Commonly used adjuvants
Antihistamines
Hydroxyzine (Vistaril, Atarax)
Diphenhydramine (Benadryl)
Antiemetics
Benzodiazepines
Moderately used adjuvants
Laxatives
Muscle relaxants
Neuroleptics
Anticonvulsants
Antidepressants
Corticosteroids
Rarely used adjuvants
Analeptics
Alpha-2-adrenergic agents
Clonidine (Catapres)
GABA agonists
Baclofen (Lioresal)
Gabapentin (Neurontin)
Others

Table XVII lists the adjuvant analgesics used to treat sickle cell pain. They have been arbitrarily divided in three major classes according to their frequency of use (Ballas 1993; Shapiro 1993). These adjuvants are usually administered as coanalgesics in certain types of pain, to reduce or counteract the adverse effects of opioid analgesics, or to treat the psychological complications of pain syndromes. Adjuvant analgesics have been widely useful in cancer pain, and their role in the management of sickle pain needs further study.

COMMONLY USED ADJUVANTS

Antihistamines

The antihistamines most commonly used as adjuvants in treating sickle cell pain include hydroxyzine (Vistaril) and diphenhydramine (Benadryl). The former is a piperazine antihistamine and the latter, like other first generation antihistamines, is an H1-receptor antagonist. Single-dose studies of hydroxyzine, diphenhydramine, and other antihistamines have demonstrated their analgesic effect in cancer pain (Campos and Solis 1980; Hupert et al. 1980; Stambaugh and Lance 1983), but no similar studies were conducted in sickle pain. High doses of parenteral hydroxyzine can have an analgesic effect similar to several milligrams of morphine sulfate. The coanalgesic effect of hydroxyzine was evident in controlled trials when used parenterally in high doses with no evidence of analgesia from oral doses (Beaver 1984). Side effects of antihistamines include sedation and dry mouth. They seem to be most useful in patients whose pain is associated with anxiety, pruritus, or nausea. They can potentiate the sedating effects of opioids and, possibly, their analgesic effects.

Antiemetics

Hospitalized patients with acute sickle cell painful episodes often complain of nausea and vomiting. These symptoms may be manifestations of a painful crisis involving the gastrointestinal tract, side effects of opioid analgesics, or both. Opioids can cause nausea by stimulating the chemoreceptor trigger zone in the central nervous system. Opioid-induced constipation also can cause nausea with or without vomiting. Altered gastric emptying produces vomiting, preceded by mild or transient episodes of nausea. Gastric stasis caused by opioids and associated with reduced gastric emptying can result in large-volume vomiting in some patients.

In most hospitalized patients complaining of nausea the coadministration of the antihistamines mentioned above controls the problem. In some patients, nausea and vomiting may be severe and require the use of potent antiemetics such as prochlorperazine (Compazine), haloperidol (Haldol), metochlorpramide (Reglan), scopolamine, or ondansetron (Zofran). Ondansetron is highly selective and non-sedating, but expensive. Intractable nausea with or without vomiting may, occasionally, be seen in a pregnant patient with sickle cell anemia in association with acute painful episodes and the use of opioids during the first trimester. In general, nausea and vomiting in sickle cell disease are not as major a problem as in cancer pain.

Benodiazepines

The role of these medications (Table XVIII) in pain in general and in sickle cell disease is controversial. Nevertheless, many of these agents are commonly used by many providers and liked by many patients. Although benzodiazepines have no analgesic or coanalgesic effects, they have other properties that may be useful in certain clinical situations and in selected patients. The ones commonly used in sickle cell disease include alprazolam (Xanax), diazepam (Valium), flurazepam (Dalmane), and temazepam (Restoril).

Table XVIII
Clinical pharmacology of commonly used benzodziazepines

Brand Name	Generic Name	Half-life (h)	Daily Dose (mg)	Time to Peak Plasma Level (h)
Ativan	Lorazepam	15	1.5–6	1–6
Dalmane	Flurazepam	72	15–30	0.5–1
Halcion	Triazolam	3	0.125–0.5	0.5–2
Klonopin	Clonazepam	34	0.5–3	1–2
Librium	Chlordiazepoxide	18	15–60	0.5–4
Restoril	Temazepam	11	7.5–30	2–4
Serax	Oxazapam	8	30–60	2–4
Traxane	Clorazepate	65	7.5–15	1–2
Valium	Diazepam	60	4–40	0.5–2
Xanax	Alprazolam	12	0.25–4	1–2

Flurazepam (Dalmane) and temazepam (Restoril) are often used to treat insomnia, primarily in the outpatient setting. Alprazolam (Xanax) and diazepam (Valium) are useful in the management of recurrent or stuttering priapism in combination with analgesics (Dorn 1983). Diazepam is useful in the treatment of anxiety that accompanies the early stages of acute painful episodes, as an adjunct in seizure disorders, in controlling opioid-induced myoclonus, and relieving muscle spasm (Singh et al. 1981; Stimmel 1983; Portenoy 1993). Clonazepam (Klonopin) is sometimes used for seizure disorders in sickle cell disease, and lorazepam (Ativan) for the short-term relief of symptoms of acute anxiety or panic attacks in hospitalized patients with sickle cell disease.

Major side effects of benzodiazepines include the potentiation of the sedating effects of opioid analgesics. Alprazolam (Xanax) may induce episodes of mania, hypomania, hostility, anger, and suicidal ideation (Drug Fact and Comparisons 1997).

MODERATELY USED ADJUVANTS

Laxatives

Contrary to expectations, constipation does not seem to be a major problem in patients with sickle cell disease despite the chronic use of opioid analgesics. Unlike patients with cancer pain who receive around-the-clock laxatives when treated with opioid analgesics, hospitalized patients with sickle pain usually take laxatives as needed (p.r.n.) (Ballas 1995a). The laxatives commonly used include: (1) saline laxatives such as milk of magnesia, citrate of magnesia, and fleet phosphosoda; (2) fecal softeners such as docusate sodium (Colace); and 3) stimulant laxatives such as senna (Senokot) and bisacodyl (Dulcolax). An occasional hospitalized patient may experience severe constipation with secondary nausea and vomiting and may require disimpaction and repeated enemas until clear. A few patients with sickle cell disease who take opioids frequently as outpatients may take laxatives on a chronic basis.

Muscle relaxants

These centrally acting compounds are marketed either singly or in combination with other agents such as acetaminophen or aspirin. With the exception of diazepam (Valium), these agents are rarely used in the management of sickle cell pain. A few outpatients may occasionally require the use of cyclobenzaprine (Flexeril), which is effective for short periods not exceeding three weeks. It loses its effectiveness if used longer. Carisoprodol is a congener of meprobamate and has a high addictive potential, especially if used in conjunction with alcohol, central nervous system depressants, or psychotropic drugs.

Neuroleptics

Neuroleptics used to manage pain are listed in Table XIX. The role of these compounds in the management of sickle pain is unknown and is limited in the management of cancer pain. Only methotrimeprazine, used parenterally, can produce analgesia comparable to morphine in nontolerant patients (Lasagna and DeKornfeldt 1961; Montilla et al. 1963; Beaver et al. 1966; Oliver 1985). Because it exerts its effect via α-adrenergic blockade, a mechanism different than that of opioids, methotrimeprazine has a potential analgesic role in both opioid-tolerant and intolerant patients in addition to its potent antiemetic effect (Breitbart and Hollant 1990). The phenothiazines,

Table XIX
Neuroleptics used in pain management

Class	Trade Name	Generic Name
Phenothiazines	Chlorpromazine	Thorazine
	Fluphenazine	Prolixin, permitil
	Methotrimeprazine	Levoprome
	Perphenazine	Trilafon
	Prochlorperazine	Compazine
	Thioridazine	Mellaril
	Trifluperazine	Stelazine
Thioxanthenes	Chlorprothixene	Taractan
Butyrophenone	Haloperidol	Haldol

Table XX
Side effects of neuroleptics

Desirable side effects
Sedation (in some patients)
Antiemesis
Potentiation of analgesic effect of opioids

Undesirable side effects
Sedation (in some patients)
Dystonia
Tardive dyskinesia
Akathisia
Neuroleptic malignant syndrome
Orthostatic hypotension and dizziness
Anticholinergic effects

which are often used in patients with sickle pain, include prochlorperazine (Compazine) and haloperidol (Haldol). Both can be used as antiemetics. Haloperidol may also be useful in the management of patients with severe agitation and hyperexcitability.

The side effects of neuroleptics are substantial (Table XX). Some are desirable, such as the potentiation of the analgesic effect of opioids and anti-emesis. Sedation may be desirable in some patients but not in others, depending on the clinical situation. Extrapyramidal effects (pseudoparkinsonism) include mask facies, tardive dyskinesia, festinating gait, and pill-rolling tremor. Tardive dyskinesia is characterized by involuntary oral, buccal, or facial movement, lip smacking, and tongue arresting. Akathisia (Meradante 1995) is characterized by severe and tense restlessness that may be reduced by ambulation and moving around. It may occur with the use of haloperidol or fluphenazine. Neuroleptic malignant syndrome (NMS) is a rare complication characterized by extrapyramidal effects, hyperthermia, and autonomic abnormalities. It is most commonly associated with haloperidol (Haldol) and fluphenazine (Prolixin, Permitil), but may occur with other neuroleptics. Onset varies from hours to months after the initiation of drug therapy, but once started it escalates rapidly within one to three days. NMS is potentially fatal. Its management includes immediate discontinuation of the neuroleptic in question, and aggressive and intensive symptomatic therapy. Dantrolene may be beneficial in controlling NMS in some patients.

Anticonvulsants

Anticonvulsants are often used in patients with sickle cell disease, not as adjuvant analgesics per se but to treat seizure disorders that may complicate the clinical picture of sickle cell disease (Greer and Schotlend 1962; Portnoy and Herion 1972; Sarjeant 1992). In a retrospective study Liu et al (1994) reported that seizure occurred in 21 of 152 patients (14%) with sickle cell disease. Meperidine-associated seizures were estimated to occur in about 7% of the patients treated with meperidine, which is greater than the nearly 1% to 3% reported in other hospitalized patients (Miller and Jick 1978; Kaiko 1983). The reported incidence of seizures in patients with sickle cell disease related to the use of meperidine varied between 1% and 12% (Targ et al. 1980; Liu et al. 1994; Nadvi et al. 1995). About 12% of patients with sickle cell disease seem to have seizure disorder not related to meperidine use but to the disease itself (Liu et al 1994).

The anticonvulsants most commonly used in sickle cell disease include phenytoin (Dilantin), 100 to 200 mg orally t.i.d., and carbamazepine (Tegretol), 200 mg orally b.i.d to q.i.d. The serum level of these agents can be measured and the dose adjusted to achieve therapeutic levels. Side effects of phenytoin include gingival hyperplasia, hirsutism, somnolence, mental clouding, diplopia, dizziness, lymphadenopathy, maculopapular rash, ataxia, and megaloblastic anemia (Ramsay et al. 1983). The last complication is unlikely to occur in patients with sickle cell disease provided they take folic acid daily.

Side effects of carbamazepine include sedation, ataxia, confusion, leukopenia, and thrombocytopenia (Hart and Easton 1982). Aplastic anemia and hepatotoxicity are rare complications of carbamazepine therapy (Flegel and Cole 1977; Hart and Easton 1982). Liver function tests and routine blood counts should be periodically checked in patients taking anticonvulsants. An anecdotal report indicates that carbamazepine is effective in the management of neuropathic pain complicating sickle cell disease (Asher 1980).

Antidepressants

Further studies are needed to determine the role, if any, of antidepressants (Table XXI) in the management of sickle cell pain. Anecdotes of the beneficial effect of amitriptyline (Elavil) in sickle pain have been reported (Ballas et al. 1995b). Sinequan (Doxepin) may be useful as a coanalgesic in the patient with insomnia. Imipramine has beneficial effects in children with enuresis.

However, care should be exerted in the use of antidepressants in sickle cell disease. Some side effects such as priapism, seizure disorders, and urine retention are also complications of sickle cell disease. Antidepressants may be contraindicated for patients with a history of these complications or should be used with caution and frequent monitoring.

The role of selective serotonin reuptake inhibitors (SSRIs) in the comprehensive management of sickle cell pain is unknown. The risk/benefit

Table XXI
Antidepressants commonly used as adjuvants

Class	Generic Name	Brand Name
Tricyclics	Amitriptyline	Elavil
	Desipramine	Norpramin
	Doxepin	Sinequan
	Imipramine	Tofranil
	Nortriptyline	Pamelor
SSRIs	Fluoxamine	Luvox
	Fluoxetine	Prozac
	Paroxetine	Pexil
	Sertraline	Zoloft
Atypical	Bupropion	Wellbutrin
	Trazodone	Desyrel
	Venlafaxine	Effexor
MAOIs	Phenelzine	Nardil
	Tranylcypromine	Parnate

Abbreviations: SSRIs = selective serotonin
reuptake inhibitors; MAOIs = monoamine
oxidase inhibitors.

ratio, side effects, and interaction with other medications must be considered in this patient population, and safety is a major issue. One possible mechanism by which SSRIs contribute to tissue damage in patients with sickle cell disease is vasoconstriction. Although serotonin has a vasodilatory effect on normal arteries, it produces vasoconstriction in damaged endothelium (Golino et al. 1991; McFadden et al. 1991). It is possible that SSRIs might enhance vasoconstriction by increasing the availability of serotonin at damaged sites (Sheline et al. 1997).

Corticosteroids

The role of corticosteroids in sickle pain is unknown and, to some extent, controversial. Because many of the features of acute sickle cell painful episode have an inflammatory component, we would expect that corticosteroids, known to have anti-inflammatory effects, may be of value in pain management. Patients with active avascular necrosis of a large joint, for example, may experience pain relief after the intra-articular injection of corticosteroids. Griffin et al. (1994) conducted a placebo-controlled, double-blind study of the effects of intravenous methylprednisolone in children and adolescents with sickle cell disease who were hospitalized with severe pain. They found that a short course of high-dose methylprednisolone decreased the duration of severe pain. The patients who received methylprednisolone, however, had more rebound affects after therapy was discontinued than did the placebo group. Haung et al. (1994), however, reported two adult patients with sickle cell disease whose clinical picture deteriorated and experienced worse pain after the administration of corticosteroids. Although the use of methylprednisolone in children seems to be promising, further trials are needed to elucidate its role in sickle pain.

RARELY USED ADJUVANTS

Analeptics

These psychostimulants include methylphenidate (Ritalin), dextro-amphetamine, and caffeine. Single-dose studies of these drugs showed that they have analgesic effects (Forrest et al. 1977; Cantello et al. 1988; Laska et al. 1984). The administration of oral methylphenidate to patients with advanced cancer improved analgesia and reversed opioid-induced sedation (Bruera et al. 1987). By analogy, it is possible that methylphenidate may have the same effects in patients with severe sickle pain who are heavily sedated.

Alpha-2-adrenergic agonists

Clonidine (Catapres) is the prototype of this group of compounds with antinociceptive effect (Quan and Wendres 1993). It is marketed in oral and transdermal forms. Sedation and hypotension are major side effects. The combined use of controlled-release agonists and transdermal clonidine have been implicated in precipitating fatal acute chest syndrome in two patients with sickle cell anemia (Ballas 1994a).

GABA agonists

Baclofen (Lioresal) is the prototype of this group of compounds. Because of its reported efficacy in trigeminal neuralgia it has been used to treat lancinating neuropathic pain (Fromm et al. 1984; Fromm 1989). It can also be useful in ameliorating the symptoms of spasticity. Patients with sickle cell disease and residual spasticity following cerebrovascular accidents may benefit from Baclofen. Sedation and confusion are its major side effects.

Gabapentin (Neurontin) is structurally related to the neurotransmitter GABA but it does not interact with GABA receptors. It is a GABAergic anticonvulsant with strong anecdotal support for analgesic efficacy when used for neuropathic pain.

ILLUSTRATIVE CASES

CASE 9.1

During one of her hospital admissions, a 41-year-old African American woman with Hb SC disease received meperidine 100 mg i.m. every two hours and ibuprofen 400 mg p.o. every six hours for acute sickle cell pain. This regimen achieved adequate pain relief. Her biochemical profile on admission was within normal limits (Table XXII) and examination of the urine showed +1 proteinuria. About three weeks after starting ibuprofen she developed diffuse erythematous maculopapular rash and severe itching. At the same time her serum albumin decreased, serum cholesterol, creatinine, and blood urea nitrogen increased, and she developed 3+ proteinuria. Sickle nephropathy, systemic lupus erythematosus, systemic vasculitis, and drug reaction were considered as possible causes. The combination of nephrotic syndrome and rash favored a collagen disease. Kidney biopsy showed tubulointerstitial nephritis with reactive glomerular changes consistent with abnormalities described with NSAIDs. Ibuprofen was discontinued. The rash resolved within a few days and her renal function gradually returned to baseline values. The patient was instructed not to take any NSAIDs in the future.

Table XXII
Renal function of the patient described in case 9.1
before and after treatment with ibuprofen

	Serum				
Time	Albumin (g/dl)	Cholesterol (mg/dl)	Cr (mg/dl)	BUN (mg/dl)	Urine Protein
Before ibuprofen					
Baseline	4.4	168	0.9	9	1+
-3 days (admission)	4.1	179	0.9	9	1+
After starting ibuprofen					
21 days	2.8	247	1.8	ND	>300
22 days	2.3	ND	2.0	29	ND
23 days	1.9	ND	2.4	37	3+ *
After discontinuing ibuprofen					
1 week	1.9	ND	1.3	7	ND
3 weeks	3.1	388	1.0	ND	3+
7 weeks	3.2	241	0.9	6	3+
3 months	3.9	209	0.9	8	2+
6 months	4.1	188	0.9	8	1+

Abbreviations: Cr, creatinine; BUN, blood urea nitrogen; ND, not done.
*The 24-hour urine protein was 17,056 mg at this time (not measured at other times).

Comments on Case 9.1

Nephropathy is one of the side effects of NSAIDs. This patient developed mild renal failure associated with nephrotic syndrome about three weeks after starting ibuprofen. She also developed skin rash as a side effect of ibuprofen. The combination of skin rash and renal failure suggested a systemic disease such as lupus erythematosus in addition to her sickle cell disease. Kidney biopsy clarified the etiology, and discontinuation of ibuprofen resolved the complications. Noteworthy is that the skin rash resolved first after the discontinuation of ibuprofen but it took about six months for the proteinuria to decrease to baseline values. Moreover, this patient received meperidine 100 mg i.m. every two hours during her entire 41-day hospitalization, with no apparent neurological side effects of this opioid.

CASE 9.2

Fig. 2 shows an ulcer in the right thigh of a 33-year-old African American man with sickle cell anemia. The ulcer was secondary to sloughing of the skin following the inadvertent subcutaneous injection of 125 mg of meperidine during treatment in the emergency department. Meperidine may be given orally, intravenously, or intramuscularly, but not subcutaneously.

CASE 9.3

Fig. 3 shows skin abrasion complicated by infection and abscess formation over the left forearm of a 21-year-old African American man with sickle cell anemia. The abrasion was due to severe itching secondary to morphine sulfate.

CASE 9.4

A 22-year-old African American woman with sickle cell anemia was given meperidine 100 mg i.m./i.v. every two hours during one of her hospital admissions for the management of a severe acute painful episode. After three days of this regimen, 10 mg of prochlorperazine (Compazine) i.m./p.o. every six hours was added for nausea and vomiting. After receiving three doses of prochlorperazine she experienced a weird and scary feeling in her face. She said that she felt as if someone was pulling her jaw and part of her face out of her body, and that her face was jumping, contracting, and pulling involuntarily. She also lost control of her face, which turned to the right uncontrollably. She had numbness and tingling over her face but no pain, burning, or itching. She was restless and anxious. Thorough neurological

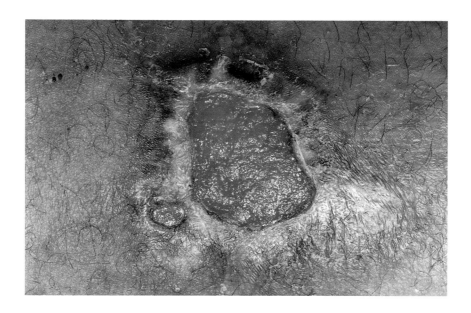

Fig. 2. An ulcer over the right thigh secondary to skin sloughing due to the subcutaneous administration of meperidine.

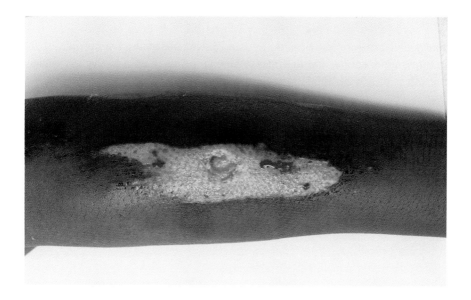

Fig. 3. An abscess over the left forearm complicating skin abrasion due to intense itching caused by morphine sulfate.

work-up including neurological examination, EEG, and CAT scan of the head showed no abnormalities. Meperidine and prochlorperazine were discontinued and she was given diazepam (Valium) 2 mg i.v. The signs and symptoms of this bizarre episode disappeared within a few hours. Meperidine was replaced with hydromorphone. On further questioning she indicated that in the past she had experienced a similar episode of unusual symptoms where she lost control of her tongue and felt as if she was swallowing it. She was advised never to take prochlorperazine and other phenothiazines, especially while receiving opioids in general and meperidine in particular. She was also advised to avoid meperidine and to use morphine or hydromorphone to manage her acute sickle cell pain.

Comments on Case 9.4

The bizarre signs and symptoms experienced by this patient suggest akathisia due to the combined administration of an opioid and a phenothiazine. Akathisia is a distressing extrapyramidal disorder characterized by restlessness, a compulsion to move, a feeling of inner tension, myoclonus, tremor, and rigidity. It may occur after treatment with drugs that possess an antidopaminergic activity, including opioids and phenothiazines. The combination of the last two classes of drugs increases the chances and severity of its occurrence. The patient described above received meperidine alone on several occasions in the past with no problems. Only when prochlorperazine was given concomitantly with meperidine did she develop akathisia. It is likely that prochlorperazine alone could have caused the occurrence of the extrapyramidal signs and that meperidine contributed an additive or enhancing effect of this complication.

10

Pharmacologic Management
of the Patient with Sickle Cell Pain

Pleasure is nothing else but the intermission of pain.
—John Selden, 1584–1654

For all the happiness man can gain
Is not in pleasure, but in rest from pain.
—John Dryden, 1631–1700

Several controversies surround the pharmacologic treatment of sickle cell pain. Exceptions to the rules established to treat cancer pain and post-operative pain abound when these rules are applied to sickle cell pain. For example, meperidine rather than morphine is the opioid analgesic most frequently used to treat acute sickle cell pain (Ballas et al. 1995a), and oral opioid analgesics are rarely used as the sole modality to manage acute painful episodes in the emergency department or the hospital. These exceptions may reflect the unique nature of sickle cell pain and suggest the need to establish specific management guidelines. The disease process and genetic background of the patients with sickle cell disease may play important roles in the pharmacokinetics of opioid analgesics and contribute to the apparent disparity with other groups of patients in response to treatment. This chapter will review current knowledge about the pharmacologic management of sickle cell pain and define areas that need further research and development.

PAIN ASSESSMENT

PAIN ASSESSMENT IN ADULTS

Prior to treating a painful episode, the clinician should evaluate the patient for other medical problems that could cause or complicate the pain and should assess psychosocial status. Patients with sickle cell disease experience a variety of painful medical problems, some related to and others unrelated to the underlying disease. The most prevalent problems include acute infections, cholelithiasis, osteonecrosis, delayed transfusion reactions, headaches, and abdominal emergencies (Milner and Squires 1987; Serjeant 1992). Evaluation encompasses a clinically directed search for medical problems and includes history, physical examination, and appropriate laboratory studies. Patients often can differentiate their usual vaso-occlusive pain from pain caused by other medical processes.

Pain has sensory and affective dimensions. Assessment of these dimensions is a critical initial step in the successful management of pain. These two dimensions account for most of the heterogeneity in self-reports of pain among patients and in the same patient during different painful episodes. Failure to relieve a patient's pain may result from lack of proper assessment of the patient's perception of pain and the failure to monitor the results of therapy (American Pain Society 1993). A comprehensive protocol for assessing pain in adults with sickle cell disease should include the following components (Shapiro 1993, 1997).

An objective tool for self-assessment of pain and activity

A *verbal pain scale* (0 = no pain, 10 = worst pain imaginable) should be employed during periods of acute pain when patients may be unable or unwilling to give a written response. Verbal responses are most useful in the emergency department or during the initial day of hospitalization and aid in determining analgesic efficacy during titrated loading doses of medication. Several studies have used a *written assessment of pain*, e.g., a visual analog scale (VAS), to examine pain relief in sickle cell disease (Walco and Dampier 1990; Ballas and Delengowski 1993). These reports confirm that patients continue to have moderate pain at the time of discharge and suggest that they continue to cope with pain as outpatients. Moreover, a daily diary noting activity, medication use, and presence or absence of pain provides information regarding the ability of patients to cope with pain as outpatients (Gill 1989).

Other single-dimension self-report measures

These measures include pain relief scale, mood scale, and sedation scale (Fig. 1). For the pain relief scale patients indicate the amount of relief (0–100%) from pain at the time of assessment compared to the previous day or to their first day of hospitalization. For the mood scale patients circle a number from 0 (worst mood) to 10 (best mood) that indicates mood at the time of assessment. The examiner also grades sedation on a scale from

Patient Name: _____   Patient ID#: _____

PAIN ASSESSMENT FORM
VISUAL ANALOG NUMERICAL SCALES

Date: _____   Time: _____

1. Please Circle The Number That Best Describes Your **Pain**.

| 0 | 1 | 2 | 3 | 4 | 5 | 6 | 7 | 8 | 9 | 10 |

No Pain   Worst Possible Pain

2. Please Circle The Number That Best Describes Your **Relief** Of Pain.

| 0 | 1 | 2 | 3 | 4 | 5 | 6 | 7 | 8 | 9 | 10 |

No Relief   Complete Relief

3. Please Circle The Number That Best Describes Your **Mood**.

| 0 | 1 | 2 | 3 | 4 | 5 | 6 | 7 | 8 | 9 | 10 |

Worst Mood   Best Mood

4. Please Circle The Number That Best Describes How **Drowsy** You Feel.

| 0 | 1 | 2 | 3 | 4 | 5 | 6 | 7 | 8 | 9 | 10 |

Not Drowsy   Asleep

PAINFUL SITES
5. Shade the figure where you feel pain.
6. Mark an X where you hurt most.

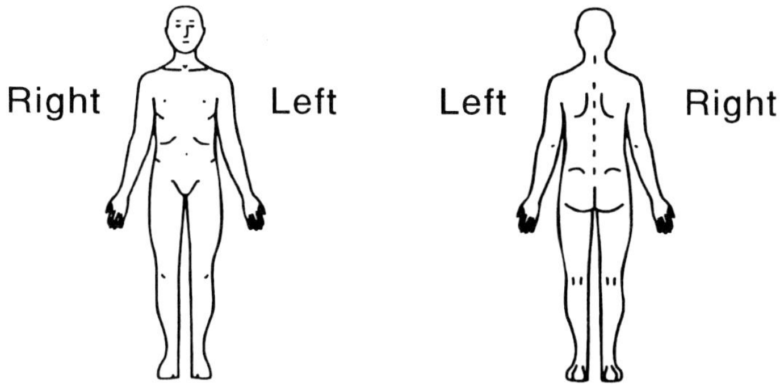

Right   Left   Left   Right

Observer: (MD/RN)
Initials:_____

Fig. 1. Pain assessment tool (adapted from American Pain Society 1993 and Jacox et al. 1994).

0 (fully awake) to 10 (deep sleep). Patients are also asked to give a verbal description of their pain and to indicate whether the pain is similar to their usual crisis pain. Pain that is not typical of crisis is a signal to conduct a thorough search for other causes.

Location of pain

The spatial distribution of pain is documented by asking the patient to mark the area of pain on a scaled drawing of the body. Fig. 1 represents a scheme where single-dimension self-report measures and the location of pain are documented at least once per day.

An objective assessment of coping strategies

Coping strategies should be assessed through structured interview techniques or a standard questionnaire (e.g., Coping Strategies Inventory; Tobin et al. 1989). These assessments are best performed in an outpatient setting rather than during hospitalization for a concurrent crisis.

Social and environmental factors that may influence the pain experience

Sickle cell disease affects the entire family. A multidisciplinary approach to pain management should assess the role of the spouse and other family members in the patient's response to treatment and their understanding of the pain and its management (Shapiro 1993, 1997). Factors for assessment include marital satisfaction, satisfaction with social support elements, performance at school or work, and participation in activities of daily living and social interactions. As with assessing coping strategies, examination of social and environmental factors should occur during pain-free interludes. The health care system itself should also be assessed, especially in difficult pain problems (Shapiro 1997). This aspect of assessment is often neglected. Such assessment should systematically review the entire network treating the patient, including physicians, nurses, and social workers (Shapiro 1997). This approach reinforces the mutual responsibilities inherent in doctor-patient relationships. Case 13.2 in Chapter 13 is an example wherein assessment of the health care system led to resolution of a difficult pain problem.

Indices of health care utilization

Patients with a high-risk behavior for frequent use of medical services should be identified. Patterns of high-risk behavior include increasing medication usage, failure in school or employment, increasing hospitalizations, and adversarial relationships with health care providers (Shapiro 1993). The frequency of painful episodes, number of emergency department visits, frequency and duration of hospitalizations, and need for analgesic medication also should be assessed.

Assessment of pain behavior

In an effort to find a tool to assess pain behavior during episodes of sickle cell pain, Gil et al. (1994) examined the utility of a brief behavioral observation method to quantify pain behavior among outpatients. They tested the method on 31 patients with sickle cell disease first seen in the clinic for a painful crisis. The methods used included observed pain behaviors, physician rating of patient pain on a 0 to 10 scale, patient rating of pain on a 0 to 10 scale, and patient pain report from the McGill Pain Questionnaire. Their data showed high reliability among raters for the brief behavioral observation, and the observed pain behavior correlated significantly with the physician ratings of pain. Although preliminary, this study suggests that a brief and reliable tool could be used in the outpatient clinic to assess and quantify sickle cell pain behavior. Such a tool is an important prerequisite to determine the efficacy of a therapeutic modality, especially the nonpharmacologic approach to treatment of sickle pain.

PAIN ASSESSMENT IN CHILDREN

Sickle cell pain in children represents an aversive stimulus that likely has a detrimental effect (Walco and Dampier 1990). Children deserve pain relief, but the assessment of sickle cell pain in children presents some unique challenges. Such pain occurs across the pediatric age group from infants to adolescents and can occur in many different parts of the body and in many different clinical contexts. The concomitant behaviors that these patients may display are likely to be age specific, as is their ability to provide meaningful self-reports of their pain experience (McGrath 1990; Shapiro et al. 1990; Weisman and Schechter 1992). The following review discusses pediatric patients in four age groups: adolescents (13–20 years), school-age children (6–12 years), preschool children (3–5 years), and infants (0–2 years).

Adolescents

Adolescents share many of the features of young adult patients. Several studies have shown the validity and reliability of a variety of self-reports of pain intensity, including typical visual analog scales (VAS) and verbal categorical scales of 0–10 or 1–100. Adolescents also use body diagrams appropriately to locate their pain. The ease of use of adjectives to describe a painful experience will likely depend on educational level. In general, most such scales for adolescents have selected a subset of words from adult questionnaires or have asked them to volunteer their own descriptors.

Little or no data exist on the type of pain behaviors typically displayed by adolescents during pain episodes. In general, they report engaging in less motor activity (e.g., sports and going to school) when in pain. The degree to which severe pain limits their ability to engage in daily living activities, or causes them to display typical pain behavior (grimacing, vocalization, guarding, etc.) varies with personality and coping styles, as it does in adult patients. Some adolescent patients may be particularly anxious about their pain experience, especially if their sickle cell disease previously had been less symptomatic. Other adolescents may engage in controlling types of behavior, which can be a particularly important issue at this stage of life. Some adolescents may become severely depressed as they begin to realize how much their pain and underlying disease may interfere with the lifestyle they desire. Thus, interpretation of an adolescent's self-report of pain and pain-related behavior will be assisted by understanding them as individuals and what the pain experience means in the context of their lives. Such enhanced understanding can be obtained with psychological testing using standardized methods.

School-age children

Pain assessment becomes complicated in this age group. The use of VAS and categorical scales with many intervals requires a concept of relative line length and other related elementary arithmetic concepts. These scales may not be useful for the younger children in this age group, but with appropriate explanations and practice, the older children can use them in a valid and reliable fashion. The use of words to describe pain characteristics also may be problematic for the younger children because of limited ability to read and a limited expressive vocabulary. To communicate with these younger children effectively, it is particularly important to understand what words or expressions are used at home to express levels of pain or discomfort.

Interpreting pain-related behavior in this age group is similarly difficult. Some older children may have issues similar to those of adolescent patients, while for the younger children fear and anxiety about the hospital experience itself may be a dominant feature. They may not want to report pain because they expect that doing so may lead to further venipuncture or intramuscular injections, procedures that may seem worse than their sickle cell pain because of the associated anxiety.

Preschool children

There have been no published studies of pain assessment of sickle cell pain in this age group. We must assume that tools developed to assess the intensity of postoperative or arthritis pain will be similarly valid for sickle cell pain. These tools consist of small-interval categorical scales (3–4 intervals), often with visual markers. One such scale uses poker chips to represent amounts of pain or "hurt," while another popular tool asks the child to use several different colored crayons to shade on a body outline the location of the pain and how much it hurts. Some of these tools may also be useful for the youngest school-age children. Some preschoolers may do better using a categorical scale based on a series of drawings of faces of ethnically appropriate infants with pain—the "oucher" scale. A methodologic difficulty of such scales is the inability to separate intensity from affective experience, but that may not be a clinically useful distinction in this age group. All these scales require considerable patience and understanding and a relatively cooperative subject. Assessment of pain-related behavior is difficult. Clinicians often must rely on the parents' judgment of how their child's behavior is different from their usual activity or temperament.

Infants

Assessment tools for pain unrelated to procedures are not available for this age group. Several observational scales have been documented for behavior associated with procedures such as heal lancing and immunizations, but their application to other pain states is doubtful. Similarly, acute changes in some physiologic variables such as heart rate and blood pressure may have some validity in these situations as indirect measures of the intensity of the infant's pain experience. Sickle cell pain in this age group typically involves the hands and or feet, so we often use motor ability in these areas (walking, weight bearing, gripping a bottle) as indirect measures of pain. Similarly, global changes in infant behavior as observed by a parent may have some validity.

OUTPATIENT MANAGEMENT OF SICKLE CELL PAIN

Management of patients with sickle cell disease in the outpatient clinic or office is the fulcrum on which the success of comprehensive care is balanced. Because they are not in severe acute pain, patients in the clinic are receptive to counseling, education, and reinforcement of good habits by nurses, technologists, social workers, and physicians. Ideally, patients should be followed by the same personnel to maintain continuity of care. The clinic or office is where the steady state of disease is defined clinically, hematologically, and biochemically, and where a multidisciplinary approach to care is maintained by regular checkups and appropriate consultations.

EDUCATION AND COUNSELING

Patients, parents, and other family members are instructed about what to expect from sickle cell syndromes by making them aware of the signs and symptoms of infection, including pain crises. The adoption of good health habits is reinforced, and the avoidance of situations and factors that could precipitate a painful crisis is encouraged. Parents are instructed to recognize the signs and symptoms of acute splenic sequestration, hand-foot syndrome, and signs of infection in infants. They are also taught how to measure temperature and administer medications.

MANAGEMENT OF PAIN AT HOME

Acute painful episodes. Table I lists the three major principles of treatment of acute painful episodes. Modification of the source of pain should include a thorough search for an infectious process that might have precipitated the crisis. Specific organ involvement should be systematically evaluated. Patients are the best authority on their pain. If the pain they describe is not typical of their usual crises, then other causes should be sought. If the initial evaluation reveals an uncomplicated painful episode, proper assessment of the pain should ensue. The aim of treatment should be to interrupt the transmission of painful stimuli along peripheral fibers and to alter the perception of pain in the central nervous system (Table I). Providers usually consider visits to the emergency department or hospitalization an indicator of significant painful episodes. Most painful episodes, however, especially in children and adolescents, are managed at home (Shapiro et al. 1995). Visits to the clinic, emergency department, or hospital seem to be determined by numerous factors besides pain severity, such as hospital experience, availability of oral medications, family support, and psychosocial factors.

Treatment of acute painful episodes at home is empiric and depends on the severity of pain and the presence or absence of complications of the disease. Painful episodes of mild severity ideally are treated at home with nonpharmacologic measures including bed rest, hydration, massage, relax-

Table I
Principles of treatment of acute painful episodes

Principle	Method of Treatment
Modify the source of pain	Treat precipitating factors (e.g., infection) if identified. Bed rest and local measures such as heating pad may be helpful
Interrupt the transmission of painful stimuli along nociceptors	Anti-inflammatory agents; salicylates, acetaminophen, and other NSAIDs
Alter the perception of pain at the CNS level	Narcotic analgesics, biofeedback, self-hypnosis

Source: Adapted from Ballas 1995a with permission.

ation, diversion, heating pads, tub baths, self-hypnosis, and motivation. Patients often sense an impeding painful crisis, and early treatment with analgesics may abort or ameliorate an evolving episode. Home treatment of pain should follow the three-step analgesic ladder (Table II) proposed by the World Health Organization (1986). This approach involves the use of analgesics in escalating potency. These medications are given alone or in combination, initially on an "as needed" followed by an "around the clock" administration for moderate to severe pain. This model controls pain in 90% of cancer patients (Jacox et al. 1994).

Chronic Pain Syndromes. Chronic pain associated with sickle cell disease includes arthropathies, aseptic necrosis, vertebral body collapse, and leg ulcers (see Chapter 6). Moreover, some patients almost always experience crisis pain. These chronic pain syndromes may be treated with one of the weak or strong opioids, depending on the severity of pain. A long-acting opioid such as methadone or oral controlled-release morphine (MS Contin, Oramorph) or oxycodone (Oxycontin) is ideal for chronic pain (Khojasteh et al. 1987; Jaffe and Martin 1990). The use of TENS may be of value in reducing the pain intensity of these syndromes, especially if associated with

Table II
Pharmacologic home management of sickle
pain using the WHO three-step analgesic ladder

Step I: Mild Pain
Nonopioid ± adjuvant

Step II: Moderate Pain
Weak opioid ± nonopioid ± adjuvant

Step III: Severe Pain
Strong opioid ± nonopioid ± adjuvant

leg ulcers. The use of fentanyl transdermal patches also are of potential value (Rowbotham et al. 1989; Payne 1992). Fever and the application of heating pads over these patches increase the absorption of fentanyl through the skin and may lead to the accumulation of toxic plasma levels.

Issues pertinent to the outpatient management of sickle cell pain

Choice and amount of analgesics. Failure to prescribe opioids for home use may cause the patient unnecessary hardships and suffering and prompt more emergency department visits, because the frequency and severity of crises are unpredictable (Charache 1981; Melzack 1990). Moreover, if not treated promptly, crises of mild to moderate severity may progress to severe pain because of the associated fear, panic, and stress. Detailed records of the number of tablets prescribed should be kept in the patient's file. It is advisable to give patients prescriptions for nonopioid, opioid, and adjuvant medications so that the patient may follow the analgesic ladder described in managing pain at home. Patients who suffer from chronic pain syndromes and frequent attacks of acute pain may need prescriptions for both long-acting and short-acting opioids. Patients should have sufficient medications to last at least one week. Frequent prescriptions for a limited amount of opioids are preferable to infrequent prescriptions for large amounts.

Brand-name vs. generic analgesics. Brand-name analgesics are more expensive than generic ones, but many patients with sickle cell disease indicate that the latter are not as effective. In many cases, increasing the amount of the generic opioid may solve the problem. In some patients, however, generic preparations cause severe nausea, vomiting, rash, or itching. Prescribing antiemetics and antihistamines may alleviate these side effects in some patients. A few patients may need the brand-name drug to achieve pain relief with no adverse effects.

Differences in the efficacy between brand-name and generic analgesics may pertain to therapeutic equivalence formulations. Specifically, drug products are considered pharmaceutically equivalent if they contain the same active ingredient(s), are of the same dosage form, and are identical in strength or concentration and route of administration (Drug Information for the Health Care Professional 1992). Pharmaceutically equivalent drugs, however, differ in characteristics such as shape, packaging, color, flavor, preservatives, expiration date, and, within certain limits, labeling. Thus, although preparations X and Y may contain the same amount of oxycodone, a patient may experience severe pruritus, nausea, or vomiting with one preparation but not the other due to sensitivity to the excipients (coloring agents, flavors, or additives) specific to that preparation.

Prescription refills. Given the unpredictable nature of painful episodes, patients with sickle cell disease may consume the prescribed opioids before their next clinic or office appointment. Consequently, they often call their provider to supply them with new prescriptions for a specific type and amount of opioid. Unfortunately, some providers overestimate the prevalence of addiction in patients with sickle cell disease (Shapiro et al. 1997) and stereotype such callers as abusers showing drug-seeking behavior. In such situations, a provider who knows the patient and who has experience in pain medicine and sickle cell disease should handle the phone request. If the conversation reveals that the patient's complaints are typical of the usual pain, then a prescription for enough opioid to last until the next visit is justified. If the conversation indicates that the patient has fever, shortness of breath, new severe headache, or weakness, then arrangements must be made to examine the patient either in the office or in the emergency department.

Hoarding and hopping. These actions may be signs of inadequate pain management of outpatients. Patients often hoard pain medications at home in case painful episodes occur unexpectedly at night, during bad weather, or times of financial hardship. Hoarding is practiced more frequently by patients who have experienced past difficulty in obtaining analgesics from their providers. Some providers consider hoarding a sign of maladaptive behavior even though many people hoard food whenever there is a forecast of a snow storm or bad weather, and even though hoarding is instinctive and widespread in the animal kingdom (e.g., storing food for the winter). Hopping from clinic to clinic may also be a sign of inadequate pain management associated with prescribing less analgesics than the patient needs. By seeking several prescriptions each for a limited amount of opioids, patients feel satisfied in securing the actual amount they need based on their past experience.

Route of administration. Most patients with sickle cell disease treat their pain at home with oral analgesics. The rectal route is rarely used. The transdermal use of fentanyl may be of potential value in patients with chronic pain syndromes. A few patients have learned to give themselves intramuscular opioid analgesics. In general, this approach should be avoided but may be considered in selected patients with adequate family and psychosocial support. Selected patients may be able to use patient-controlled analgesia (PCA) at home (O. Castro, personal communication). Its advantages include fewer visits to the emergency department and fewer hospitalizations. These new approaches to the home management of sickle pain need properly conducted controlled trials.

Chronic use of opioid analgesics. Treatment of chronic pain syndromes with opioids necessitates the long-term use of these agents, which traditionally has been discouraged because of the fear the patient would develop tolerance, physical dependence, and addiction. Fear of addiction has adversely limited the rational use of opioids in patients with sickle cell disease (Shapiro et al. 1997; Payne 1997), even though few patients receiving opioid analgesics for medical reasons develop psychological dependence or addiction (Levine 1984). Chronic treatment with opioids has become standard therapy for patients with cancer pain (Saunders 1967; Twycross 1974; Twycross and Wald 1976; McGivney and Crooks 1984), few of whom develop abuse behavior or significant toxicity. This success challenges traditional concepts about long-term management and suggests that a similar approach may be warranted in management of chronic nonmalignant pain (Taub 1982; Tennant and Uelman 1983). In one report 38 patients with nonmalignant chronic pain were treated with long-term opioid analgesics for up to seven years (Portenoy and Foley 1986). Most patients described acceptable or fully adequate pain relief, and a few attributed gainful employment or improved social function to the institution of opioid therapy. No toxicity was reported, and management became a problem in only two patients with a history of prior drug abuse. In another study of 11,882 hospitalized patients who received at least one opioid preparation, only four became addicted (Jiak et al. 1970). These studies suggest that maintenance opioid therapy can be a safe and more humane alternative to no treatment in patients with chronic nonmalignant pain syndromes. For more information on the subject of opioid therapy for chronic nonmalignant pain the reader may wish to refer to a recent review by Portenoy (1996).

PAIN MANAGEMENT IN THE EMERGENCY DEPARTMENT

SPECIFIC TREATMENT

Emergency department management should follow the specific sequence of: (1) evaluation and assessment, (2) appropriate treatment, and (3) proper disposition as illustrated in Fig. 2. Evaluation and assessment requires a thorough history and physical examination, including a search for signs and symptoms of infection. Hematologic determinations should include a reticulocyte count with a comparison to steady-state values. Systematic evaluation should assess potential involvement of specific organ systems, including the central nervous system, cardiopulmonary, hepatobiliary, genitourinary, and musculoskeletal systems. Patients are the best authority on their pain; if it is not typical of the usual crises, other causes of pain should be investigated aggressively and managed according to the specific findings.

When the initial evaluation suggests an uncomplicated painful episode, further assessment of the pain should ensue as described above. Pain of mild

PRECIPITATING FACTOR(S)

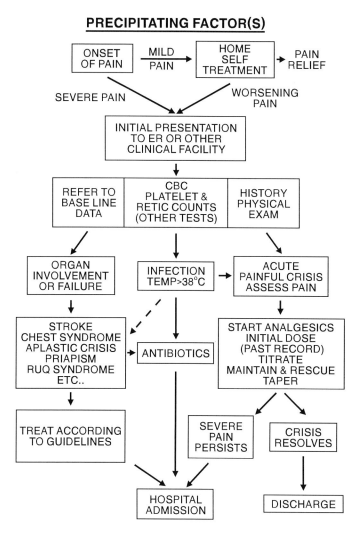

Fig. 2. Flow chart for management of painful episodes in patients with sickle cell disease (from Ballas 1994b with permission).

severity may be treated with oral nonopioid analgesics or weak opioids according to the three-step ladder described above. Most adults, however, come to the emergency department only after these measures have failed at home, so their treatment entails the parenteral use of strong opioid analgesics directed at relieving pain promptly. The specific opioid analgesic varies from patient to patient, time to time, and center to center.

Other measures may include hydration (oral or intravenous) or treatment with a heating pad or other nonpharmacologic methods. Fever or vomiting justify intravenous hydration. There is no evidence that oxygen inhalation reduces the intensity or duration of pain, and its use should be reserved for those patients who have pulmonary complications resulting in hypoxemia (Payne 1997; Zipursky et al. 1992).

Adjuvants are used in conjunction with the opioid analgesics to enhance the analgesic effect and prevent or ameliorate pruritus (see Chapter 9). Opioid analgesics (morphine, hydromorphone, or meperidine) should be given regularly, usually i.m. or i.v. every two to four hours depending on the patient's complaint. The intravenous route is the preferred method of opioid delivery, particularly in children. The intramuscular route may be necessary in patients with poor vascular access or those who insist on i.m. injection because of past habit. The best guide for the initial amount is the dose the patient required in the past.

Patients should be reassessed periodically after the initial dose of the opioid analgesic. With parenteral administration, reassessment should occur 30 minutes after the initial dose. If there has been absolutely no pain relief or sedation, 50% of the initial dose can be repeated 30 minutes after the previous dose. If a patient is mildly sedated and still has significant pain, then 25% of the dose should be repeated 30 minutes after the previous dose. Close monitoring of vital signs and the availability of a physician experienced in the use of opioids are essential for the success of this approach. Monitoring of respiratory rate is most important in averting potential serious side effects. A rate of less than 10 per minute is a sign of respiratory depression and an indication to discontinue opioids temporarily and reduce the subsequent dose.

The disposition of the patient in the emergency department depends on the results of the management described above, evaluation, assessment, and specific treatment. The opinion of the patient regarding the need for hospitalization may provide helpful guidance for prompt disposition. If the pain is tolerable, the patient may be discharged with a few tablets or a prescription for a limited amount of opioid analgesics to treat resolving pain. Failure to achieve adequate pain relief after treatment for six to eight hours in the emergency department (Table III) is an indication for hospital admission. Suspected infection and organ involvement may necessitate prompt hospital admission.

Problems associated with pain management in the emergency department

Dose of opioid analgesic. The initial treatment for a patient with acute sickle cell pain is often a standard dose of an opioid analgesic. For an

Table III
Guidelines for effective management of acute episodes
of sickle cell pain in the emergency department

Believe the patient.

Identify precipitating factors if possible and treat accordingly (example: antibiotics for infection.

Conduct thorough clinical assessment periodically, including documentation of pain severity, pain relief, and mood.

Select the appropriate opioid analgesic and its dose based on previous history.

Administer opioid analgesics parenterally on a regular basis (maintenance dose).

Monitor sedation and vital signs with special attention to the respiratory rate (RR).

Titrate the maintenance dose of opioid analgesic (taper or escalate).

Give rescue doses (¼–½ maintenance dose) for breakthrough pain every 30 minutes.

Decrease or skip maintenances dose if RR < 10/minute or if severely sedated.

Give nonopioid analgesics and adjuvant analgesics in combination with opioid analgesics.

If the acute painful episode is broken and pain is relieved to tolerable level the patient may be discharged from the emergency department.

Give limited amount of analgesic medication or a prescription for pain medication to treat resolving pain.

Design a discharge plan and arrange for outpatient follow-up by the primary physician.

Failure to achieve adequate pain relief after aggressive therapy for six to eight hours is an indication for hospital admission.

opioid-naive patient the chosen dose may lead to excessive sedation or, at worst, respiratory depression. Conversely, the dose may be insufficient for an opioid-tolerant patient, who continues to suffer. The medical staff assumes that the patient is manifesting drug-seeking behavior (Shapiro et al. 1997) because an apparently appropriate dose did not resolve the pain complaints. By individualizing the quantity of loading doses, based on the patient's past experience, and by employing objective scales to confirm pain relief, medical staff can expeditiously control acute pain due to vaso-occlusive crises.

Lack of coordinated care. Unlike the clinic, where coordinated management of patients provides the basis for rational care, the emergency department has other priorities that may necessitate a different agenda. Patients have described their visits to the emergency department as a dehumanizing experience, and many prefer to have a sufficient supply of opioids at home to treat themselves overnight or over the weekend until the office or clinic reopens. Nevertheless, the severity of pain compels most patients to seek emergency department care when their painful episodes do not resolve after a trial of home treatment.

In contrast with the clinic hematologist who is familiar with a patient's clinical profile and disease complications, the emergency department physician is less focused on the special nature of sickle cell disease. The absence of objective signs of painful crisis in about 50% of patients (Ballas et al. 1988) compounds the situation. Patients may wait hours before receiving analgesic therapy. Moreover, some physicians who harbor misconceptions about the need for narcotic analgesics in sickle cell disease may consciously or unconsciously convey a negative attitude to the patient. These factors aggravate patients, increase their stress, exacerbate their painful episodes, and thus may increase the likelihood of hospital admission. In actuality, only a few patients demonstrate drug-seeking behavior and abuse the system. Such patients should be treated according to specific guidelines (see Chapter 13) and their behavior should not be generalized to the majority.

Emergency department hopping. Hopping from one medical facility to another may be a sign of inadequate pain management. Unlike hopping from clinic to clinic during daytime, emergency department hopping carries with it another dimension of unnecessary suffering. Such hoppings are associated with acute episodes of pain, occur usually late at night, and often are complicated by unfavorable weather conditions (which may precipitate painful episodes), especially cold and snowy nights in some geographic regions. Patients who are released from one emergency department with little or no treatment have to arrange for their own transportation to another facility under unfavorable conditions that may further aggravate painful episodes. Patients are usually brought to the emergency department by ambulance or police, but transportation from the emergency department is the patient's responsibility. The problem is compounded for patients who come alone to the emergency department. It is unfortunate that some providers unknowingly inflict so much suffering on patients who have an inherited disease characterized by recurrent episodes of pain.

POSSIBLE SOLUTIONS

Different sickle cell disease centers have developed programs to improve the emergency department management of patients with acute painful episodes. Educating the staff and enhancing communication among providers, patients, and advocates is a contribution to improving the situation. Three specific approaches are described below.

The Georgia Sickle Cell Center at Grady Memorial Hospital in Atlanta adopted a *24-hour acute care center* (Platt and Eckman 1990). Such a center has at least two prerequisites: a large number of patients (> 500) and abundant funding from local, state, and federal sources. The center is staffed 24 hours a day, seven days a week by physician assistants and nurse practitioners and is supervised by attending hematologists and house staff. Physicians follow established guidelines in evaluating and treating patients. This approach ensures continuity of care and precludes most of the aforementioned problems associated with the emergency department. Patients are treated promptly by personnel who are familiar with them. Benefits include a decreased frequency of hospital admissions, early assessment of complications, centralization of medical information, and a positive provider-patient relationship.

The Bronx Comprehensive Sickle Cell Center at Montefiore Medical Center in the Bronx, New York established a *day hospital* (Benjamin and Nagel 1991). Open Mondays through Fridays from 9 A.M. to 5 P.M., it provides consistent and individualized clinical management of pain coupled with supportive attitudes. Although this approach is less ideal than the 24-hour acute care center, it has the advantage of being amenable to implementation by smaller sickle cell disease centers with limited budgets. The success of a day hospital requires effective communication with the emergency department, where patients receive care when the day hospital is not open.

Individual guidelines can be established for treating patients in vaso-occlusive crisis (Ballas 1990b). The patient carries a wallet-sized, plasticized card that includes demographic and hematologic data, known complications of disease, other medical problems, the recommended analgesic, its dose, route, and frequency of administration, and the name and address of the hematologist or health care provider who knows the patient best (Fig. 3). The patient presents this card to the physician in the emergency department or hospital. The card system requires only a Polaroid camera and a laminator and thus can be implemented by any sickle cell disease center irrespective of its size or budget.

MANAGEMENT OF SICKLE CELL PAIN IN THE HOSPITAL

TREATMENT OF ACUTE PAINFUL EPISODES IN THE HOSPITAL

Failure to break the painful crisis in the emergency department is an indication for hospital admission. Management of pain in the hospitalized patient is essentially a continuation of the process of evaluation, assessment, and titration of the opioid dose to achieve adequate pain relief. This process can occur through either parenteral administration of opioid analgesics on fixed schedule with rescue doses, or patient-controlled analgesia (PCA) as follows.

Front:

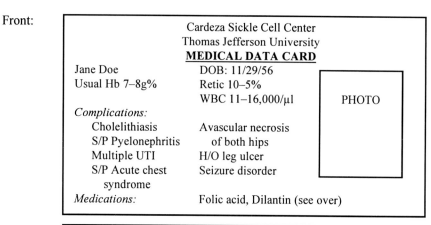

Back:

USUAL PAIN TREATMENT

Outpatient: Dilaudid p.o. p.r.n.
                    Acetaminophen 500 mg p.o. q6h p.r.n.
Inpatient: Dilaudid 4–6 mg i.v., i.m., or s.c. q2h
                    Vistaril 50 mg i.m. q4h
                    Acetaminophen 500 mg p.o. q6h
                    Doxepin 100 mg p.o. q hs

Attending physician: Samir K. Ballas, M.D.

Fig. 3. Example of a wallet-sized plasticized ID card that lists pertinent hematological and clinical data and recommendations for treatment of sickle cell pain (from Ballas 1994b with permission).

Fixed schedule of parenteral opioids with rescue doses

Pain therapy during the first two to three days of hospitalization should be aggressive with regular assessment of pain intensity and titration of the opioid dose to achieve pain relief (Table IV). Analgesics should be given parenterally on a fixed schedule (usually every two hours) rather than "as needed." The pain should be assessed every 30 to 60 minutes and the dose of the opioid titrated with rescue injections equal to 25–50% of the initial dose. If three or more rescue doses are needed within 24 hours or less to achieve adequate pain relief, the initial dose should be increased by 25–50% and the process repeated until adequate pain relief is achieved. Sedation and vital signs should be monitored as described above.

After two to three days of this aggressive parenteral therapy the loading dose may be decreased by 25% every 24 hours and replaced by an oral equianalgesic dose (see Chapter 9) on a fixed schedule. It is advisable to use the same opioid parenterally and orally whenever possible. If pain assessment shows continued improvement, proceed with decreasing the parenteral opioid analgesic by 25% every day and replace with an equianalgesic oral dose. After 24 to 48 hours the oral opioid may be given as needed. If pain relapses escalate the dose to the previous level of administration. Table V provides an example of a comprehensive regimen for managing severe episodes of sickle cell pain in the hospital.

Patients may be ready for discharge if they are pain free or if their pain is adequately controlled with oral analgesics. Give enough medication upon

Table IV
Guidelines for the treatment of acute episodes of sickle cell pain in the hospital
Method A
Fixed schedule of parenteral analgesia with rescue doses

Believe the patient.

Periodically conduct thorough clinical assessment, including documentation of pain severity, pain relief, and mood.

Select the appropriate opioid analgesic, its dose and frequency of administration based on previous experience.

Administer regular doses of opioid analgesics, usually every two to four hours in adults (maintenance dose) given parenterally (preferably i.v.).

Give nonopioid analgesics and adjuvant analgesics in combination with opioid analgesics. NSAIDs are contraindicated in the presence of impaired renal and/or hepatic function and history of gastropathy.

Monitor sedation and vital signs with special attention to the respiratory rate (RR).

Assess pain severity every 30 minutes.

Give rescue doses (25–50% of maintenance dose) for breakthrough pain every 30 minutes if adequate pain relief is not achieved.

If three or more rescue doses are needed in 24 hours or less increase the maintenance dose by 25–50% and follow the same procedure of assessment and dose adjustment.

Decrease or skip maintenances dose in the presence of severe sedation or if RR <10/minute.

After two to three days of therapy decrease the maintenance dose by 25% every 24 hours and replace with an oral opioid in regular divided doses.

After 24–48 hours the oral opioid may be given as needed. If pain relapses, escalate the dose into its previous level of administration.

Patients may be discharged if pain free with no comorbid condition or if pain is adequately controlled with oral analgesics.

Design a discharge plan with follow-up as an outpatient.

Table V
A comprehensive regimen to manage severe episodes
of sickle cell pain in the hospital

Maintenance therapy with opioid analgesic
Morphine sulfate, 0.1–0.2 mg/kg i.v., i.m., or s.c. q2-3h, *or*
Meperidine, 1.5 mg/kg i.v. or i.m. q2–3 h, *or*
Hydromorphone, 0.02–0.04 mg/kg i.v., i.m., or s.c. q2-3h

Nonopioid analgesic
Ibuprofen, 600 mg p.o. q6h, *or*
Ketorolac (Toradol), 60 mg i.m. initially followed by 30 mg i.m. q6h for a maximum
  of 5 days

Rescue therapy for breakthrough pain
One-fourth to one-half the maintenance dose of the opioid analgesic given parenterally
  30–60 minutes after the maintenance dose

Adjuvant therapy
Diphenhydramine (Benadryl), *25–50 mg i.m. or i.v. q4-6h, *or*
Hydroxyzine (Vistaril), *25–50 mg i.m. or i.v. q4-6h

Anxiolytics/muscle relaxants
Diazepam (Valium), 2–10 mg p.o. q8h p.r.n.

Antiemetics
Prochlorperazine (Compazine), 5–10 mg p.o. or i.m. q6h p.r.n. (not recommended with
  meperidine)

Laxatives
Magnesium citrate 8 oz p.o. qd p.r.n.

Other supportive measures
Hydration (oral or intravenous)
Heating pads
Hydrotherapy
Biofeedback
Relaxation
Diversion

---

*Not FDA approved for this indication.

discharge to treat resolving pain and to last until the next office appointment
with their primary care physician.

Patient-controlled analgesia (PCA)

PCA gives patients an active role in managing pain through a program-
mable pump that allows a patient to self-administer intravenous or subcutaneous opioids within set limits for the infusion level (lockout interval) and
number of possible doses per time period. In addition, the system can deliver
a continuous baseline dose of an opioid and boluses for breakthrough pain.
For most sickle cell patients, PCA may be an ideal method for treating acute

pain (Payne 1989b; Shapiro 1993; Shapiro et al. 1993). After an effective loading dose of an opioid analgesic, the patient can obtain an analgesic bolus by activating a demand switch that prompts delivery of a preset dose of opioid if a predetermined time (lockout interval) has elapsed since the previous dose. Thus, PCA allows patients considerable control over the experience of pain and produces an overall improvement in analgesia without significant increase in sedation.

The standard PCA infusion pumps allow limitation of cumulative doses over one to four hours. Patient-administered doses, lockout intervals, and four-hour limits must be based on the required loading dose and on opioid tolerance. Experience with postoperative patients has demonstrated that they will titrate themselves to minimally effective analgesic concentrations and will not overdose to produce significant adverse effects such as sedation or respiratory depression.

One method employing PCA to manage acute sickle cell pain in adults (Table VI) entails recording an initial verbal pain score and loading with small boluses of either morphine (2.5–10 mg), hydromorphone (0.5–2 mg), or meperidine (2.5–10 mg) every 10 minutes intravenously (Cantees et al. 1995). The verbal pain score is assessed following each bolus. Loading boluses are continued until the patient is comfortable, the pain scale has decreased 50%, or the patient is sedated. This approach individualizes each loading regimen of opioid analgesics and avoids overtreatment of opioid-naive patients and undertreatment of those who are opioid tolerant.

Following the rapid relief of acute pain by the individualized loading procedure, the patients continue to control their pain by boluses of opioids of the same dosage employed for loading. The lockout interval is set at six minutes to permit more rapid pain relief. Continuous intravenous infusions are not used during the day. Patients receive reinforcement that they are in control of their pain management and can deliver 10 PCA doses each hour if needed. However, a portion (66%) of their daytime hourly opioid use by PCA is given as a continuous infusion from 10 P.M. to 8 A.M. to ensure adequate rest at night. In the morning they resume control of their pain management by using only PCA boluses.

A four-hour cumulative opioid dose delivery limit may be set as a precaution until the staff become familiar with the PCA delivery system. However, if a continuous infusion is used, an appropriate allowance for PCA boluses must be permitted to avoid patient frustration if they trigger the PCA device without obtaining pain relief.

Appropriate dosing of analgesics using PCA can be titrated by allowing each patient to control his or her own pain. Conversion to either morphine or hydromorphone, and thus avoiding the risk of seizures due to the

Table VI
Guidelines for the treatment of acute episodes of sickle cell pain in the hospital
Method B
Patient-controlled analgesia (PCA)

Believe the patient.
Assess patient's perception of pain by employing a verbal pain scale (0–10).
Administer intravenous boluses of either morphine (2.5–10 mg) or hydromorphone (0.5–2 mg) every 10 minutes. Meperidine (10–25 mg) is used only in patients who are truly intolerant of morphine or hydromorphone.
Reassess the patient's perception of pain with the verbal pain scale after 10 minutes. Continue to administer intravenous boluses every 10 minutes until either the pain scale is decreased 50%, the pain is relieved, or the patient is sedated. The total loading dose of opioid should be recorded to document tolerance to opioids to facilitate appropriate loading during the next episode of acute pain.
Begin PCA by using 20% of the quantity of opioid bolus that was used in loading the patient to be delivered with a six-minute lockout interval. Reassess the patient's perception of pain every 30 minutes initially and less frequently later, by using either a verbal or a visual analog pain scale.
Encourage patients to control their own pain by reinforcing the quantity of opioid that they can deliver as needed and the equivalent potency when converting from meperidine to morphine or hydromorphone.
Determine the hourly use of opioid during the day and give 66% of the hourly dose as a continuous infusion at night to ensure rest.
On day 2 or 3 of hospitalization replace with an equivalent oral dose of opioid analgesic (preferably the same as the one used in PCA) on a fixed schedule around the clock and decrease the PCA dose by 25% every 24 hours.
After 24–48 hours, the PCA can be discontinued. Oral breakthrough doses can be administered between fixed doses of oral analgesics.
Patients may be ready for discharge if they are pain free or if their pain is adequately controlled with oral analgesics.
Taper the opioid after discharge over the following one to two weeks to prevent symptoms of the abstinence syndrome.
Resume control of chronic pain using the three-step analgesia ladder if indicated.

accumulation of normeperidine, can be facilitated by educating the patient about equivalent doses to allay fear or mistrust as this change occurs. Emphasizing to the patient the total quantity of analgesic that they can self-administer if needed to relieve pain also transfers the control of pain to the patient. Finally, negative interactions between the medical staff and patients regarding the control of opioids and judgments of the veracity of their pain by a second party can be avoided.

Table VII presents an example of a comprehensive regimen to manage severe sickle cell pain in the hospital by PCA. The schedule can be modified

Table VII
Example of a comprehensive regimen to manage severe sickle cell pain
in the hospital by using patient-controlled analgesia (PCA)

Opioid medication	Hydromorphone (Dilaudid) 0.5 mg/ml
Mode of opioid delivery	PCA only
Parameters	PCA dose 1 ml Lockout interval (delay) 10 minutes One-hour dose limit 8 ml
Continuous basal rate (if applicable)	None
As-needed nursing boluses	1 ml i.v. or i.m. q30min p.r.n.
Continuous i.v. solution	0.9% saline at 42 ml/h
Monitor respiratory rate, pain level, sedation	q30min after initialization of PCA × 2, then q60min × 2, then q4h for duration of therapy. In addition, if a bolus is given monitor parameters q15min × 2.

to include basal administration of opioids or to change the dose or the mode of delivery at night as needed. Other aspects of treatment such as nonopioid analgesics and adjuvants are the same as was described above for the fixed dose regimen.

ISSUES ASSOCIATED WITH MANAGEMENT OF SICKLE CELL PAIN IN THE HOSPITAL

Continuity of care

Ideally, the team that knows the patient should follow care during hospitalization to maintain continuity and minimize management problems. Admission of patients to a general medical service staffed by rotating personnel is destined to interrupt continuity (Benjamin 1989; Ballas 1990b) and weakens comprehensive management. Physicians at all levels should receive education about sickle cell disease in general and about pain and its management in particular.

Choice of opioid

Despite reservations (Pryle et al. 1992; Grundy et al. 1993; Davis and Bevan 1996; Forbes et al. 1996; Meltzer 1996; Simni 1996; Ward 1996), meperidine is the most commonly reported opioid in the treatment of hospitalized patients with sickle cell disease both in the United Kingdom and the United States (Davies and Brozovic 1989; Pegelow 1992; Grundy et al.

1993; Ballas et al. 1995a; Shulman et al. 1995). In contrast, morphine is the most commonly used opiate for cancer pain. Meperidine is familiar to many patients with sickle cell disease and, often, it is their drug of choice for the treatment of severe painful episodes. Its fast onset of action, euphoric effect, past habit, and relatively low incidence of severe pruritus, nausea, and vomiting contribute to its common use in sickle cell disease. The association of seizure with the prolonged administration of meperidine limits its use in some patients. Mitchell et al. (1991) reported the death of a patient in sickle cell crisis during grand mal seizure after two days of taking continuous i.v. meperidine at a high dose of up to 150 mg per hour. His serum concentration of meperidine was 2.2 mg/l (upper limit of therapeutic range 2 mg/l) and his serum normeperidine concentration was 5.2 mg/l at the time of death (upper limit of therapeutic range 1.5 mg/l). Meperidine may be suitable for the treatment of painful episodes in patients who experience infrequent crises that last less than two to three days. Long-term treatment with high doses of meperidine should be discouraged.

Brookoff and Polomano (1992) have reported that using intravenous and controlled-release oral morphine instead of intramuscular meperidine reduced the frequency of hospital admissions of patients with painful episodes and their length of stay. The decrease in hospital admissions, however, perhaps occurred because some patients transferred their care to other hospitals in the area (Ballas et al. 1992) after the institution of the morphine-only policy. Unfortunately, this report gave the wrong message to providers (especially the nursing and house staff), who thought that morphine is the *only opioid* to be used to treat acute sickle cell painful episodes. I have emphasized that pain management should be individualized (Ballas et al. 1992). Moreover, there have been reports of fatal pulmonary failure with the use of morphine in patients with sickle cell disease (Gerber and Apseloff 1993; Ballas 1994a). Physicians who replaced meperidine with morphine in their protocols to treat acute painful episodes noted a higher incidence of acute chest syndrome with morphine (Mallouh, personal communication; Ballas and Gay, unpublished observations). In addition, morphine, like meperidine, is contraindicated in the presence of renal failure (see Chapter 9).

Table VIII summarizes published reports of studies that compared the efficacy of different analgesics with or without adjuvants in the treatment of acute sickle cell painful episodes in the hospital. As can be seen, there is little convincing evidence that one opioid is more efficacious than another. Oxygen inhalation had no effect on the duration of painful episodes treated with opioids (Robieux et al. 1992; Zipursky et al. 1992).

High-dose intravenous methylprednisolone therapy for acute painful episodes in children and adolescents reduced analgesic requirements in a placebo-controlled trial (Griffin et al. 1994), but a few patients who received methylprednisolone experienced rebound attacks of pain a few days after discharge. Foley and Portenoy (1994) criticized this study by indicating a serious deficiency where the authors confused the duration of analgesic use with analgesia and did not use any of the pain measurement tools to assess the outcome of therapy with methylprednisolone.

A trial of the NSAID diflunisal did not affect the outcome of treatment of painful episodes with meperidine and hydroxyzine (Perlin et al. 1988). Moreover, the patients who took diflunisal experienced more nausea than did those who took placebo. Two of three reports indicated that the co-administration of ketorolac was associated with greater pain relief, less meperidine consumption, and shorter hospital stay (Wright et al. 1992; Ernst et al. 1993; Perlin et al. 1994).

There is some evidence that adjuvants may have a beneficial effect on the outcome of treatment of painful episodes with opioids. There are anecdotes of successful pain management in sickle cell disease using oral tricyclic antidepressants in conjunction with parenteral or oral opioids and NSAIDs (Pollack et al. 1991; Sanders et al. 1992; Ballas et al. 1995b). McPherson et al. (1990) reported that the administration of hydroxyzine, an anxiolytic antihistamine, in addition to patient-controlled meperidine, gave better treatment ratings than did meperidine alone.

Route of administration of opioids

Opioid analgesics are usually administered parenterally to hospitalized patients with acute episodes of sickle cell pain. Although the intravenous route is preferred, adequate venous access may be a problem in many patients. Despite the declining acceptance of intramuscular injections of opioids, they have a good record of safety in short-term administration (Howard 1993). The i.m. administration of opioids over a long time (every 2–3 hours for one to two weeks) may be complicated by the formation of sterile abscesses, infection, and fibrosis. Morphine and hydromorphone may be given subcutaneously provided the dose can be adjusted because the equianalgesic dose given subcutaneously is 1.5 to 2 times that of the intravenous dose (Urquhart et al. 1988; Moulin et al. 1991). Venous access is often obtained by the insertion of totally implantable intravenous catheters such as peripherally inserted central catheters (PICC) or Infusaports. Infection, catheter thrombosis and venous thrombosis may complicate the use of these routes (Phillips et al. 1988). Such maneuvers to secure venous access in patients with sickle cell disease is associated with a marked increase in total complications and complications requiring catheter removal compared to patients without sickle cell disease (Phillips et al. 1988).

Table VIII
Comparative studies of analgesics used in the treatment
of sickle cell pain in the hospital

Treatment Protocol	Main Results	Reference
Randomized placebo-controlled double blind-trials		
Continuously infused morphine plus oxygen inhalation vs. morphine plus air in 34 children	No significant difference in duration of pain or appearance of new pain sites	Robieux et al. 1992
i.v. morphine plus i.v. methylprednisolone vs. morphine plus saline in 56 episodes in 36 children and adolescents	Methylprednisolone group required less morphine but were more likely to suffer recurrent episodes of pain after treatment ended	Griffin et al. 1994
Oral diflunisal plus i.m. meperidine vs. oral placebo plus meperidine in 37 episodes in 32 adults	Nausea was more common for diflunisal- treated episodes, but no significant differences in days in hospital, meperidine consumption, patient-rated pain intensity, or other adverse effects	Perlin et al. 1988
i.v. meperidine plus i.m. ketorolac vs. meperidine plus saline in 24 episodes in 18 adults	No significant difference in patient-rated pain intensity of meperidine consumption during four hours of observation	Wright et al. 1992
Opiates plus i.v. cetiedil citrate vs. opiates plus saline in 67 adults	Cetiedil group had significantly fewer painful sites, shorter painful episodes, and better overall treatment evaluations, but no significant differences in analgesics required, adverse reactions or laboratory measures	Benjamin et al. 1986
Analgesics plus i.v. pentoxiphyllin vs. analgesics plus saline in 36 adults and children	Pentoxiphyllin group had significantly shorter painful episodes and treatment, but no significant differences in analgesic consumption, additional pain sites, adverse reactions, or laboratory measures	Teuscher et al. 1989
i.v. sodium bicarbonate vs. i.v. sodium chloride in 25 episodes in 18 children	No significant difference in physician-rated symptoms half an hour after treatment	Schwartz and McElfresh 1994

(continued)

Table VIII—Continued

Treatment Protocol	Main Results	Reference
Uncontrolled trials		
Subcutaneous/i.m. nalbuphine vs. i.m. meperidine in 45 episodes in children and adolescents	Little difference in days hospitalized or overall assessments of pain relief and adverse reactions	Woods et al. 1990
Ketorolac used vs. not used in 459 episodes in 106 patients	Fewer narcotic injections needed when ketorolac was used	Ernest et al. 1993
Patient-controlled meperidine plus hydroxyzine vs. meperidine alone in 15 adult	Hydroxyzine group gave better treatment ratings	McPherson et al. 1990
Randomized double-blind trial		
i.m. butorphanol vs. morphine in 45 episodes in18 adults	No significant differences in patient-rated pain and pain relief, nurse-rated alertness, physical measures, adverse reactions, discharge rates, or global assessment of treatment	Gonzalez et al. 1988
Placebo-controlled trial		
i.m. meperidine plus i.v. ketorolac vs. meperidine plus saline in 21 patients	Ketorolac group required 33% less meperidine, had significantly shorter treatments, and had significantly better patient-rated pain relief over five days	Perlin et al. 1994

Source: Adapted from Elander and Midence 1996 with permission.

Yaster et al (1994) reported that epidural analgesics with local anesthetics were effective in children whose sickle cell pain did not respond to conventional analgesia. Moreover, this approach was life-saving in some of their patients with acute chest syndrome by providing adequate analgesia without hypoventilation. Epidural analgesia in sickle cell disease, however, is controversial, and controlled studies are needed to define its role in the management of sickle cell pain.

Friedman et al (1986), Powers (1986), and Conti et al (1996) advocated the use of oral opioids to manage acute sickle cell painful episodes in the emergency department in uncontrolled trials involving a small number of adult patients. In an important advance, Christensen et al. (1996) reported encouraging results for the transdermal fentanyl administration in children and adolescents with painful crises. Table IX summarizes published reports that compared various methods of administration of opioids to patients with acute episodes of sickle pain.

Table IX
Comparative studies of the route of administration of opioids
in the treatment of sickle cell pain in the emergency department (ED) or hospital

Treatment Protocol	Design	Main Results	Reference
Management protocol with emphasis on oral rather than parenteral opiates vs. standard ED care in five very frequent adult ED users	Before and after comparison	Number of ED visits, mean length of ED stay, frequency and doses of parenteral opiates all significantly reduced after the change in management protocol	Powers 1986
Protocol based on oral morphine vs. parenteral meperidine protocol in 15 frequent adult ED users	Retrospective before and after comparison	No change in rate of ED visits but significant reductions in hospital admissions, amount of opiates dispensed, and number of analgesic injections	Friedman et al. 1986
PCA meperidine vs. fixed-schedule injections in 20 children	Uncontrolled retrospective comparison between random sample of 10 children treated by each method	Time in hospital and duration of therapy were similar, but meperidine doses were greater for PCA	Holbrook 1990
PCA meperidine vs. fixed-schedule i.m. meperidine	Randomized trial	No significant differences in meperidine consumption, patient-rated pain intensity, and pain relief.	Perlin et al. 1993

PCA morphine vs. intermittent i.v. morphine in 45 adults	Randomized trial	No significant difference in amount of morphine administered, patient-rated pain, nurse-rated pain, nurse-rated alertness, adverse reactions, duration of treatment, or overall nurse-rated and patient-rated treatment evaluations.	Gonzalez et al. 1991
Continuous i.v. morphine vs. intermittent i.v. or i.m. opiates in 66 children and adolescents	Prospective comparison	Significantly shorter duration of patient-rated severe pain for continuous infusion, but no significant difference in morphine equivalent dose, days in hospital, or days with opiates. Drowsiness significantly more common for continuous i.v. morphine but no significant differences in other adverse reactions	Robieux et al. 1992
Continuous i.v. meperidine or morphine vs. intermittent i.v. meperidine in 98 episodes in 38 children	Retrospective case comparison	Significantly greater analgesic consumption and much more common adverse reactions for continuous treatment (which was used selectively for more severe pain)	Cole et al. 1986

Source: Adapted for Elander and Midence 1996 with permission.

Studies examining methods of opioid administration have focused on direct comparisons between PCA and intermittent or fixed-schedule injections of opioids, and also comparison of continuous i.v versus intermittent i.v. or i.m. opioids. Comparisons between PCA and intermittent or fixed-schedule injections did not show positive findings (Table IX). The groups showed no significant difference in time spent in the hospital or duration of analgesic therapy (Holbrook 1990; Gonzalez et al. 1991; Perlin et al. 1993). In one study (Holbrook 1990), patients treated with PCA used larger quantities of meperidine than did those treated with fixed-schedule injections. Two other studies (Gonzalez et al. 1991; Perlin et al. 1993), however, showed no difference in the amounts of opioids consumed between the PCA and fixed-schedule/intermittent group (Table IX). Advantages of PCA included the active participation of the patients in their own treatment and the reduction in the number of intramuscular injections. Shapiro et al. (1993) retrospectively reviewed the medical records of 46 hospitalized children and adolescents with sickle cell disease who used patient-controlled analgesia (PCA) 92 times for the management of vaso-occlusive pain. Patients varied widely in the drug administered, use of basal infusion, individual dose, and total amount of drug received. The average maximum hourly dose was equivalent to 0.09 mg/kg of morphine. Of the 46 patients studied, 15 (33%) had problems with PCA: 11 patients disliked it, two families disapproved the technique after it was started, one patient had respiratory compromise, and one patient tampered with the machine in an attempt at suicide. The relatively high dissatisfaction rate with PCA in this report may represent the uncertainties that surround a new, unfamiliar modality of pain control. Carefully designed prospective studies are needed to define the role of PCA in the management of sickle cell pain.

Comparisons between continuous intravenous injections and fixed-schedule or intermittent injections of opioids showed that: (1) continuous infusion controlled pain in a more stable way than did intermittent bolus injections (Ives and Guerra 1987; Sartori et al. 1990); (2) the duration of severe pain was shorter with continuous infusion than with intermittent morphine (Robieux et al. 1992); and (3) side effects and complications including lethargy, acute chest syndrome, abdominal distention, and wheezing were more common with continuous infusion of opioids (Cole et al. 1986).

In summary, data in the English literature suggest that the administration of opioid analgesics either by PCA (Table VI) or by fixed-schedule injections (Table IV) is effective, safe, and entails the consumption of comparable amounts of opioids. Continuous infusion of opioids, although effective in achieving adequate pain relief, seems to be associated with undesirable side effects and may not be advisable for routine use.

Side effects of opioids

Sedation, respiratory depression, nausea, vomiting, constipation, and pruritus are anticipated side effects of all opioids. Prophylactic use of an antihistamine (hydroxyzine or diphenhydramine) can decrease pruritus in patients who have experienced this side effect from morphine. Similarly, the empiric use of an antiemetic (transdermal scopolamine or an oral phenothiazine) and a stool softener can obviate the nausea or constipation in most patients. Large-volume vomiting in a sedated patient may be associated with aspiration pneumonia and can be fatal in a patient with compromised pulmonary function. Severe sedation may be avoided by the coadministration of stimulants such as 5 mg of oral methylphenidate each morning. Given that each opioid may not produce the same (crossover) side effects, trying a different opioid may lessen symptoms. Alternatively, changing the dosing regimen (e.g., decreasing the concentration of each intravenous bolus while shortening the time interval) may abate side effects.

All patients should have naloxone readily available for treatment of respiratory depression. However, in contrast to the use of naloxone in the emergency department to quickly reverse a suspected drug overdose, a dilute solution of naloxone (one ampule of 0.4 mg diluted with saline to 10 ml) should be available for titration. This solution should be administered at 0.5 ml i.v. every two minutes to avoid the precipitation of profound withdrawal, seizures, and severe pain (American Pain Society 1993).

CONCLUSIONS

Severe sickle cell pain necessitates the use of strong opioid agonists. The intravenous route is the ideal method of administering opioids, followed by the subcutaneous route. The intramuscular route should be avoided if possible, especially in patients who require opioid analgesia for prolonged periods, but may be unavoidable in a subset of patients who have difficult venous access and who refuse the insertion of ports. The subcutaneous administration of opioids entails increasing the dose because the s.c./i.v. ratio, at least for hydromorphone, is 1.5 to 2. Transdermal fentanyl patches are being widely used for outpatients with pain in general, and their use in patients with sickle cell disease is increasing. One or two fentanyl patches (100 µg each) every three days seem to be effective in some patients with chronic sickle cell pain. Short-acting opioids given orally as needed may also be needed for breakthrough pain (O. Castro, personal communication, 1997). One potential problem with fentanyl patches is that fever may accelerate the absorption of fentanyl to toxic levels. Again, controlled prospective studies are needed to optimally tailor pain management to the satisfaction of individual patients.

These new routes of administration of opioids, such as the transdermal, intrathecal, and epidural, require further study. Meperidine should be avoided whenever possible, especially in patients who require opioid analgesics for several days or weeks. A subset of adult patients have been treated with large doses of meperidine for lengthy periods with no apparent serious effects. Both morphine and meperidine should be avoided in renal failure. The side effects of morphine in adults with sickle cell disease need more study. Administration of opioids via PCA or fixed schedule seems to be associated with less serious side effects compared to continuous i.v. infusions. The choice of opioid, dose, and route of administration should be individualized case by case.

In conducting studies of various therapeutic interventions with opioids it is extremely important to collect comprehensive data including treatment by centers and providers other than those conducting the study. Thus, a facility that uses only oral opioids to treat acute painful episodes may report fewer admissions and less opioid consumption because their patients, when in severe pain that required parenteral analgesics, might have seek medical help in other facilities. The Multicenter Study of Hydroxyurea in Sickle Cell Anemia (Charache et al. 1995, 1996) considered that factor and found that patients are often treated in facilities other than those of the principal investigators, especially in large urban communities. The other studies mentioned in this chapter did not seriously consider this factor in analyzing their data.

ILLUSTRATIVE CASES

CASE 10.1

Our sickle cell center was consulted in the management of a 38-year-old African American woman with sickle cell anemia who was admitted to the gynecological service with pelvic pain. She complained of pain in her low abdomen that was not typical of her usual crisis pain. The pain was constant, dull, deep, and crampy with an intensity score of 10 on a scale of 10. In contrast, her usual crisis pain was throbbing and involved her low back, chest, arms, and legs. Her obstetrical history was significant for one spontaneous abortion and one spontaneous vaginal delivery at eight months and dilatation and evacuation for retained products of conception. She had laparoscopic tubal ligation and left oophorectomy two weeks prior to admission. Complications of her sickle cell disease included more than four severe painful episodes per year that were usually treated with hydromorphone

(Dilaudid) 3–4 mg i.m. every two to three hours. Milder episodes of pain were treated at home with oxycodone and acetaminophen (Percocet). Other complications included history of recurrent pneumonia, acute chest syndrome, cholecystectomy, and alloimmunization (five clinically significant alloantibodies) secondary to multiple transfusions for severe anemia. Her baseline hemoglobin was 5–6 g%.

Physical examination showed a sick woman complaining of severe low abdominal pain. Her temperature was 39.2°C, respiratory rate 26/min, and pulse 100/min. She had diffuse abdominal tenderness that was most severe in the low abdomen, worse on the right than the left. Pelvic examination was difficult to assess due to guarding. Her hemoglobin decreased to a level of 4.7 g% and her white blood count was 36,400/µl.

Management consisted of hydration, antibiotics, and blood transfusion. Pain was initially treated with Dilaudid 4 mg i.m. every two hours and then morphine sulfate 6 mg i.v. every two hours when venous access became available. She complained that she experienced no pain relief with morphine sulfate.

Recommendations included increasing the dose of morphine to 20 mg i.v. every two hours and continuing pain assessment and monitoring. With 15–20 mg of morphine i.v. she experienced 40–50% pain relief comparable to that experienced with 4 mg of hydromorphone i.m. She continued, however, to complain of the unusual nature of her pain and insisted that "something is wrong with me" other than the sickle crisis. She continued to have fever and did not respond to antibiotics. MRI of the pelvis showed bilateral adnexal masses that were suggestive of tubo-ovarian abscesses. Consequently, exploratory laparatomy revealed a large pelvic abscess in the cul-de-sac with multiple bowel adhesions. The abscess was drained and the adhesions were lysed. Cultures grew *Enterococcus* species.

Following surgery she improved gradually and became afebrile by the third postoperative day. Pain intensity decreased gradually, opioids were tapered gradually, and she began receiving oral Percocet 10 days after surgery and was discharged from the hospital four days later.

Comments on case 10.1

This case illustrates two important points in the management of patients with acute painful episodes. The first pertains to equivalent dosing of analgesics. Replacing one opioid with another must consider equianalgesic doses: 6 mg of morphine are not equivalent to 4 mg of hydromorphone, and the morphine dose had to be increased. Alternatively, the same dose of hydromorphone could be given either i.v. or i.m., although the former is preferable. The second issue in this case, persistent or worsening pain despite adequate management, suggests progression of the nociceptive process. Moreover, the patient's own assessment that the pain was unusual compared to her typical crises should suggest an aggressive search for other causes. In this case pelvic abscesses caused the progressive nociception that was relieved with drainage followed by antibiotic therapy.

CASE 10.2

A 43-year-old African American man with Hb SO Arab disease complained of low back pain that was not typical of his usual crisis pain of about one week duration. The pain was sharp and lancinating and had a score of 8 of 10. It radiated to both buttocks (left worse than right) and to the left lower extremity. It was associated with numbness and tingling over the left thigh but with no burning. He also noted weakness in his left lower extremity and difficulty walking. Past medical history revealed frequent acute painful episodes (about 10 per year) that were usually treated in the emergency room with hydromorphone i.m. The pain of these episodes involved his low back, arms, thighs, knees, and legs. The pain was usually sharp and throbbing. Mild episodes of pain were treated at home with oral oxycodone and acetaminophen (Percocet). Known complications of his disease included history of pneumonia, cholecystectomy, and a penile implantation for impotence due to priapism.

Physical examination revealed tenderness over the lumber spine and the paraspinal area. Pinprick sensation was decreased over the lateral aspect of the left thigh, and the motor power of the left lower extremity was weaker than the right. Straight-leg raising was positive on the left side. He walked with a limp to the left side. The deep tendon reflexes were intact in the upper and absent in the lower extremities.

Multiple radiographs of the lumbar spine compared with examinations in previous years showed loss of height, disk space narrowing, and osteophyte production at L3–L4 compatible with progressive degenerative disk disease at this level (Fig. 4). Tests revealed no evidence of endplate destruction. The remainder of the lumber spine showed anatomic alignment without evidence of fracture or subluxation. Surgical clips were noted in the right upper quadrant and a penile prosthesis reservoir was noted in the left pelvis. All osseous structures showed coarsened trabeculae indicative of diffuse infarcts due to his sickle cell disease.

Magnetic resonance imaging of the lumber spine showed severe degenerative disk and endplate change at L3–4. At this level a broad-based central disk herniation caused a moderate central stenosis. Lateral extension of the

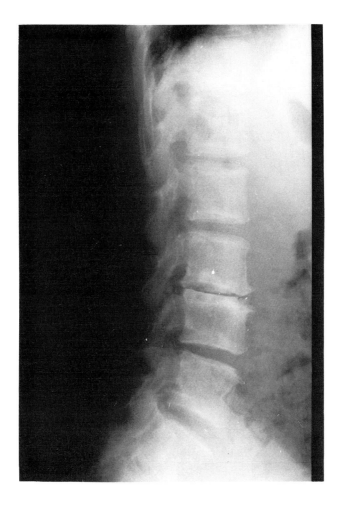

Fig. 4. Radiograph of the lumbar spine of the patient described in Case 10.2 shows loss of height, disk space narrowing, and osteophyte production at L3–L4 compatible with degenerative disk disease.

degenerative process and disk bulge caused bilateral foraminal stenosis that was severe on the left side (Fig. 5). At the L4–5 level the MRI showed a smaller, broad-based disk herniation with mild central stenosis and a mild to moderate bilateral foraminal stenosis. Small central disk herniation was noted at L2–3. The conus had normal signal and caliber.

This patient was first treated symptomatically with bed rest, opioid analgesics (Percocet, 2 tablets p.o. q2–3h p.r.n.), and NSAIDs (ibuprofen, 800 mg p.o. q8h p.r.n.) with no improvement. His symptoms continued to worsen

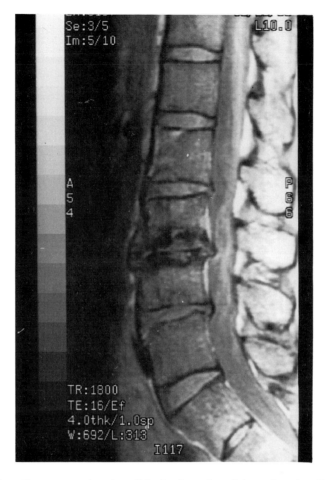

Fig. 5. Magnetic resonance imaging of the lumbar spine of the patient described in Case 10.2 shows severe degenerative disk and endplate changes at L3–L4.

and eventually he had laminectomy with excision of L3–4 disk and L4–5 disk and foraminotomy at L3–4 and at L4–5.

Immediately following surgery he complained of worsening pain in his low back and both lower extremities, probably due to a painful crisis precipitated by the stress of surgery. A few weeks later, however, the neurological signs and symptoms in the left lower extremity improved significantly, but with residual occasional numbness over the left thigh.

Comments on case 10.2

This case emphasizes the need to thoroughly evaluate patients with sickle cell disease whenever they present with new or unusual signs and symptoms. A thorough history and physical examination is mandatory. It is advisable not to assume that any pain in a patient with sickle cell disease is a form of usual crisis pain. An unusual aspect of this patient, given his age, is the severe degenerative disk changes and central stenosis. Tissue damage due to recurrent infarctive crises may have contributed to these findings. Such unusual findings may be more common in the future as better general medical care lengthens the lives of patients with sickle cell disease. This case also demonstrates that the stress associated with surgery may precipitate acute painful episodes. In such situations the combination of postoperative pain and crisis pain aggravates symptoms and may necessitate an aggressive approach to pain management.

Part IV
Alternatives to Pharmacologic Therapy

11

Nonpharmacologic Therapy of Sickle Cell Pain

Happiness is not being pained in body or troubled in mind.
— Thomas Jefferson, 1743–1826

The art of life is the art of avoiding pain; and he is the best pilot, who steers clearest of the rocks and shoals with which it is beset.
— Thomas Jefferson, 1743–1826

The therapeutic goals of nonpharmacologic techniques are to reduce pain and alleviate stress in both acute and chronic pain, and to increase activity and normal function. Some patients with sickle cell disease have discovered on their own the beneficial effect of modalities such as diversional methods (e.g., watching television, playing cards), self-motivation (e.g., setting goals to be achieved within a certain period), application of heating pads to painful areas of the body, massage, and mechanical stimulation. Table I lists some nonpharmacologic strategies often used by patients with sickle cell disease.

These modalities may be underutilized in sickle cell disease because of noncompliance by patients and a failure by caretakers to communicate effectively with patients (Shapiro 1991). Moreover, reported studies on the efficacy of behavioral and cognitive therapy (Shapiro 1991) did not always employ appropriate control groups, so success rates are uncertain.

On a positive note, Pegelow (1992) sent a questionnaire on pain management therapy for children with sickle cell disease to 32 physicians listed as principal investigators for clinical studies of sickle cell disease sponsored by the National Institutes of Health. Twenty-one of the 32 physicians contacted (66%) responded. The respondents estimated they provide care for 3500 children with sickle cell disease.

Table II lists the nonpharmacologic methods used by the respondents. Seventeen indicated that their programs included child life workers, 20 used play therapists, and 20 used schoolteachers. Two used TENS, one used

Table I
Nonpharmacologic strategies often used
by patients with sickle cell disease for
self-induced pain management

Cognitive coping strategies
   Directive prayer
   Diversion, distraction
   Coping self-statements
   Comparing self to others
   Goal setting
   Positive planning

Cognitive motor strategies
   Rocking
   Pacing
   Stair climbing
   Pushups
   Dancing

Autonomic relaxation techniques
   Visual imagery
   Relaxation breathing
   Nondirective prayer
   Meditation

behavioral modification, one used self-hypnosis, and five used video games, video cassettes or television for distraction. The schoolteachers were also, in part, instrumental in diverting the children's attention from their pain. Fifteen physicians thought that their regimen was very effective in controlling severe pain, and 12 believed that their regimen decreased the frequency and duration of hospitalizations. Only five respondents, however, thought that their regimen reduced the amount of analgesic medications administered to control pain. Although the data are uncontrolled, this survey suggests that nonpharmacologic pain control methods may be used at institutions having a special interest in providing medical care for children with sickle cell disease.

    An important issue that pertains to the efficacy of nonpharmacologic therapy of sickle cell pain is the neurobehavioral status of patients with sickle cell disease in the steady state and during acute or chronic painful episodes (Gil 1989). The success of cognitive behavioral therapy, for example, requires that the patient have adequate neurobehavioral coping skills. Again, few reports address this aspect of sickle cell disease. Early reports on the psychosocial impact of the painful episodes were descriptive (Whitten and Fischhoff 1974; Kumar et al. 1976; Nash 1977; Conyard et al. 1980) and based on the clinical impressions of health care providers. Nevertheless, these important pioneering reports paved the way to a more empirical ap-

Table II
Nonpharmacologic therapeutic modalities
reportedly used by pediatricians

Modality	Number of Pediatricians Using It
Physical Measures	
Local heat	15
Warm baths	11
Early ambulation	16
Increased fluids	20
Distraction	
School teacher	14
Video games	5
Other Therapies	
Child life workers	17
Play therapists	20
Behavior modification	1
Hypnosis	1

Source: Adapted from Pegelow 1992, with permission.

proach to the study of sickle cell pain. Wasserman et al. (1991) found that a group of 43 children and adolescents with sickle cell disease had a higher incidence of neuropsychological deficits on visual-motor tasks (writing, reading, memory, arithmetic, etc.) than did their socioeconomically matched siblings. Comparing adolescents to younger children, Fowler et al. (1988) reported increased deficits in visual-motor skills as patients with sickle cell disease matured. Bentz and Ballas (1994) reported compromised cognitive functioning in 11 adult patients with sickle cell anemia that was independent of the abnormalities demonstrated by MRI, CT, or EEG. The compromised function, however, may be the result of limited motivation due to the pain and fatigue associated with a chronic disease process. Additional testing, with a larger population, and other instruments could expand and confirm these observations.

CLASSIFICATION OF NONPHARMACOLOGIC THERAPEUTIC MODALITIES

EDUCATION AND COUNSELING

All therapeutic modalities should be preceded by patient education and counseling (Turk and Rennert 1981). In particular, nonpharmacologic therapy entails the active participation of the patient, so education plays an extremely important role in these treatment modalities. An educated patient is more likely to be compliant and thus to secure a positive outcome. Patient education should include, in lay language, details of the new therapy including its advantages, disadvantages, duration, expected results, and side effects, if any. The provider must answer all questions posed by the patient and allay fears, and the patient has the right to decline the proposed method. Education sessions may include friends, family, or other relatives if the patient agrees to their presence.

CUTANEOUS THERAPIES

Stimulation analgesia

Stimulation analgesia includes the use of transcutaneous electrical nerve stimulation (TENS), vibration, massage, heat or ice packs, and menthol cream rubs. These methods are, essentially, counterirritants. Most reports of their use in sickle cell pain are anecdotal. TENS provides pain relief by inhibiting pain transmission at the level of the dorsal horn via selective stimulation of large-diameter myelinated afferent fibers, according to the gate control theory (Fields 1987; Wall and Melzack 1994). These fibers are preferentially activated because they have the lowest threshold to externally applied electrical stimuli; the much higher electrical threshold of the small-diameter myelinated and unmyelinated primary afferent nerve fibers renders TENS a painless procedure. It is ideal for patients with localized chronic pain such as occurs in avascular necrosis of a joint or leg ulcers (Ballas et al. 1995b). Patients must be well instructed on the use of the TENS device to derive optimal benefit from this modality.

Spinal cord and brain stimulation are invasive procedures that evolved from the successes of TENS. They entail surgical implantation of electrodes over the dorsal column or in the periventricular gray matter (PVG) (Fields 1987; Wall and Melzack 1989) to modulate pain intensity by inhibition. The author is unaware of studies of these methods in sickle cell disease.

In a randomized placebo-controlled double-blind trial Wang et al. (1988) treated 60 acute painful episodes in 22 adolescents and adults with TENS versus a sham TENS procedure with no current (Table III). The trial showed nonspecific benefit in that the patients reported finding the treatment helpful, but pain ratings were similar for the TENS and placebo groups.

Mechanical stimulation is based on the same principle as TENS, but uses mechanical rather than electrical stimuli. It entails activation of low-threshold primary afferent nerve fibers by the cutaneous application of a vibrator. This method may be beneficial in alleviating localized muscle or bone pain.

Table III
Comparative studies of nonpharmacological therapeutic modalities
in the treatment of sickle cell pain

Treatment Protocol	Design	Main Results	Reference
Combined relaxation, biofeedback, cognitive strategies, and self-hypnosis in 15 adults	Before and after comparison	Emergency department visits reduced by 38%, admissions by 31%, inpatient days by 50%, and analgesic use by 29%	Thomas et al. 1984
EMG and thermal (digital) biofeedback in 8 children and adolescents	Before and after comparison	Self-reported headaches, pain intensity, days when analgesics used, self-treated painful episodes, and anxiety all reduced significantly over the 12-week training period, but no significant reduction in emergency department visits and admissions at six-month follow-up	Cozzi et al. 1987
TENS vs. Sham TENS procedure with no current in 60 episodes affecting 22 adolescents and adults	Randomized, placebo-controlled, double-blind trial	Significantly higher proportion of TENS patients reported finding the treatment "helpful" (74% vs. 39%) but no significant difference in patient-rated pain or analgesic requirements	Wang et al. 1988
Acupuncture at one pain site vs. non-acupuncture needling at another (two pain sites per episode were treated) in 16 painful episodes affecting 10 adults	Placebo-controlled double-blind trial	Patient-reported but no examiner-reported responses to treatment were significantly better for sites treated with acupuncture	Co et al. 1979

Source: Adapted from Elander and Midence 1996, with permission.

Acupressure

Acupressure refers to the application of finger pressure to anatomical points that correspond to meridians used in acupuncture (Kenyon 1988). It is similar to the use of trigger point massage in Western medicine (Simons and Travel 1989). The meridians, according to the Chinese, are channels in which the body's vital energy circulates (Kenyon 1988). Balanced flow of energy is synonymous with health. The flow of energy along the meridians is directional and acupressure must be applied in the direction of the meridian's flow. Interestingly, Melzack et al. (1977) found that about 70%

of trigger points correspond to acupuncture sites. The efficacy of acupressure in sickle cell pain has not been reported. Anecdotally, however, some patients with sickle cell pain often report that the application of pressure to the painful area renders the pain more bearable.

PHYSIOTHERAPY

The following physiotherapeutic modalities are often used as an adjuvant in the management of sickle cell pain, but the literature includes no reports on their patterns of use or efficacy.

Thermotherapy

Therapeutic heat applied to a painful area provides temporary analgesia and is one of the oldest forms of analgesic intervention. Therapeutic benefits of heat include increased distensibility of tissues, local and systemic relaxation, and tone reduction (Lehman and de Lateur 1982, 1989; Basford 1988). Heat therapy is ideal for soft tissue inflammation and is contraindicated in areas of decreased sensation or decreased circulation.

Therapeutic heat may be used superficially or deeply. Superficial heat penetrates less than 1.5 cm into tissue and may be administered with hot packs, heating pad, heat lamp, or hydrotherapy. Hydrotherapy allows buoyancy and non-weight-bearing activities. Common devices for hydrotherapy include the whirlpool and the Hubbard tank. The former is used for limb immersion, whereas the latter accommodates the whole person. Besides temporary pain relief, whirlpool therapy is useful for wound debridement and particularly for debridement of the leg ulcers that complicate sickle cell disease (see Chapter 7).

Deep heat penetrates more than 1.5 cm and may be achieved with ultrasound, microwave units, and short-wave diathermy. Ultrasound is the safest modality; and the other two are contraindicated in the presence of metal (e.g., plates, pacemakers) or fluid (e.g., cysts, ascites).

Cryotherapy, the therapeutic application of cold, is used commonly in rehabilitation medicine. Its effects include amelioration of inflammation, reduction in muscle spasm, and temporary analgesia (Lehman and de Lateur 1982, 1989). Cryotherapy may be achieved by the direct application of cold packs or ice massage. It may also be administered via vapocoolant sprays such as fluromethane or ethylchloride. Cryotherapy is contraindicated in anesthetic tissues and in patients with peripheral vascular disease or cold hypersensitivity (Lehman and de Lateur 1982, 1989)

Therapeutic exercises

These exercises include passive or active stretching to improve the range of motion of stiff joints, isotonic or isometric strengthening, and graded general conditioning. They also include training in transfer, ambulation, and coordination. They may be administered at the bedside or in a hospital gym.

BEHAVIORAL THERAPY

Operant behavioral therapy focuses on the behavior generated by the pain experience. Pain is not directly treated; instead, the clinician emphasizes the actions or behaviors of patients and their families. Such therapeutic programs may help patients change certain behaviors so as to improve function. Techniques include increasing physical activity and involving family members in reinforcing healthy behavior and withholding reinforcements of disability and maintenance of the pain behavior. Management usually addresses excessive drug use, pain behavior, reduced activity, lack of social behavior, absence of vocational or recreational activities, and inappropriate family responses.

Salutary results of behavior modification can be achieved by setting goals that are within the patient's capacity. Specific approaches to achieve these goals include homework, modeling, role playing, rehearsal, and graded task management. In this manner success can be measured and reinforced.

Two studies reported that operant behavioral therapy was associated with reduced levels of sickle cell pain. Vichinsky et al. (1982) surveyed 152 adult and adolescent patients at a comprehensive multidisciplinary center. Their data showed that involvement in job, school, and group activities, and family and community relationships, were associated with more effective outpatient management of sickle cell pain. Less social support and less involvement in activities were associated with more frequent hospital visits and higher opioid consumption. Gil et al. (1989) examined pain coping strategies in 79 patients by using a structured interview to assess pain, activity level, and the use of health care facilities during painful episodes. Coping strategies were important predictors of pain and adjustment. Thus, patients who scored high on negative thinking and passivity had more severe pain, were less active, more depressed, and used more health care services during painful episodes than did patients who scored high on coping attempts.

COGNITIVE BEHAVIORAL THERAPY

These methods provide pain relief by acting at the level of the cerebral cortex, limbic system, and reticular formation; that is, they modulate the affective response to painful stimuli (Fields 1987; Fishman and Lascalzo 1987). A multidisciplinary pain management program that used psychotherapy, self-hypnosis, support groups, psychosocial assessment with follow-up, home visits by nurses, and a 24-hour hot line reported that emergency department visits decreased by 58% and hospital admissions decreased by 48% (Vichinsky et al. 1982). Self-hypnosis, biofeedback, relaxation, and cognitive methods have been used to treat the pain of sickle cell disease, as will be discussed below. The effectiveness of any one of these techniques as compared with another or with standard medical therapy remains unknown. Moreover, these strategies provide adjuncts, not alternatives, to medical treatment.

Relaxation methods

Methods such as diversion, imagery, autogenic statements (examples: "I feel quite well"; "My crisis will resolve soon"), progressive muscle relaxation, rhythmic breathing, and meditation are often applied by patients with sickle cell pain; however, controlled studies of their efficacy are lacking.

Biofeedback

Biofeedback treatment (Table III) trains a patient to modify physiologic activity. Variables such as skin temperature and muscular activity are measured and reported to the patient, who attempts to change thoughts or behavior to produce a more quiescent physiologic state. One study (Cozzi et al. 1987) examined biofeedback in sickle cell pain by using electromyography and finger temperature biofeedback in eight children and adolescents during 12 weekly training sessions. Significant physiological changes occurred during the biofeedback procedure, and self-reported headaches, pain intensity, anxiety, and frequency of analgesic use decreased significantly over the 12-week training period. At the six-month follow-up the salutary effects had decreased significantly, which suggests that the technique may be effective only for mild episodes of pain.

Training in biofeedback to increase finger temperature was effective in reducing the frequency of hospitalization for acute sickle cell painful episodes and decreasing the analgesic requirement of a 9-year-old girl (Hall et al. 1992). She resumed regular school attendance, but follow-up training was needed because the patient relapsed to persistent pain one year after the initial intervention.

Thomas et al. (1984) reported a small group trial of combined relaxation, biofeedback cognitive strategies, and self-hypnosis in 15 adults with before and after comparisons. The data showed that emergency room visits decreased by 38%, hospital admissions by 31%, and time spent in the hospital by 50% during the six months after training compared with a previous period. Self-reported benefits included improvements in self-efficacy, mood, and analgesic use, and eight of the 15 patients returned to work or began studies.

Hypnosis and self-hypnosis

Zeltzer and colleagues successfully used self-hypnosis in the management of two adolescent males with sickle cell disease characterized by frequent hospitalization and complicated by narcotic abuse and habituation in one and illicit analgesic and tranquilizer use in the other (Zeltzer et al. 1979; Zeltzer 1986). Hypnosis was induced readily through eye fixation and progressive relaxation techniques. Both patients were described as excellent hypnotic subjects and these simple techniques were sufficient to induce a somnambulistic hypnotic state. Both patients were able to induce verifiable peripheral vasodilation and increased skin temperature during training sessions in self-hypnosis when they were instructed to feel satisfaction of feeling warm and to visualize vasodilation. One patient was monitored for four months and the other for eight months after the training. Emergency department visits decreased from 17 to two and from 37 to one during those periods compared with the previous 12 months, and neither patient was admitted to the hospital during the follow-up period. Opioid use decreased significantly in one patient and was eliminated completely in the other. Secondary benefits encompassed social activity, education, and employment.

ACUPUNCTURE

Co et al. (1979) conducted a placebo-controlled double-blind trial to determine the efficacy of acupuncture in the management of 16 painful episodes in 10 adult patients (Table III). Acupuncture at one pain site was compared to nonacupuncture needling at another (sham) site; two pain sites per sickle cell episode were treated. When acupuncture needling was applied to standard acupuncture sites and "sham" sites, patients' and observers' ratings of pain showed a favorable response for both acupuncture and sham sites, but only the patients' ratings differed significantly between authentic and sham treatments. In that study, however, the two forms of treatment were used during the same episode of pain for each patient, so that the evaluation took the form of a comparison between responses at separate local pain sites during the same painful episode. This approach differs from the other evaluations reported here, where patients or painful episodes were the units of analysis.

SUPPORT GROUPS

The following information about the organization, function, and other issues related to support groups was obtained from the Psychological Research Division of the Duke University/University of North Carolina Comprehensive Sickle Cell Center (Nash et al. 1992).

Purpose of support groups

Support groups have developed from a human need for emotional support in times of stress and crisis. The traditional support provided by family, friends, and community life has greatly decreased in the past 20 years. Meanwhile, the pace of daily life has increased. New stresses—economic, educational, environmental, political, and social—have added to the feelings of isolation and helplessness experienced by many Americans. Because there are no easy solutions, especially for problems or illnesses that are lifelong, many persons are seeking and finding emotional support in groups dedicated to helping people help themselves (U.S. Department of Health and Human Services 1987).

There is evidence that mutual help groups assist people in staying well, speed the recovery of those who are ill, and improve the quality of life in those for whom a full recovery is not possible (U.S. Department of Health and Human Services 1987). Mutual help groups are vital care giving systems that allow interactions among participants and provide them with opportunities to increase social support and knowledge.

The increase in the number of mutual help groups reflects their importance as an alternative means of care. It is estimated that half a million support groups are operating in the United States and providing a wide range of services for more than 10 million Americans (U.S. Department of Health and Human Services 1987). Within the mutual help movement, the African American community has played an active and vital role as evidenced by the number of sickle cell mutual help groups across the United States. Within these groups members are finding support and learning how to cope with an inherited disease that primarily affects the African American community.

Any person who wishes to start a mutual help group or to enhance an existing one should consider several issues. Organizers or leaders should constantly evaluate the needs and goals of the group's members. When starting a mutual help group, organizers should consider location, time, and length of meetings and should focus on development of a belief system to guide group actions and discussion. When striving to conduct a successful group, leaders should focus on developing opportunities for the members to assume the leadership role. The membership should develop a goal and needs calendar that provides specific targets that can be measured monthly. In this way members learn the process of evaluation in a practical manner. Communication between members and between leaders and members becomes crucial for group success. Other factors such as fundraising and publicity about the group's existence and goals may contribute to its effectiveness.

Activities of support groups

The activities of mutual help groups vary. Some groups focus on social activities, while others meet to discuss effective coping strategies for dealing with a problem or illness. The group also provides an excellent network for sharing pertinent information. Members who have a great deal of experience in dealing with a problem or illness can be helpful to those who are just encountering the problem. In addition, mutual help groups may invite speakers or professionals to meetings to increase their knowledge about specific problems or illness. Other groups strive to combine all these activities to effectively meet the needs of members.

One of the most valuable aspects of mutual help groups is the socialization that takes place. As members share information, experiences, and feelings, new friendships are often formed. These relationships become a vital part of a person's support network and may prove very helpful to those experiencing difficult periods in their lives.

Professional involvement in support groups

The study on factors that hinder or promote group formation suggested that successful groups are likely to emerge when professionals assist in their formation or contribute leadership without assuming total control (Nash et al. 1992). Most professionals in these groups tended to be social workers, nurses, psychologists, or other health care professionals. Their knowledge of group development, dynamics, and goal attainment facilitates group formation. In addition, research affirms that groups appear to thrive when professionals assist in their initial formation and gradually move into an indirect, nonauthoritarian role as consultant to group members.

Factors that hinder group formation and development

All groups encounter obstacles as part of organizational and growth processes. Some common barriers cited by the sickle cell mutual help groups in the Duke/UNC study (Nash et al. 1992) are as follows:

- illness or death of members or leaders
- lack of direction within the group
- irregular attendance of group members
- distance to meetings is too far
- dominating and controlling members
- dominating and controlling leaders
- time constraints of group members
- conflicting agendas and priorities.

Factors that promote group success

Although it is expected that all groups will encounter problems, there is no need to let these problems overwhelm the group. Some key factors that may help promote success in mutual help groups are as follows.

- development of a common goal
- member commitment to group goal attainment
- mutual concern and support among all members
- a committed group with the ability and willingness to motivate other members to attend and participate in the group
- an abundance of social activities and/or group projects
- prayer and religious faith.

Source of information

The Duke/UNC Comprehensive Sickle Cell Center collected information on the location and type of sickle cell mutual help groups across the United States and Canada; 158 groups participated in this data collection. The information was published in the national Sickle Cell Mutual Help Directory and distributed in fall 1994. Of these 158 groups, membership was mixed in 76, while 25 groups were for parents; 20 were for adults only; and 17 were for adolescents. Additional in-depth group-level and individual-level information was derived from a 1990–1991 data collection that revealed much variety among group members in income, educational level, and employment. Group leaders tended to be more affluent and to have received more formal education than group members.

The Sickle Cell Mutual Help Group booklets and the National Sickle Cell Mutual Help Directory can be obtained free of charge from the Psychosocial Research Division of the Duke University/University of North Carolina Comprehensive Sickle Cell Center, Chapel Hill, NC 27599, USA (Tel: 919-966-5932; Fax: 919-962-0890).

SPIRITUAL INTERVENTIONS

These interventions include prayer and reading a patient's favorite passage from Scripture or other inspirational readings. Ohaeri et al. (1995) reviewed the psychosocial problems among 170 patients with sickle cell disease in Ibadan, Nigeria, and found that patients frequently resorted to prayers as a method of coping. Pastoral care services should be provided to those patients who derive actual or potential support from spiritual resources (Stiles 1990; Emblen and Halstead 1993). Care providers, chaplains, or social workers can assist patients and families to identify and use temple- and church-sponsored programs that minister to the sick.

OTHER THERAPIES

Recently a variety of unorthodox and unconventional modalities to treat pain have gained widespread acceptance by the patient population (Parris 1997). These include ayur veda, herbal medicine, homeopathy, Native American medicine, Asian traditional medicine, antioxidizing agents, reflexology, rolfing, crystal therapy, therapeutic touch, and oxidizing agents (such as hydrogen peroxide and ozone). Various colleges, institutes, organizations, and societies that provide alternatives to medical care approved some of these modalities, thus enhancing their popularity and giving them a seemingly conventional status. Controlled trials to evaluate their efficacy treating pain in general and sickle cell pain in particular are not available. To clarify the role of these modalities in a scientific manner, the United States government in October 1991 created the Office of Alternative Medicine (OAM) within the National Institutes of Health (NIH) under a special appropriations bill. The involvement at a federal level is a salutary step that will provide unbiased evaluation of these alternative modalities to treat pain.

CONCLUSION

Elander and Midence (1996) reviewed pain management in sickle cell disease and the factors that affect its quality. They indicated that nonpharmacological therapeutic modalities of pain have been applied in a limited way to the management of sickle cell pain, with mixed but generally encouraging results. Nonpharmacologic modalities have the potential to lessen reliance on conventional analgesia and promote greater individual autonomy in pain management. They may not, however, be suitable for everyone and may not be effective for severe episodes of pain or for use during the acute phase.

12

New Therapeutic Modalities

We must all die. But that I can save (a person) from days of
torture, that is what I feel as my great and even new privilege.
Pain is a more terrible lord of mankind than even death itself.
— Albert Schweitzer, 1875–1965

Despite impressive "quantum leaps" in our understanding of the pathophysiology of sickle cell anemia, a specific, safe, and nontoxic curative
therapy has not yet been identified—with the possible exception of bone
marrow transplantation. Nevertheless, the overall medical care of patients
with sickle cell disease in developed countries has improved such that their
life expectancy has almost doubled since 1951 (Platt et al. 1994). At the
present there are at least four major approaches for the treatment of sickle
cell disease: (1) symptomatic treatment, (2) supportive treatment, (3) targeted therapy to special situations, and (4) molecular and cellular therapy
(Table I). This chapter will address the new molecular and cellular modalities for the treatment of sickle cell disease and pain.

PRIMARY MOLECULAR AND CELLULAR THERAPY

PREVENTIVE THERAPY

The goal of preventive therapy is to ameliorate the clinical picture of
sickle cell disease in general and to decrease the frequency and severity of
acute painful episodes in particular. For many years the major goal of primary therapy for sickle cell disease was to identify an antisickling agent that
would prevent or reverse the polymerization of sickle hemoglobin in red
cells. Sodium cyanate inhibited polymerization of Hb S in vitro but was not
beneficial in vivo at levels that provide acceptable toxicity (Stevens et al.
1981b). As was mentioned in Chapter 7, the use of sodium cyanate was
associated with peripheral neuropathy and subcapsular cataracts that prevented its use as an antisickling agent. Although the search for beneficial
antisickling compounds continues, the most promising approach to prevent

Table I
Types of therapy used in sickle cell disease

Symptomatic treatment
  Pain management
  Transfusion for symptomatic anemia
  Antibiotics for infection
Supportive therapy
  Folic acid
  Vaccination
  Penicillin prophylaxis
  Psychosocial support program
  Other modalities
Targeted therapy
  Exchange transfusion/chronic transfusion
    Stroke in children
    Acute chest syndrome
    Hepatic cholestasis (hepatic crisis)
  Iron chelation therapy
  Special approach to surgery and anesthesia
  Other approaches
Primary molecular and cellular therapy
  Preventive therapy
  Curative therapy

the polymerization of Hb S has been the use of compounds that increase the production of Hb F. In recent years, hydroxyurea proved effective in decreasing the frequency of painful crises, and thus renewed interest in the quest for modalities to ameliorate clinical symptoms. The following sections review the status of these attempts.

Induction of fetal hemoglobin (Hb F)

High levels of Hb F have a beneficial effect in patients with sickle cell anemia. Platt et al. (1991) demonstrated a significant inverse correlation between the frequency of painful crises and Hb F levels greater than 4%, i.e., the higher Hb F, the milder the disease. Hb F interferes with the polymerization of Hb S; the higher (and the more pancellular) the Hb F level, the lower the intracellular concentration of Hb S. Exceptions to this rule, however, include some patients with high Hb F level and severe disease, and vice versa (Ballas 1991). Agents that increase the level of Hb F in humans are listed in Table II. Among these, hydroxyurea, used alone, seems to be the least toxic and most effective.

Hydroxyurea. This cell-cycle-specific cytotoxic agent inhibits ribonucleotide reductase. The molecular mechanism(s) by which hydroxyurea increases the production of Hb F is(are) unknown. Possible mechanisms include perturbations in cellular kinetics or recovery from cytotoxicity (Stamatoyannopoulos et al. 1990; Stamatoyannopoulos and Nienhius 1992, 1993), recruitment of early erythroid progenitors, and recruitment of primitive erythroid progenitors (BFU-E) that lead to production of Hb F-containing reticulocytes (F-reticulocytes). Charache et al. (1992) reported that long-term hydroxyurea therapy with maximum tolerated dose (mean dose 21.3 ml/kg), with respect to myelosuppression, raises Hb F to as high as 15 to 20% (mean 14.9%, range 1.9 to 26.3%). In a randomized, placebo-controlled, double-blind study (Charache et al. 1995) among 299 adult patients with sickle cell anemia with three or more painful crises per year, hydroxyurea caused a significant ($P < 0.001$) reduction in the incidence of painful crises, acute chest syndrome, and transfusion requirement. There was no difference between the placebo and hydroxyurea groups in the incidence of death, stroke, and hepatic sequestration. Maximum tolerated doses of hydroxyurea were not required to reduce the incidence of painful episodes. In another, smaller study (Voskaridou et al. 1995) with 25 to 36 weeks of follow-up, hydroxyurea also decreased the incidence of painful episodes in sickle cell-β-thalassemia and increased Hb F levels to nearly 23% ± 7.7 (mean ± SD). Scott et al. (1996) treated children with sickle cell disease with hydroxyurea in an open trial and reported significant decrease in the number of hospitalizations for painful episodes in children who took hydroxyurea

Table II
Agents capable of augmenting
fetal hemoglobin production

Cell-cycle-specific agents
  5-Azacytidine
  Cytosine arabinoside
  Myleran
  Hydroxyurea

Short-chain fatty acids
  Intravenous agents
    Arginine butyrate
  Oral agents
    Isobutyramide
    Phenylacetate
    Phenylbutyrate
    Valproic acid

Recombinant human erythropoietin (rHuEPO)

Combination therapy
  Hydroxyurea + rHuEPO
  Other combinations

for at least one year. Ferster et al. (1996) conducted a single-blind, crossover clinical trial of hydroxyurea administered for six months to 25 children with severe sickle cell anemia. The data of the 22 who could be evaluated showed that treating children and young adults with hydroxyurea is feasible, well tolerated, and significantly improves the clinical course of sickle cell anemia. Although an increase in Hb F seems to be the obvious and logical explanation for the salutary effects of hydroxyurea, other reasons for its beneficial effects include changes in red cell volume, cellular hydration, and the cell membrane, and a direct effect on endothelial cells (Ballas et al. 1989a; Adragna et al. 1994).

Side effects of hydroxyurea are listed in Table III. Toxic effects are dose and time dependent, but can be prevented by careful monitoring of the blood counts every two weeks after starting treatment. The frequency of monitoring blood counts and blood chemistries can be decreased to once every one to two months once the patient is in a stable condition and receiving an acceptable maintenance dose. Anemia is a rare toxic effect of hydroxyurea; in most patients hemoglobin level increased (Charache 1993; Charache et al. 1995). Some patients experienced the idiosyncratic effects of hydroxyurea, but the incidence was similar between those taking placebo and hydroxyurea in the randomized double-blind study reported by Charache et al. (1995). In animal studies, hydroxyurea showed carcinogenic and teratogenic effects. To date, however, no carcinogenic effect has been reported in humans treated with hydroxyurea for polycythemia vera and erythrocytosis due to congenital heart disease (Fruchman et al. 1994; Triadou et al. 1994).

Use of hydroxyurea to prevent painful crises in patients with sickle cell disease has the following limitations: (1) to date, the U.S. Food and Drug

Table III
Side effects of hydroxyurea

Toxic side effects
Myelosuppresion
Leukopenia
Thrombocytopenia
Anemia
Idiosyncratic side effects
Nausea
Vomiting
Pruritus
Skin rash
Hair loss
Effects reported in animals
Carcinogenesis
Teratogenesis

Administration has not approved hydroxyurea for the prevention of crises; (2) the long-term effects of hydroxyurea in patients with sickle cell disease are not known; and (3) some patients do not respond to hydroxyurea. Studies are evaluating methods to identify these nonresponders to improve the selection process for hydroxyurea therapy (Yang et al. 1996). In some patients combining hydroxyurea with other agents that augment Hb F production may be indicated (see below).

Short-chain fatty acids. Butyrate analogs were proposed as potential inducers of Hb F synthesis based on the observation that the normal fetal-to-adult hemoglobin switch does not occur normally in infants who have high plasma levels of α-aminobutyric acid in the presence of maternal diabetes (Perrine et al. 1985). This finding led to the discovery that butyric acid, sodium butyrate, and α-aminobutyric acid inhibit the normal progress of hemoglobin switching in developing animals (Perrine 1988) and stimulate the production of Hb F in adult animals (Constantoulakis et al. 1989). Butyrate seems to exert its effect through sequences near the transcriptional start site to induce the activity of the human γ-globin-gene promoter (McDonagh and Nienhuis 1991; Perrine et al. 1991).

In a small phase I/II study three patients with sickle cell anemia and three patients with β-thalassemia who were treated with intravenous arginine butyrate showed significant and rapid increase in fetal globin synthesis to levels that can ameliorate clinical symptoms (Perrine et al. 1993). These promising results, however, could not be reproduced by Sher et al. (1995). The demonstration of specific neuropathological lesions in baboons receiving extended infusions of butyrate at four-fold the human dose raised safety concerns about the use of butyrate in humans (Blau et al. 1993).

The prolonged use of butyrate is limited because it must be given intravenously and is rapidly metabolized by the liver. These factors prompted efforts to find oral butyrate analogs to induce Hb F. Isobutyramide, a butyrate derivative, has been produced as an oral alternative and has increased Hb F production (Saleh et al. 1995). Sodium phenylbutyrate, an analog of butyric acid, is an investigational drug being used in a phase III trial for the treatment of patients with inherited disorders of the urea cycle (Brusilow and Horwich 1989). One study found that nonanemic patients taking phenylbutyrate had high levels of Hb F (Dover et al. 1992). Moreover, Dover et al. (1994) reported that phenylbutyrate rapidly increased Hb F level in patients with sickle cell anemia. Furthermore, phenylacetate, a metabolite of phenylbutyrate, also increases the production of Hb F in vitro (Fibach et al. 1993). Because butyric acid and its analogs are short-chain fatty acids, other compounds that belong to this category were considered as potential inducers of Hb F; for example, nonanemic patients receiving valproic acid for epilepsy had increased levels of Hb F (Collins et al. 1994). With the exception of arginine butyrate, the analogs mentioned above (isobutyramide, phenylbutyrate, phenylacetate, and valproic acid) are available in oral form.

Available data thus suggest that short-chain fatty acids may play a role in the primary treatment of sickle cell disease by increasing Hb F production. Their precise role alone or in combination with other agents, however, awaits controlled phase III clinical trials.

Erythropoietin. Hematopoietic growth factors such as interleukin-3 (IL3), granulocyte-colony stimulating factor (G-CSF), and granulocyte-monocyte-colony stimulating factor (GM-CSF) can augment Hb F levels in erythroid cell cultures and in experimental animals, but such use in clinical trials has not been reported. Recombinant human erythropoietin (rHuEPO) increases Hb F levels in erythroid cell cultures and in nonanemic baboons and macaques (Al-Khatti et al. 1987; Fibach et al. 1994). The molecular mechanism by which rHuEPO augments Hb F level seems to involve recruitment of F-positive progenitor cells, primarily CFU-E derived from an influx of the more primitive BFU-E compartment. In clinical trials patients with sickle cell anemia who received high doses of rHuEPO along with iron supplementation showed an increase in the percentage of F-reticulocytes and Hb F (Nagel et al. 1993). Rodgers et al. (1993) found that rHuEPO exerts an additive effect when given with hydroxyurea in alternating doses.

Cellular rehydration

As was mentioned in Chapter 4, polymerization of deoxy Hb S creates a vicious cycle by causing cellular dehydration, which increases the intracellular concentration of Hb S and leads to further polymerization. A major mechanism by which water is lost from sickle cells is the Ca^{2+}-activated K^+ channel (Gardos channel). Activation of this channel results in K^+ and water loss from sickle erythrocytes with consequent dehydration. A decrease in the intracellular concentration of Hb S, even small decreases, can slow the polymerization of Hb S to a point where erythrocytes can exit from the capillaries (decreased transit time) before the Hb S polymerizes (increased delay time for polymerization). Hydroxyurea achieves this goal by decreasing the effective concentration of Hb S and diluting it with Hb F, which does not participate in polymerization. Another approach to inhibit polymerization is to rehydrate sickle erythrocytes and restore their normal water content.

Attempts to rehydrate sickle erythrocytes included hypotonic swelling with water loading, vasopressin, and a low-sodium diet (Rosa et al. 1980). Although this approach resulted in cell swelling, decreased Hb S concentration, and decreased sickling, maintaining hyponatremia at dangerously low levels posed practical difficulties. Moreover, Charache and Walker (1981) could not reproduce these findings. Recently, Brugnara et al. (1996) has used oral clotrimazole in a more selective approach to specifically inhibit the Gardos pathway. Five patients treated with 20 mg/kg per day of clotrimazole showed inhibition of the red cell Gardos channel, increase in cell K^+ content, rehydration of red cells, and a very modest increase in hemoglobin levels. Compared to hydroxyurea, however, clotrimazole produced only modest cellular rehydration. Nevertheless, the advent of clotrimazole offers a novel therapeutic approach and warrants a larger long-term clinical trial to determine its efficacy in the primary treatment of sickle cell disease. Furthermore, a combination of hydroxyurea and clotrimazole may produce an additive beneficial effect in ameliorating the clinical symptoms.

CURATIVE THERAPY

Allogeneic bone marrow transplantation

Bone marrow transplantation (BMT) is the only curative therapy now available for sickle cell disease (Kirpatrick et al. 1991). In 1994 there were reports of 42 bone marrow transplantations in Europe (Vermylen et al. 1994) and 5 in the United States (Johnson et al. 1994). After this slow start, another 23 bone marrow transplantations were performed in the United States: Kalinyak et al. (1995) reported one and Walters et al. (1996) reported 22.

Table IV
Outcome of 70 reported patients with sickle cell disease
who were treated with allogeneic bone marrow transplantation

Status of Patient	Belgium	France	USA	Total
Alive	27	14	26	67
Dead	1	0	2	3
Cured	25	13	21	59
Rejection/failure	3	2	5	10
Second transplant	1	1	1	3
Acute GVHD*	9	4	3	16
Chronic GVHD	4	2	1	7
Stable chimerism	0	0	1	1
CNS complications†	0	0	3	3
Total number of patients	28	14	28	70

*Graft versus host disease
†The indication for bone marrow transplantation in these patients was cerebrovascular accidents. They were cured of sickle cell anemia but the neurological complications recurred.

Table IV summarizes the outcome of allogeneic bone marrow transplants in the 70 reported patients with sickle cell disease. Of these, three patients died (4.3%), one of cerebral hemorrhage and two of graft versus host disease. In 10 patients (14%) engraftment was followed by bone marrow rejection; three of these patients (4.3%) had a successful second transplant. Thus, 59 patients (84%) were cured; one patient had stable mixed chimerism with no symptoms. In addition to sickle cell disease, two patients from the United States had other indications for allogeneic bone marrow transplantation: one had acute myeloid leukemia and the other had Morquio's disease. Among the 15 patients from the United States who had stroke before transplant, 11 had sustained engraftment and three of these (27%) had subsequent recurrence of neurological events. This finding suggests that progression of neurological pathology and recurrence of clinical symptoms in the presence of normal rheologic parameters may be due to worsening of the already damaged cerebral vessels by the bone marrow transplantation conditioning program (Kalinyak et al. 1995).

Inclusion and exclusion criteria for eligibility for bone marrow transplantation in children with sickle cell disease are listed in Tables V and VI, respectively. In the multicenter study reported by Walters et al. (1996) only 6% of the patients with sickle cell anemia who were less than 16 years old

Table V
Inclusion criteria for bone marrow transplantation in children with sickle cell disease

Sickle cell disease (sickle cell anemia, sickle cell-hemoglobin C disease, or sickle cell-β-thalassemia)
Age less than 16 years
HLA-identical related donor
One or more of the following:
Stroke or central nervous system event lasting longer than 24 hours
Acute chest syndrome with recurrent hospitalizations or previous exchange transfusions
Recurrent vaso-occlusive pain (two or more episodes per year for several years) or recurrent priapism
Impaired neuropsychological function and abnormal cerebral MRI scan
Stage I or II sickle lung disease
Sickle nephropathy (moderate or severe proteinuria or a glomerular filtration rate 30 to 50% of the predicted normal value)
Bilateral proliferative retinopathy and major visual impairment in at least one eye
Osteonecrosis of multiple joints
Red-cell alloimmunization (two or more antibodies) during long-term transfusion therapy

Source: Walters et al. 1996, with permission.

Table VI
Exclusion criteria for bone marrow transplantation in children with sickle cell disease

Age greater than 15 years

Lack of availability of HLA-identical donor*

One or more of the following:

Karnofsky or Lansky functional performance score <70[†]

Acute hepatitis or evidence of moderate or severe portal fibrosis or cirrhosis on biopsy

Severe renal impairment (glomerular filtration rate <30% of the predicted normal value)

Severe residual functional neurologic impairment (other than hemiplegia alone)

Stage III or IV sickle lung disease

Demonstrated lack of compliance with medical care

Seropositivity for the human immunodeficiency virus

Source: Walters et al. 1996, with permission.
*Patients with HLA-matched related donors with the sickle-cell trait were not excluded.
[†]The Lansky performance score is a measure of functional status in children.

and followed in the collaborating centers met the inclusion criteria for transplantation. By the time the patients were selected, many already had organ damage and severe vasculopathy that might have predisposed them to adverse events after transplantation. The authors hypothesized that bone marrow transplantation early in the course of sickle cell disease might be associated with fewer complications.

The inevitable question is whether bone marrow transplantation is justifiable in sickle cell disease (Platt and Guinan 1996). The death rate among children who undergo bone marrow transplantation for nonmalignant disease is 10% and is unlikely to decrease without a major breakthrough. In contrast, the overall death rate for children with sickle cell disease is about 1% in the first decade of life. Furthermore, hydroxyurea seems to be as effective in ameliorating the symptoms of sickle cell disease in children as in adults, as was mentioned above. Thus, the selection of candidates for bone marrow transplantation must follow stringent criteria associated with meticulous and scrupulous case-by-case analysis of the risk/benefit ratio.

Umbilical cord blood transplantation

Umbilical cord blood transplantation from related and unrelated donors (Gluckman et al. 1997) in children with sickle cell anemia is a possibility in the future. Reports of children with hemoglobinopathy who received umbilical cord transplantation are encouraging. Moreover, ethnic umbilical cord blood banks for transplantation across human leukocyte antigen (HLA) barriers are another future possibility.

Gene therapy

Gene therapy, in simple terms, is the introduction of new functioning genes into healthy or abnormal cells either in vitro or in vivo. One potential approach to curing sickle cell anemia is to introduce a functional β^A-globin gene into hematopoietic stem cells of the affected person to replace the defective β^S-globin gene (Forget 1994). Approaches to achieve the goals of gene therapy in sickle cell anemia include: (1) the transfer of normal β^A-globin genes into hematopoietic cells (gene addition) via retroviral vectors or adeno-associated viruses that have been modified and crippled so they do not become infective; (2) targeted insertion of the transferred gene into the endogenous globin locus by homologous recombination (gene replacement) so that the transferred β^A-globin gene is located in the proper chromosomal environment and expressed at the same level as endogenous β-globin genes; and (3) chimeroplasty or gene repair by targeted mutagenesis that introduces chimeric oligonucleotides composed of DNA and modified RNA residues into stem cells to direct correction of the mutation in the β^S gene (Cole-Strauss et al. 1996).

Gene therapy in sickle cell anemia is limited at the present to transgenic mouse models and to investigational laboratory procedures to determine the most effective and safe method of altering the genetic information in hematopoietic stem cells. Transgenic knockout mouse models of sickle cell anemia (Paszty et al. 1997; Ryan et al. 1997) are currently used to understand the pathophysiology of sickle cell disease and to test new approaches to therapy, including gene therapy. Transgenic mouse technology allows the introduction of exogenous genes into the mouse genome to inactivate mouse genes to produce human disease. Research in this area has advanced at a faster rate than previously expected, and gene therapy soon may be available for trial in selected patients with sickle cell disease.

ILLUSTRATIVE CASE

CASE 12.1

A 24-year-old African American woman was diagnosed with sickle cell anemia at the age of one year after voluntary screening by the family because her older brother had the disease. Major manifestations included a painful episode every four to eight weeks that required treatment in the emergency department or hospital. The pain usually involved her low back and knees, was throbbing, and had an intensity score from 6/10 to 10/10. Mild and moderate episodes of pain were treated at home with ibuprofen or codeine with acetaminophen (Tylenol #3). Severe pain had first been treated with meperidine and later with hydromorphone. Severe crises that required hospitalization lasted up to seven days. Known complications included history of recurrent pneumonia in childhood.

Treatment with hydroxyurea began in 1992, and over six to eight months the dose was gradually increased to a maximum of 2500 mg per day. As shown in Table VII, the anemia improved and the frequency of painful crises decreased significantly to a current rate of fewer than one per year.

Comments on case 12.1

This case illustrates the beneficial effects of hydroxyurea as a treatment to prevent acute sickle cell painful episodes. The frequency of crises progressively and significantly decreased in this patient. The beneficial effects of hydroxyurea may be due to its induction of Hb F production, although other mechanisms are possible. Nevertheless, hydroxyurea is both a carcinogen and a teratogen. This patient has been advised to practice safe sex to avoid becoming pregnant while she is taking this agent. Her health care providers routinely reinforce these facts during follow-up. The long-term effects of hydroxyurea are unknown, so patients should be regularly followed and monitored.

Table VII
Hematological and clinical parameters of case 12.1
before and after treatment with hydroxyurea (HU)

Parameter	Before HU	After HU	
		2 Years	4 Years
Hb, g/dl	8.0	9.8	10.2
Hct, %	22.0	28.8	29.5
MCV, fl	96.0	121	115
MCH, pg	34.0	41.0	39.6
MCHC, %	35.6	34.0	34.5
Retic, %	15.4	6.8	10.0
Platelets, $10^3/\mu l$	537	591	456
WBC, $10^3/\mu l$	15.8	8.6	10.3
Hb F, %	6.1	22.9	24.1
Crisis rate/year	9.0	1.5	0.5

NEW APPROACHES TO ANALGESIA

POTENTIAL NEW ANALGESIC AGENTS

Recent advances in understanding the molecular neurobiology of pain suggest a novel approach to identify new analgesic agents. Potential candidates include: (1) selective inhibitors of cyclo-oxygenase-2 (COX2), as mentioned in Chapter 9; (2) capsaicin analogs that block sensitization of peripheral nociceptors but are not associated with the initial burning pain caused by capsaicin; (3) selective blockers of the N-methyl-D-aspartate (NMDA) receptor and other non-NMDA receptors; and (4) antagonists to bradykinin and other mediators of inflammation (anticytokine therapy).

CELL THERAPY FOR PAIN

The systemic administration of catecholamine (serotonin and norepinephrine) reuptake inhibitors, such as the tricyclic antidepressants, amplifies the activity of endogenous peptides capable of inhibiting the conduction of painful afferent sensory impulses within the central nervous system (Yaksh and Malmberg 1994). A novel approach to increase the concentration of these peptides involves the transplantation of adrenal chromaffin tissue into the subarachnoid space as a new therapy for chronic malignant and non-malignant pain states (Sagen et al. 1991; Winnie et al. 1993). Extensive animal data and limited human data support this hypothesis. The source of adrenal chromaffin tissue can be human organ donors or animals. Bovine adrenal chromaffin (BAC) cells are encapsulated into a permeability-selective membrane prior to implantation in the lumbar subarachnoid space. The encapsulation process allows the flow of nutrients into the donor cells and enables the egress of analgesic peptides and catecholamines into the subarachnoid space of the host. Controlled human trails are in progress in Europe and are pending in the United States

SURFACTANT THERAPY OF ACUTE PAINFUL EPISODES

To date there is no effective treatment to terminate the sickle cell painful episode. Hydroxyurea decreases the frequency of painful episodes, but its effect on the severity, duration, and consumption of narcotic analgesics has not yet been analyzed. Adams-Graves et al. (1997) reported that in a pilot study poloxamer 188, formulated as RheothRx (a nonionic surfactant) seemed to reduce the severity and duration of painful episodes of hospitalized patients with SCD. The role of this agent in shortening painful crises needs further investigation.

The mechanism of action of this agent is not well understood. It is hypothesized that it blocks hydrophobic regions of cells, thus providing a hydrated barrier that seems to block hydrophobic interactions (cell-cell, protein-protein, and cell-protein) in the blood. Consequently there is reduction in blood viscosity, erythrocyte aggregation, adhesion to vascular endothelium, and improvement in microvascular blood flow (Hunter et al. 1990).

Part V

Miscellaneous Aspects of Sickle Cell Pain

13

The Adult "Difficult" Patient with Sickle Cell Pain

Pain is real when you get other people to believe in it.
If no one believes in it but you, your pain is madness or hysteria.
— Naomi Wolf, 1962–

There is no real evil in life except great pain. All others are in
your imagination and depend on the way one thinks of things.
All other evils find their remedy either in time or in moderation
or in strength of mind – reflection, devotion, philosophy can
soften them.
— Marie Marquis de Sevigne, 1626–1696

With the advent of prenatal diagnosis, newborn screening, prophylactic antibiotic therapy, and better general medical care, the number of children with sickle cell disease (SCD) who survive into adulthood is gradually increasing. The clinical picture of SCD changes with age and emergence of chronic complications such as avascular necrosis and leg ulcers. The frequency and severity of painful episodes may increase in many adult patients and lead to physical dependence on and tolerance to opioid analgesics. Unlike children, adults with SCD often lack a supportive environment and face frequent stressors of daily living that lead to depression, isolation, loneliness, and the precipitation of more painful events. A subset of patients with sickle cell disease (about 10–15% of all patients in a given center) are often referred to as "problem" or "difficult" patients. The problems include suspicion of drug seeking behavior, overuse of health care facilities, dependence on opioid analgesics, and evidence of antisocial personality disorder. The patients, however, frequently indicate that some of these problems are the result of negative attitudes by some providers, improper pain management, and delay in initiating analgesic therapy (Ballas and Riddick 1995).

DEFINITION OF TERMS PERTINENT TO OPIOID USE

A major issue that is associated with the "difficult" or "problem" patient pertains to the use of opioid analgesics. Precise definition of the terms related to this subject is important so that health professionals can communicate effectively and avoid making harmful value judgments that may adversely influence patient care. Every patient must be treated with patience, respect, and compassion and given the benefit of the doubt. Sickle cell disease is an incurable ailment that inflicts a heavy toll on the lives of those afflicted, particularly as they get older. Table I defines terms pertinent to this subject (Kanver and Foley 1981; Newman 1983; Stimmel 1983; Payne 1989a,b; Schug et al. 1991).

Physical dependence, addiction, and tolerance may become confused and used interchangeably because these three conditions may occur together in the active drug abuser. Drug-seeking behavior is rare in patients taking opioids under medical supervision, and the incidence of iatrogenic addiction

Table I
Definition of terms pertinent to chronic users of opioid analgesics

Physical dependence
A state characterized by the physiologic need to consume continuously a drug to prevent signs and symptoms of withdrawal

Psychological dependence (or addiction)
A state characterized by an intense craving for the drug and which produces drug-seeking behavior

Drug-seeking behavior
A compulsive and intentional behavioral drive exhibited by patients to obtain and administer narcotics for reasons other than pain relief, usually outside of accepted medical circumstances; it may include manipulation of the medical system, acquisition of drug from other sources, forgery and theft of prescriptions, alleged loss of the drug, sale of prescribed drugs, and unapproved use of other illicit drugs

Drug abuse
Same definition as drug-seeking behavior

Drug misuse
The unintentional use of a drug in a manner other than its accepted one

Habituation
A state characterized by a patient who continues to consume opioids for their desired effects, but does so infrequently enough to avoid physical dependence

Tolerance
A physiologic need to increase the consumption of an opioid to achieve the same effect; it may be associated with physical dependence or habituation

Pseudoaddiction
A syndrome of behavior and attitudes that emerges in patients who are not being provided with adequate analgesics

is small (Pescor 1939; Jiak et al. 1970). Few formal studies have examined the prevalence, incidence, and long-term effects of these complications in sickle cell disease.

CHARACTERISTICS OF THE "DIFFICULT" PATIENT

Patients with sickle cell disease who seem to overuse hospital services and who use large amounts of opioid analgesics create the most difficult management problems for hospital staff and other patients with sickle cell disease. This group is a small subset of those affected, yet they account for most emergency department visits and hospital admissions. Schraeder et al. (1993) have compared the pattern of hospitalization of 39 patients characterized as high users of care with 32 patients characterized as low users during 1991. The high-user group comprised 33% of inpatients with sickle cell disease but accounted for 70% of admissions for acute painful episodes, 96% of hospital days for treatment of acute pain, and 73% of the cost of care. The mean number of admissions was 11.3 per year for the high-user group and 0.8 for the low-user group. The average length of hospital stay was 10 days for high users and 6.9 days for low users. The high-user group was significantly younger in age, poorer, less likely to be employed, less active socially and physically, and had more medical interactions, need for opioid analgesics, and interpersonal strife. To describe these groups, house staff have developed such terms as the "good sickler" or low user and the "bad sickler" or high user. It is from this relatively small group of high users that the medical staff formulate their opinions of drug-seeking behavior. This stereotyping results in inadequate treatment of pain in other sickle cell disease patients. The perception of widespread drug abuse in this patient population hampers appropriately aggressive management of sickle pain with opioid analgesics (Schecter et al. 1988).

Most patients with sickle cell disease who are characterized as problematic are young adult males. In three large studies (Powars et al. 1990b; Baum et al. 1987; Platt et al. 1991) that analyzed use of health services by age and gender, the average frequency for men rose to a peak for patients in their twenties before falling by age 35 years to the lower and more stable level of women. In another preliminary study of 308 patients (Ballas and Riddick 1995), 34 of 45 problem patients (76%) were men with a mean age of 32 years and the remaining 11 patients were women with a mean age of 28 years. Most of the interpersonal problems occurred between the problem patients and female Caucasian members of the nursing staff who were of comparable age. Mortality among the problem patients was high, with

20 deaths (44% of this group) during 15 years of follow-up compared to 36 deaths among 263 nonproblem patients (14%) during the same period.

The pathophysiologic reasons why age and gender affect the frequency of crises are unknown. One possibility pertinent to gender may be that hemoglobin level is higher in males than in females with sickle cell anemia (Ballas et al. 1982). As was mentioned in Chapter 5, hemoglobin levels show positive correlation with the frequency of acute painful episodes (Baum et al. 1987; Platt et al. 1991). Other possibilities may reflect the psychosocial behavior of young men in that they engage in stressful situations or activities that precipitate acute painful episodes. Another possibility, though unlikely, is that young men are more apt to seek medical intervention when in crisis pain than are women.

Understanding the diversity within this subgroup of "difficult" patients may help in formulating the most appropriate plan of management. Thus, the "difficult" patient may belong to any of the following subclasses:

Undertreatment. Pain that is undertreated or managed inadequately can lead to drug-seeking behavior. A patient whose report of pain is not believed may resort to manipulative or exaggerated pain behavior to obtain adequate analgesics. Such behavior is an example of pseudoaddiction that can be construed as evidence of drug-dependency or addiction (Weissman and Haddox 1989).

Secondary gain. Some patients rely on medical services because of social, financial, or psychological problems. They are often admitted but use minimal pain medication, while their other needs are being met.

Convenience. Some patients find it easier to use the emergency department frequently than to make and keep regular outpatient visits.

Maladaptive behavior. In regard to demographics, patients with sickle cell disease might be considered at a relatively high risk for drug addiction. Many reside in inner cities and are socioeconomically disadvantaged compared to the general African American population (Brozovic and Anionwu 1984; Farber et al. 1985). Patients who frequently use health care facilities for painful crisis tend to be young men who might have been exposed to illicit drugs through peers or social contacts. Recurrent attacks of acute pain, chronic pain, and exposure to prescription opioids may also constitute risk factors for addiction (Maruta et al. 1979) that are compounded by the coexistence of adjustment and affective disorders that are more common among adult patients with sickle cell disease than among groups with other types of chronic illness (Midence and Elander 1996).

Despite the above-mentioned risks for addiction, several reports note that addiction among patients with sickle cell disease is the exception rather than rule, although the reports did not specify the criteria applied to detect drug addiction. Only six of 20 clinical research centers that use parenteral opioids to treat painful episodes in children reported addiction as a side effect (Pegelow 1992). Morrison (1991) reported only one case of addiction among 198 children and adolescents with 423 admissions for administration of intravenous opioids. Vichinsky et al (1982) reported an incidence of drug addiction of 3% among 101 patients who received opioid analgesics and noted that another seven patients were drug dependent. Brozovic et al (1986) noted no incidence of iatrogenic drug addiction in 610 patients with sickle cell disease in London. Payne (1989b) reported that 14 of 160 patients (9%) with sickle cell disease demonstrated maladaptive behavior including history of illicit drug use, excessive use of hospital services with discrepancies between pain reports and pain behavior, tampering with drug delivery systems in the hospital, or involvement with the police or the courts through drug-related activities. Ballas and Riddick (1995) noted maladaptive behavior (defined by the use of illicit drugs, recurrent aberrant behavior despite counseling and education) in seven of 308 patients (2.3%) with sickle cell anemia.

The relatively few patients with sickle cell disease who are addicted to opioids or illicit drugs should be considered to suffer from two chronic diseases: sickle cell disease and addiction. O'Brien and McLellan (1996) indicated that addiction is a chronic disorder due to changes in brain pathways caused by the addicting drugs. These changes are chronic and persist after the discontinuation of the inciting drugs. Detoxification is a symptomatic treatment of addiction and not a cure. It cleanses the patients of drugs and withdrawal symptoms but does not address the underlying disorder, and thus is not a curative treatment (O'Brien and McLellan 1996). A single course of detoxification, therefore, is not a guarantee to cure addiction, and the former addict continues to be at great risk of relapse. These facts should be taken into consideration in the long-term management of patients who suffer from sickle cell pain and addiction. The treatment of the latter should not exclude rational management of the former—that is, the administration of opioid analgesics to treat painful episodes may be controlled but not withheld after detoxification.

MANAGEMENT OF THE "DIFFICULT" PATIENT

Approaches to effective management of the "difficult" adult patient with sickle cell disease include identifying the source of the problem and formulating an interdisciplinary plan with intensive counseling, psychiatric evaluation, rehabilitation, and alignment with a drug rehabilitation unit. For the undertreated group, approaches directed to providers should impart a rational basis for the treatment of sickle pain with adequate opioid analgesics as needed.

Managing other subgroups of "problem" or "difficult" patients, especially those associated with maladaptive behavior, is both difficult and time consuming. It requires extreme patience and clear communication. Clinicians should not expect overnight miracles, and desired results usually proceed with a sluggish pace. These patients must not be denied opioid analgesics to treat their pain. Often, despite all efforts, some patients continue to be resistant to all forms of management.

In an effort to manage conflict between nursing staff and "problem" or "difficult" patients, Malloy et al. (1993) conducted a series of educational sessions involving a group of 39 patients who overused the health care system. An issue that surfaced during a session focused on communication skills was the frequency of conflicts between patients and staff. Sources of conflict identified by patients included cultural differences, communication styles, management of pain, and hospital policies. Patients were encouraged to express their feelings and process situations through group discussion. They were taught communication techniques designed to promote understanding and constructive change. The patients enthusiastically received the techniques and have reported some success in using them.

Recognizing that negative staff attitudes and communication styles contribute to escalation of conflicts, two psychiatric clinical nurse specialists offered a series of sessions to assist in avoiding and handling potential conflicts. The sessions focused on exploring the source of conflicts, changing communication patterns, identifying the meaning of behavior, and breaking vicious cycles. Staff participated in creative exercises to facilitate understanding and expression of their feelings about caring for patients with sickle cell disease. They shared and practiced suggestions for resolving interpersonal conflicts and dealing with challenging behaviors. Staff eagerly participated in the exercises and discussion and have begun to apply principles learned and to look more objectively at behavioral issues. To maintain this reported success, however, such sessions ought to be conducted regularly to reinforce newly learned skills and to educate new patients and nurses who join the program.

The following recommended guidelines address the management of problem or difficult patients (Fultz and Senay 1975; Tennant and Uelmen 1980; Hartrick and Pither 1995):

- Keep accurate count of the amount of opioid analgesics prescribed to each patient.

- Set limits of consumption per unit time. It is advisable to prescribe weekly to avoid rapid consumption of large amounts and premature requests for more.
- Designate a specific physician to be the primary care provider in charge of each patient. Having several providers with different treatment plans sends confusing messages to the patient who, in turn, can play off one provider against another.
- Avoid opioid agonist-antagonists that may precipitate withdrawal signs and symptoms.
- Reduce the amount of prescribed opioid analgesic gradually, for example, by one tablet a week or a month, depending on the individual situation.
- Encourage patients to set goals for themselves, for example, a decrease in consumption by 25% within six months. Reinforce good habits.
- Establish an individualized case management plan where the manager coordinates the services needed to address the biopsychosocial aspects of sickle cell disease.
- Encourage patients to enroll in detoxification programs if indicated. However, enrollment in a detoxification program may present problems. Typical substance abuse clinics and programs require abstinence from opioids as a condition for continued treatment. The sickle cell patient may not be able to adhere to this requirement during an acute painful episode.
- Obtain the patient's agreement to a contract that lists the above points, with the understanding that the contract may be revised periodically at the request of either party (Perlman 1988; Burghardt-Fitzgerald 1989). Other items that may be mentioned include: (a) a pledge not to use illicit street drugs; (b) a pledge not to seek prescriptions from physicians other than those mentioned in the contract; (c) an agreement for periodic random urine drug screens to document the use of the prescribed opioids; (d) an agreement to report to the police the loss or theft of opioid medications or prescriptions and to obtain a copy of the police report if replacement is to be requested (however, repeatedly lost, stolen, or destroyed prescriptions will not be replaced); and (e) a pledge to fill opioid prescriptions at one pharmacy.

Issues pertaining to contracts

Treatment contracts designed to set limits are associated with some controversies. Providers must view these contracts as letters of understanding rather than legal documents. Unfortunately, providers who do not recognize this distinction may levy severe and unwarranted punishment on patients who breach certain aspects of the contract. Such contracts are usually reviewed by the legal counselor of the institution where the providers deliver health care. The patient usually does not have a medicolegal advisor review the contract.

The ultimate goal of the contract must be clear. If the goal is to terminate care in an institution or expel the patient from a program then the contract is neither legal nor ethical as it may encourage some providers or ancillary personnel to provoke patients in pain so that they demonstrate antisocial behavior that may justify their expulsion. "Corrective" measures for breach of contract may include withholding prescriptions for a certain period of time, decreasing the amount prescribed, or prescribing nonopioid analgesics until the conflict is resolved. To the contrary, repetitive violation of the contract (more than two times) calls for more interdisciplinary education and counseling to revise the contract and establish a new one. A breach of a contract should not be an excuse to withhold pain treatment in the emergency department or admission to the hospital for patients experiencing acute painful episodes. Maladaptive behavior in a patient with sickle cell disease may often be a cry for help and not a justification for dismissal. Hospitals that ban problem patients from receiving care at their facilities and refer them to other institutions do not solve the problem but export it to others. This approach may prove more costly to the overall health care system. A committed care provider considers a problem patient a challenge rather than a nuisance.

Treatment contracts may be more enforceable if others, in addition to the patient in question, are involved in their construction. These participants include, but are not restricted, to the following:

1. *Persons providing the immediate social support for the patient (e.g., spouse, parents, children).* Pain due to sickle cell disease affects the entire family, so family members should be involved in the development of a pain treatment contract. They can be instructed in the home management of pain and in behavioral modification techniques that the patients can employ to improve their ability to cope with a chronic pain syndrome. In addition, expectations for treatment of pain in the emergency department and during hospitalizations can be solidified among the family, the patient, and the medical staff by involving the family at the inception of a contract.

2. *Other patients with sickle cell disease or patient advocates within the community.* Some patients with sickle cell disease fail to realize that their behavior affects the care administered to other patients. To make them aware of this fact, a pain management contract encourages patients who frequently

use hospital services to become involved in sickle cell and other community programs. These programs can provide social and recreational activities to improve a patient's ability to cope with pain. The involvement of selected patients or patient advocates also ensures that the care outlined in the contract is reasonable and not overly punitive.

3. *The patient's primary physician.* One physician must assume the primary responsibility for the patient's continuity of care both in and out of the hospital and should be the focal point for pain management. As part of the contract, only this physician should write prescriptions for opioids to control pain. Ideally, only one pharmacy should fill these prescriptions to ensure an accurate assessment of the patient's opioid use. The physicians caring for the patient and the pharmacist filling the prescriptions must develop trust that the patient is using these medications judiciously.

4. *A member of the medical staff of the emergency department where the patient is frequently seen.* Patients with pain due to sickle cell disease are infrequently admitted directly to the hospital. More commonly, patients are initially evaluated and treated by emergency department medical staff, who also should be involved in writing the contract for a consistent pain management plan. Thus, a patient ideally consults with one primary care physician, fulfills prescriptions at one pharmacy, and seeks treatment at only one emergency department and hospital.

The goals of a contract should include relief of pain through treatment with opioids, but within the context of a consistent, coordinated plan that includes behavior modification and involvement in social support groups for patients with sickle cell disease. Such support groups often help in improving patient-physician relationships (Butler and Beltran 1993). Moreover, joint sessions with patients (when in their steady state and free of crisis), physicians, and nurses often enhance effective communication and allow setting common and realistic goals for pain treatment. Emergency department physicians and hospital nurses are often surprised how well patients with sickle cell disease look when not in crises and how well they express their feelings about their disease, family, career, and other concerns common to us all.

ILLUSTRATIVE CASES

CASE 13.1

A 34-year-old African American man was referred to our center for psychosocial and medical evaluation. The referral note indicated that he demonstrated drug-seeking behavior with hostile attitude toward providers. Past history included complaints of chronic pain in his hips and recurrent acute painful episodes of mild or moderate severity involving his low back, arms, and legs. The acute attacks occurred at a rate of one every two to three weeks. The chronic pain was described as a dull ache and the acute pain as sharp and throbbing.

He obtained adequate pain relief with oral oxycodone and acetaminophen (Percocet). He was given a prescription for 35 tablets of Percocet per week, which he usually consumed within four days. Because refills were denied, he had to go to the emergency department once or twice per week. Every three to four months he was admitted to the hospital for three or four days for the treatment of for severe pain. Because of his recurrent weekly visits to the emergency department of another hospital, he was viewed and treated as a drug seeker, and adversarial disputes with the staff there led to his expulsion. Similar problems were rapidly developing with the staff of our emergency department.

Medical evaluation indicated that he had sickle-β^0-thalassemia complicated by avascular necrosis of the left femoral head and by recurrent priapism. Psychosocial evaluation revealed that he had a supportive family, was married, had four children, and was self-employed in the painting business. He was a leader in his neighborhood, where he fought the use of illicit drugs among children .

Management included reassurance that he would receive sufficient analgesics to achieve adequate pain relief and decrease the frequency of visits to the emergency department. To that end he consumed 70–80 tablets of Percocet per week. Random determinations of serum acetaminophen showed values below toxic range. His visits to the emergency department decreased dramatically to about one visit per year for prolonged priapism. Later, he tried to set his own limits on use of Percocet, and his consumption often dropped to about 50 tablets per week. His hospital admissions also decreased significantly to about once in three years. In recent years he agreed to try long-acting opioids (controlled-release morphine or oxycodone) with Percocet for breakthrough pain.

Physical medicine evaluations indicated the need to use maneuvers to decrease weight bearing on his hip joints. He received instruction and was advised to use a cane regularly. An orthopedist recommended against surgical intervention but suggested periodic evaluation.

Later he became interested in supporting other patients with sickle cell disease. He was chosen president of a patients' committee that was charged to counsel patients with sickle cell disease and monitor the interaction between patients and providers and resolve conflicts as needed. The committee established ties with the local chapter of the Sickle Cell Disease Association of America and together functioned as patients' advocates.

Comment on case 13.1

This case is a typical example of pseudoaddiction. Undertreatment of pain resulted in "pain-relief" behavior that was misinterpreted as drug-seeking behavior. Undertreatment of pain resulted in frequent visits to the emergency department, unpleasant encounters with providers, anxiety about pain medications, and stressful situations that may have precipitated or worsened painful episodes. Adequate pain management broke the vicious cycle of unpleasant events and restored the patient's self-esteem and feeling of self-worth. Once the need for analgesics was met adequately, he could resume an independent and productive life coupled with a passion to support other patients and advocate their needs. The multidisciplinary approach in the management of this patient was essential in enhancing the quality of care.

CASE 13.2

Our social worker was consulted to resolve a dispute between the nursing staff and a 36-year-old African American man with sickle-α-thalassemia who was hospitalized for an acute painful episode involving shoulders, arms, low back, and legs. He rated his throbbing pain as 10 on the 10-point scale. Pain was treated with meperidine 125 mg i.m. every two hours as needed. Complications of his disease had included avascular necrosis of the left shoulder, leg ulcers, recurrent thrombophlebitis, pneumonia, and priapism. Physical examination revealed a well-developed, muscular young man in moderate distress. His hemoglobin ranged between 11 and 13 g%.

The nursing staff indicated that he demonstrated uncooperative, hostile, and disruptive behavior. He had stable family life and was a contractor of a construction business and was anxious to leave the hospital to resume his duties. It was also mentioned that he was verbally abusive, loud, and demanded medication before it was due. The patient, however, indicated that administration of his pain medication was usually delayed up to 30 minutes.

Further evaluation, discussion, and observation revealed a discrepancy between the time when the injection was given and the time it was recorded; for example, an injection given at 2 P.M. would be recorded at 2:30 P.M. when the nurse returned to the nursing station after lengthy rounds to many patients. Consequently, the patient expected another injection at 4 P.M. but the record indicated it should be 4:30 P.M. Repetition of this scenario escalated the problem, which could have been avoided by giving the medication on a fixed schedule (every 2 hours around the clock) or by PCA. Unfortunately, the patient was discharged before a change could be instituted.

Comment on case 13.2

This case illustrates a series of misunderstandings that may culminate in unrelieved pain, a hostile patient, and a frustrated nursing staff. This patient looked deceptively healthy. He had a hemoglobin level of 11–13 g% and was muscular and well developed. Patients with relatively high Hb level (those with Hb SC disease, sickle-α-thalassemia, or sickle-β$^+$-thalassemia) usually appear to be healthy. The relatively high Hb level, however, increases the blood viscosity associated with Hb S and thus predisposes the patient to vaso-occlusive episodes, especially avascular necrosis.

In our experience, as well as that of others, ethnic tension and friction seem to be most acute between young male patients with sickle cell disease and Caucasian female nurses of comparable age group. In other countries, such as Jamaica, where the nursing staff and patients are of the same ethnic group, the nurses share the patients' fears and concerns and realize that their own families are susceptible to the same disease process, which is of national concern and not limited to a subset of the population.

"Clock-watchers" are neither addicts nor innately hostile. They seek pain relief. This case, along with case 13.1, demonstrates that inadequate pain management is one cause of seemingly aberrant behavior. Avoiding p.r.n. dosing and giving analgesics on a fixed schedule around the clock or by PCA usually prevents unpleasant encounters between patients and providers.

14

Issues Pertinent to Sickle Cell Pain

*President J.F. Kennedy once told Billings that he would trade
all his political successes and all his money just to be out of pain.*
—Ralph G. Martin, *Seeds of Destruction*, 1995

Pain is not good without an audience.
—Chinese Proverb

As an inherited chronic illness characterized by recurrent and unpredictable acute painful episodes, sickle cell disease affects all aspects of daily living. This chapter will review certain issues that have an impact on sickle cell pain such as the interaction of patients with family, friends, providers, the health care system, and employers. Some of these issues are stressors that can have a negative effect on sickle pain whereas others can help patients cope with their disease and its sequelae.

PATIENT'S RIGHTS

Patients with sickle cell disease, like any other patients, have rights, and all hospitals should endorse a patient's "bill of rights."* Compliance with these rights contributes to effective care. Care providers should deliver pain management with an overriding concern for their patients, and, most importantly, recognition of their dignity as human beings. A modified version of the American Hospital Association's "Patient's Bill of Rights" (1993) should be conveyed by providers to all patients, including those with sickle cell disease. Patients have the right to:

- considerate and respectful care with recognition of their personal dignity;
- have their property treated with respect;
- confidentiality of their records in compliance with legal requirements;

---

*Legislation for a *pain* patient Bill of Rights is currently being considered by the California State Congress.

283

- be fully informed in advance of any change in the care or service provided to them and that may affect their well-being;
- participate in planning care and services or changes in care and services unless they are judged incompetent;
- obtain from their certified provider complete, current information concerning their diagnosis, treatment, and prognosis in terms they can reasonably be expected to understand. When it is not advisable to give such information to the patient, the information should be available to an appropriate person acting on the patient's behalf;
- receive from their certified provider information to relevant to giving informed consent prior to the start of any procedure or treatment. Such information shall include the medically significant risks associated with any procedure and probable duration of incapacitation. Where medically appropriate, alternatives for care or treatment should be explained to the patient;
- refuse any and all treatment, to the extent permitted by law, and to be informed of any of the medical consequence of such action;
- consideration of privacy concerning their medical care program, limited only by state statutes, rules, regulations, imminent danger to the patient or others;
- reasonable continuity of care;
- be informed of anticipated termination of service by the provider or of plans to transfer services to another provider;
- be advised if the clinician, hospital, clinic, etc., proposes to engage in or perform human experimentation affecting care or treatment. Patients have the right to refuse to participate in such research projects;
- voice grievances about care and services furnished by the provider (or services not furnished) without discrimination or reprisal for doing so. A grievance procedure should be provided to each patient on admission.

PATIENT'S RESPONSIBILITIES

The flip side of rights is responsibilities (Ballas et al 1996). Patients should:
- provide accurate and complete information about their disease, hospitalization, emergency room visits, medications, and other matters relevant to their health;
- treat their providers and ancillary personnel with respect;
- comply with instructions related to services and products provided;
- cooperate with all personnel (in the clinic, office, emergency depart-

ment, hospital) and ask questions if they do not understand the information or instructions given to them;

- participate in the planning of their care and services as outpatients;
- inform the clinic or office when they will not be able to keep an appointment;
- provide information and make arrangement (e.g., obtain referrals) for payment for the services rendered by their care provider;
- understand the management of pain and the need for judicious use of opioid analgesics;
- understand the importance of establishing a trusting environment between themselves and their health care providers.

COST OF CARE

Sickle cell disease can be very costly given its chronicity, recurrent hospital admissions for acute painful episodes, surgical and nonsurgical treatment of complications, use of intensive care facilities, and multidisciplinary approach to management. One report (Ballas 1992a) used six indicators to analyze the cost of health care for adult patients with sickle cell anemia: (1) hospital admissions, (2) attending physician and consultation fees, (3) clinic visits, (4) accident-and-emergency department visits, (5) cost of diagnostic procedures (e.g., laboratory, radiography, scans) and consultations for outpatients, and (6) cost of prescriptions. At 1991 rates, the total annual charge for the care of an adult sickle cell patient was about $112,350. Given that the average life span of patients with sickle cell anemia is 42 years for men and 46 years for women (Platt et al. 1994), the total charge per adult male patient would be about $2,696,400 for 24 years (between the ages of 18 and 42 years) and about $3,145,800 for a female patient. These figures do not consider the cost of care in childhood or that many patients are unemployed, disabled, or dependent on welfare and social security benefits. Moreover, hospitals, physicians, emergency departments, and laboratories receive only a fraction of the charges mentioned above in reimbursement, which discourages hospitals and physicians from routinely and regularly taking care of these patients.

Geographic differences in the pattern of hospital use and costs for patients with sickle cell disease have been reported. Davis et al. (1997) used data for 1989 through 1993 from the National Hospital Discharge Survey to estimate that in the United States there are about 75,000 hospitalizations per year of patients with sickle cell disease. The average direct cost per hospitalization (in 1996 dollars) was $6300, with a total direct annual cost of $475 million. In 66% of hospital discharge records, one of several government programs was listed as the expected principal source of payment.

Woods et al. (1997) analyzed the pattern of hospital use and costs for adult patients with sickle cell disease in Illinois during calendar years 1992 and 1993. About 97% of hospital admissions were for painful crisis, and 4% of the patients accounted for almost 25% of hospital admissions. Total hospitalization charges were more than $59 million.

Yang et al. (1995) emphasized the cost effectiveness of comprehensive care of sickle cell disease by comparing the costs to the health sector of comprehensive and episodic health care for their patients during calendar year 1989. There were major differences in the pattern of utilization and in health care costs among sickle cell patients who attended the Comprehensive Health Care Clinics and those who did not. Patients not using these clinics, although they accounted for only 33.5% of the total patients, constituted 71.4% of visits to the emergency department and 42.3% of hospital admissions. Patients enrolled in the Comprehensive Health Care Clinics used emergency departments and hospitals less frequently ($P \leq 0.6005$) and were responsible for significantly less health care cost in each category ($P < 0.03$). Total health care costs billed in 1989 were $1,494,584. Of these, $657,737 (44%) were collected. Fifteen percent of patients were responsible for 77% of the total health care costs related to sickle cell disease.

Thus, finding a cure for sickle cell disease may be cost effective. The charge for bone marrow transplantation (1991 estimate) is about $200,000. A successful bone marrow transplantation in childhood will generate substantial total savings and result in a healthy, productive individual. The cost of gene therapy, should it become available in the future, is unknown at present. We may speculate, however, that once gene therapy has been perfected, it may also generate substantial savings in the overall cost of health care delivered to patients with sickle cell disease.

BARRIERS TO QUALITY CARE

Despite recent advances in the treatment of sickle cell anemia, the quality of patient care is far from ideal. The comprehensive management of sickle cell disease, particularly in adults, raises certain difficulties. Adult patients often feel they are not believed, respected, or taken seriously, and that they are taken for granted, neglected, and abandoned. Health care providers and the medical system often fail to provide adequate relief when dealing with a patient's complaint of pain in general and sickle cell pain in particular. In recent years, standards for the management of acute pain and pain related to terminal cancer (Carr et al. 1992; Jacox et al. 1994) have been published. These manuals are good reference sources for practitioners treating these conditions. They also provide information regarding the appropriate use and monitoring of nonopioid and opioid analgesics. These manuals do not, however, consider the specific issue of the management of sickle cell pain. In contrast to conditions producing acute pain or to a disease such as cancer that generates chronic pain of short duration, the medical management of pain in patients with sickle cell disease poses unique problems because these patients face many disadvantages (Table I). Factors responsible for the generation of these disadvantages are complex and may be related to issues manifested by patients, by care providers, and by the health system as described below.

PATIENT-RELATED ISSUES

Patients with sickle cell disease often do not convey their true feelings about their management for fear of not receiving adequate treatment for pain. Those who do, however, may be considered as "problem" or difficult patients. Patients know that their conduct in seeking various avenues to achieve pain relief is often stereotyped as "drug-seeking behavior" by some care providers. The patients, however, consider their conduct as "pain-avoidance behavior" and believe that health care providers treat them with contempt and resentment. Many patients become depressed, afraid, angry, aggressive, and develop a love-hate relationship with their providers (Ballas

Table I
Barriers to effective management of patients with sickle cell disease

Sickle cell disease is inherited, chronic, and usually incurable.* It involves frequent and unpredictable attacks of acute pain that often require treatment in the emergency department or hospital

Differences in the sociocultural background between patients and health care providers

Heavy use of opioid analgesics by some patients

Failure by health care providers to distinguish between addiction, dependence, and tolerance

Overemphasis by some providers on the addictive effects of opioid analgesics

Lack of continuity of care in some institutions

Lack of adequate insurance coverage for most patients

A prevalent negative attitude among providers toward patients with sickle cell disease

Psychosocial factors as obstacles to effective management

*Cure has recently been reported after successful bone marrow transplantation in selected patients.

1990b). As a result, patients do not trust providers and the medical establishment at large.

Nevertheless, patients with sickle cell disease are not as active or as vocal as other groups of patients with chronic disease (such as cystic fibrosis, cerebral palsy, multiple sclerosis) in promoting their cause at local, state, and national levels. Many do not know their rights as citizens and as patients with a chronic disability. They tend to *react* to conflicts and disputes rather than *act* on them. Thus, a patient who perceives ill-treatment and provocation by a provider may react by demonstrating aggression, belligerence, foul language, and physical threats rather than by documenting the details of the episode and filing a complaint to appropriate personnel. Whenever a dispute arises between a patient and a provider the latter has the advantage of documenting his or her point of view in the patient's chart in a way that conveys the unacceptable behavior. Patients have only their recollection of the details of the episode, which can fade with time should the dispute culminate in future litigation. Patients should organize their efforts and channel the energy of their frustration into constructive pursuits. One approach includes reporting such episodes to support groups and community advocates. The latter may counsel providers and institutions in an effort to resolve the conflict and prevent future recurrences. Providers should avoid provocative behavior because many patients are extremely perceptive to insensitive remarks, body language that belies lack of interest, and disrespect. Moreover, documenting and recording such episodes of conflict may reveal hidden trends practiced by providers and institutions in treating patients with sickle cell disease. Such documentation, for example, revealed that one hospital expelled about 25 patients with sickle cell disease from its program, but did not take similar action against other groups of patients (Brandon and Brandon, personal communication, 1997). Community advocates are an important resource for educating patients about their rights, as will be discussed below.

PROVIDER-RELATED ISSUES

Although providers and institutions deny any negative attitude toward patients with sickle cell disease, their practices indicate otherwise (Ballas 1996). One survey of hospital staff, for example, showed that sickle cell patients were perceived to be opiate dependent twice as often as were other pain patients (Waldrop and Mandry 1995). Techniques often used by providers to avoid patients with sickle cell disease include, but are not restricted, to the following.

The blunt technique

A physician may tell patients in a straightforward, candid manner: "I do not see patients on Medical Assistance." or "I do not see patients with sickle cell disease. Try Dr. X or Dr. Y."

The selective technique

According to this method, providers retain those patients who have a mild clinical course (no more than one crisis per year) with few complications and who have "good" insurance coverage such as Blue Cross or Blue Shield. In this situation the prejudice is hidden behind a group of well-to-do patients who consume little or no opioid analgesics and who usually are employed and from middle-class families. Most patients (over 50%) in programs that use this technique have milder forms of sickle cell syndromes such as sickle-β^+-thalassemia and Hb SC disease. In an unbiased program in the United States, these diagnoses comprise less than 30% of the patients, while the remaining 70% suffer from sickle cell anemia, the most severe form of the disease.

INSTITUTIONAL AND SYSTEM-RELATED ISSUES

Race and income

Recently, Gornick et al. (1996) reported that race and income had substantial effect on mortality and use of medical services among Medicare beneficiaries. Thus, in the case of ischemic heart disease, for example, the rates among blacks for both angioplasty and coronary bypass grafting were significantly lower than those for whites, although both groups were equally affluent and had similar hospital discharge rates. Gay and Ballas (personal communication) indicated that the effects of race and income on the quality of care are not limited to Medicare beneficiaries but are also applicable to other categories of patients. Thus, the disparity in the quality of service between whites and blacks persists at the other end of the scale where Caucasians with Medical Assistance receive relatively better care than their African American counterparts. The situation is even worse for African American patients with sickle cell disease who use opioids. Other categories of patients with different disease processes and variable opioid consumption fill the rest of the spectrum, with a quality of care score between 2 and 9, and always maintain the differential service rendered to white patients.

It is unfortunate that a disease like sickle cell anemia that links molecular biology to clinical and psychosocial medicine is the target of so much circumlocution. We are inclined to conclude that providers have this negative attitude because most of the patients are minorities who are dependent on Medical Assistance, who do not pose a medicolegal threat to providers, and whose care is not cost effective. It is ironic that the first molecular disease that paved the way to gene therapy is also the first to be abandoned by its own specialists and hit hard by negativism and economic constraints (Ballas 1996a).

Medicolegal impediments

Prescribing opioids for chronic nonmalignant pain is controversial (Shealy 1997). The controversy is the result of the interaction between physicians who manage pain and officials who try to enforce drug abuse and drug diversion laws. Medical licensing agencies scrutinize physicians' patterns of prescribing these agents. Disciplinary action is often taken against physicians who prescribe inappropriate amounts of opioids for patients with chronic benign pain. In some states, federal enforcement agencies have imposed multiple-copy prescription programs (MCPP) to scrutinize the use of opioids. Given these medicolegal issues and concern about regulatory scrutiny, many physicians tend to undertreat malignant and nonmalignant pain by reducing the dose and quantity of opioids or by choosing a controlled substance in a lower schedule (Weissman et al. 1991; Angarola and Joranson 1993; Hill 1993).

PATIENT ADVOCACY

The literal meaning of advocacy is the act of pleading for intercession—speaking or writing in support of a cause. An advocate is a pleader in favor of something or a person who defends, vindicates, or espouses a cause by argument. Functionally, patient advocacy is a strategy exercised by certain persons to influence the policies that shape the delivery and the quality of care in the community. The ultimate goal of advocacy is to consider patients with sickle cell disease as partners in their own health care and acknowledge their right to make decisions and choices regarding their lives.

During hospitalization, advocacy is extremely important to patients because they are confronted with issues such as physician-patient relations, appropriate medical diagnosis, pain management, and discharge planning. During these times of ill health, patients are unable to appropriately address these concerns without experiencing undue stress, which directly affects their disease. The role of the advocate is to resolve these issues to allow the patient hospitalization with little or no stress.

Achieving self-sufficiency and being treated with respect are major concerns to a patient with sickle cell disease. If they are employed, they may be fired from their job because of frequent absenteeism due to their illness. If they pursue higher education and can't keep up with the workload, they may be forced to drop out. If they try to get medical or life insurance coverage, they often have to pay higher premiums and stay well for a defined period of time, or they are dropped due to their illness. Such situations require the intervention of advocates to resolve these conflicts fairly.

Table II outlines the methods advocates use to achieve their goals. The process is time consuming and may be successful with some but not all patients. Educating patients by providing detailed information is a major first step and should include information about their disease, their rights and responsibilities, their rights as disabled employees, and the workings of the health care system. Well-informed patients can then empower themselves through effective communication with providers, insurers, employers, and legislators. Such patients will be able to identify tasks that they can perform well and then can act effectively. Given the proper chance via advocacy, patients with sickle cell disease could become self-advocates, which would enable them to break the cycle of dependency and maintain effective control over their lives.

Table II
Role of advocates in sickle cell disease

Information
    Provide patients with detailed information about their:
        Disease
        Rights
        Responsibilities
        Rights as employees (Americans with Disabilities Act)
Empowerment
    Train patients to communicate effectively with:
        Care providers
        Employers
        Managed care companies
        Legislators
Guidance
    Help patients to:
        Identify their points of strength
        Become advocates for themselves
        Act on specific tasks they choose

NEGLECT BY THE MEDICAL PROFESSION AT LARGE

Several seminal articles about various aspects of sickle cell disease have been published in recent years (Vichinsky et al. 1990; Platt et al. 1991; Castro et al. 1994; Charache et al. 1995; Walters et al. 1996). We would expect that such an illness would be of great learning and teaching value, because almost all subspecialties in medicine could find a model of pathophysiologic events that affect their organ of interest. Unfortunately, this is not usually the case, and apathy prevails among health care providers toward patients, particularly adults, with sickle cell disease (Ballas 1996a).

CAREER AND EMPLOYMENT

Sickle cell disease has a negative impact on career development, employment, and work history. Despite anecdotal reports of exceptional success stories, for example, patients who became scientists (Ballas et al. 1995b) or physicians, most of those affected are dependent on Medical Assistance and the Social Security system (Ballas 1990b). The literature contains sparse data about career and employment in sickle cell disease (Evans 1994; Brandon 1995).

Patients with sickle cell disease are disadvantaged regarding employment. To give one specific example, aviation authorities exclude persons with sickle cell disease from flight deck duties (Hull 1988; Evans 1994). Factors such as physical stress, extremes of temperature, hypoxia, and dehydration can precipitate acute painful episodes (Franklin and Atkin 1986). Chronic complications of sickle cell disease exert a negative impact on employment. Persistent leg ulcers can interfere with regular work attendance (Franklin and Atkin 1986). Avascular necrosis of the femoral heads may restrict lifting and climbing and such restriction has been recommended for patients with hip replacement for this complication (Archibald et al. 1990). Reduced visual acuity due to retinopathy, cerebrovascular accidents with residual weakness, and progressive organ damage with age may negatively affect work and limit employment opportunities (Mann 1981; Franklin and Atkin 1986).

Brandon (1995) reported that young adults were fearful that their health would not allow them to participate in normal adult activities. Among 100 patients with sickle cell disease interviewed, 98 indicated that their health interrupted their college education and prevented them from finding and maintaining a full-time job (Brandon 1995). A major fear among patients with sickle cell disease is the probable loss of their job due to frequent absenteeism caused by recurrent crises. This fear constitutes a major stressor in precipitating painful episodes and interrupting coping skills.

In an effort to determine the pattern of employment among patients with sickle cell disease, Abrams et al. (1994) interviewed 30 patients living in North Carolina. Fifteen (eight men and seven women) reported employment in occupations including teaching, nursing, secretarial, sales, social work, managerial, postal work, public safety, machine operation, assembly work, construction, and general labor. Of the 15 unemployed patients, 13 reported past employment. The total group averaged 14.5 years of employment (range one month to 38 years). Twenty patients reported an annual income less than $15,000. Obviously, more data are needed about the pattern of work history among patients with sickle cell disease. Such information may be of value in counseling adolescents and young children and guiding them regarding avenues of employment. In the United States, advocates should make patients and their employers aware of the Americans with Disabilities Act, which defines the rights of disabled/impaired persons in the workplace. Such awareness may lessen the stress generated by fear of losing a job.

LITIGATION

Recently, the number of medical litigation cases involving patients with sickle cell disease has increased significantly (Vichinsky and Lubin 1996). Although this increase may be due to heightened community awareness of legal avenues to address concerns, the impact of managed care designed to limit costs may be a contributing factor. Thus, rationing of health services, especially in cities, decentralization of care, and reduced access to specialty care have led to significant curtailment of comprehensive care for patients with sickle cell disease. Vichinsky and Lubin (1996) noted that hematologists specializing in the care of patients with sickle cell disease frequently have been approached to function as expert witnesses to resolve disputes pertinent to quality of care issues for patients with sickle cell disease. The malpractice cases reviewed fell into six categories as follows:

- lack of evaluation or intervention for fever resulting in death from bacterial sepsis;
- failure to recognize or promptly treat CNS complications resulting in permanent neurologic deficit or death;
- inappropriate use of analgesics resulting in death;
- failure to identify or appropriately treat acute chest syndrome;
- incorrect prenatal diagnosis;
- failure to recognize transfusion reactions resulting in death.

Vichinsky and Lubin (1996) suggested that information regarding litigation in sickle cell disease could serve a useful purpose in improving the delivery of health care to patients. They recommended: (1) establishing a central agency of litigation cases; (2) providing a medical based advocacy group to patients, families, or attorneys considering litigation; (3) offering education programs to health care providers where adverse outcomes have been identified; and (4) organized efforts to prevent restriction of necessary health care intervention and to encourage outcome analysis in managed care settings.

Epilogue

Patients with sickle cell disease are an unfortunate group caught in a tangled network of complexities. They must cope not only with a morbid disease characterized by pain and suffering but with numerous barriers at every level of human interaction. Most important among these are an inadequate health care system and providers (including many hematologists) inattentive to the unique nature of sickle cell pain. In addition, some providers stereotype patients as malingerers and addicts. At least three factors contribute to the neglect of sickle cell pain and its related issues, as summarized here.

DISPARITY OF FOCUS BETWEEN HEMATOLOGISTS AND PATIENTS

The discovery that sickle cell anemia is a molecular disease generated a beehive of activity in bench research that attempted to elucidate the pathophysiology of vaso-occlusion and to identify methods to prevent it. This commendable feat aimed for primary therapy and culminated in treatment with hydroxyurea in the 1990s. Despite the availability of this primary therapy, patients and their families remain focused on pain, which is a consequence of vaso-occlusion and is the major symptom of the disease. Although potent analgesics were available in the 1950s and 1960s, no attempts were made to conduct clinical research on pain. As a result, undertreatment of pain in this disease is widespread. The natural history study sponsored by the National Institutes of Health in the late 1970s was a welcome endeavor that focused on the longitudinal progression of sickle cell disease.

INAPPROPRIATE MANAGEMENT OF SICKLE CELL PAIN

Evidence of inappropriate management of sickle cell pain and stereotyping of patients as drug seekers abounds in the literature. Hematologists not only were preoccupied with the pathophysiology of vaso-occlusion but unfairly described sickle cell pain and its management. The following quotations from hematology reference books illustrate this point.

> Patients with painful infarctive crises require analgesics, but because these crises may recur, there is a risk of addiction. If this has occurred, the patient may pretend to have a crisis solely to obtain opiates. (Williams et al. 1977)
>
> Narcotic addiction, a major complication of sickle cell anemia, is more easily prevented than treated by close surveillance of narcotic usage. (Wintrobe et al. 1981)
>
> Management of the pain of infarctive crises represents a particularly difficult problem for the physician. . . . [I]t is often necessary to use narcotics. Like patients with other diseases associated with chronic or recurrent pain, many patients with sickle cell disease have become addicted to narcotics, and those who have not may become so. (Williams et al. 1983, 1990)

Understandably, physicians, house staff, students, nurses, and others who read these books received the impression that patients with severe sickle cell disease are all potential drug addicts. Also, these quotations suggest the withholding of narcotics to treat pain lest the patient becomes an addict. This approach may have contributed to the negative attitude toward patients with sickle cell disease in urban hospitals and their emergency departments.

LACK OF AWARENESS IN THE IVORY TOWER

In 1989 I submitted a paper to the *New England Journal of Medicine* titled "Treatment of Pain in Sickle Cell Disease." It was rejected based on the comments of one reviewer who indicated that my description of the way patients are treated "has certainly not been [his/her] 20 years experience in treating sickle cell anemia patients, participating in the training of medical students and house officers, and sharing experiences with physicians all over the country, many who are part of comprehensive sickle cell centers. . . . [I]f true, [this description] reflects poorly on the quality and training of health care providers in that institution." I changed the title of the paper to "Treatment of Pain in *Adults* with Sickle Cell Disease" to ensure it did not fall in the hands of the same reviewer (whom it seems was a pediatrician), and submitted it to the *American Journal of Hematology,* where it was readily accepted (Ballas 1990b). Following its publication I received numerous calls and letters of support from the United States and abroad congratulating me for addressing a difficult subject in an open forum. This article opened the sluice-gate for several publications by others, listed in bibliography of this book, which indicated the magnitude of the problem, especially in the adult population.

I mention this anecdote for one purpose: the prestigious reviewer was *not* aware of what patients with sickle cell disease endure! Had he or she been aware, this reviewer might have used his or her influence to address sickle cell pain and its management in a serious and effective manner and hasten a rational approach to this problem.

I hope this book will enhance the awareness of providers regarding the complexities and unique nature of sickle cell pain. A goal is to bridge the gap between bench and bedside hematological research. A union of these approaches could elucidate the events that occur beyond vaso-occlusion and identify novel approaches to pain relief. This book may also bridge a gap between pain medicine at large and sickle cell pain. Researchers in pain medicine may find that sickle cell pain represents a unique model of lifelong recurrent acute pain and that its mechanisms of pain transmission, modulation, and perception are worthy of study.

Appendix A

Sickle Cell Knowledge Self-assessment for Medical Personnel

This appendix employs a question and answer format to reinforce relevant information about sickle cell pain. Medical students, residents, fellows, nurses, social workers, medical staff, and practicing physicians will find it informative and useful. The self-assessment covers the types of questions commonly encountered in: (1) the delivery of care to patients with sickle cell disease; (2) an academic environment on teaching rounds for students and house staff; and (3) clinical problem solving in the office. Questions are generally phrased in a way that provides the general picture so that the interested reader must locate the original material described in Chapters 1 through 14 to continue the educational process. Many of the questions have been designed to reflect real clinical situations in the office, emergency department, or hospital.

Although several textbooks in hematology as well as a large number of computerized learning systems in medicine are available, none of them has delved into the details of sickle cell pain and related issues. Moreover, these methods have not yet surpassed the effectiveness of Socrates' conversational approach to education in the form of question and answer dialogues in both academic and clinical settings.

ANSWERS TO QUESTIONS ARE LISTED IN APPENDIX B
(PAGE 315)

QUESTIONS 1–27: ONE BEST ANSWER

Directions: Each of the numbered questions or incomplete statements is followed by lettered suggested answers or completions. Select the *one* that is *best* in each case (circle letter).

1. Nonsteroidal anti-inflammatory drugs (NSAIDs) exert their analgesic effect by:

    A. Decreasing the synthesis of arachidonic acid due to inhibition of phospholipase.
    B. Decreasing the synthesis of prostaglandins due to inhibition of lipooxygenase.
    C. Decreasing the synthesis of prostaglandins due to inhibition of cyclooxygenase
    D. Altering pain perception at the level of the central nervous system by binding to the m receptors.

2. A 28-year-old male patient with sickle cell anemia was admitted to the hospital for elective cholecystectomy. His hemoglobin was 10.5 g%, WBC 12,000/ml, reticulocyte count 12.0%, and platelet count 350,000/ml. The surgeon consulted you to clear this patient for surgery. Your history and physical exam indicated that the patient had been taking ibuprofen (Motrin) 800 mg p.o. q8h p.r.n. The last dose was taken two hours before you saw the patient. Your advice was:

    A. Go ahead with the surgery right away as there are no contraindications for surgery.
    B. The patient may have surgery while receiving platelet transfusion.
    C. Postpone surgery for 10 days.
    D. Postpone surgery for a period of time equal to five half-lives of ibuprofen (Motrin), i.e., 12–24 hours.

3. All of the following analgesics are pure opioid agonists except:

    A. morphine sulfate
    B. hydromorphone (Dilaudid)
    C. codeine
    D. nalbuphine (Nubain)

4. The reticular formation is:

    A. the substantia gelatinosa of the dorsal horn of the spinal cord.
    B. the medial spinothalamic tract.

C. a collection of neurons in the core of the brain stem concerned with awareness and behavior.
D. the trigeminothalamic tract.

5. The pain associated with the acute sickle cell painful crisis is best described as:

A. nociceptive
B. neuropathic
C. deafferentation
D. psychogenic

6. Individuals with HbH (β_4) disease have the following α-globin genotype:

A. $--/\alpha\alpha$
B. $-\alpha/-\alpha$
C. $-\alpha/\alpha\alpha$
D. $--/-\alpha$

7. A screening test for the sickle gene such as the "sickle cell prep" is positive in all of the following diagnoses except:

A. sickle cell anemia
B. sickle trait (AS)
C. Hb SC disease
D. Hb CC disease

8. One of the following hemoglobins is nonfunctional:

A. Hb A2 ($\alpha_2\delta_2$)
B. Hb F ($\alpha_2\gamma_2$)
C. Hb S ($\alpha_2\beta^S_2$)
D. Hb Bart's (γ_4)

9. One of the following pathogens is more commonly associated with osteomyelitis in sickle cell anemia than the others:

A. *Salmonella typhimurium*
B. *Streptococcus pneumoniae*
C. *Escherichia coli*
D. *Clostridium welchii*

10. Acute sickle cell painful episodes may involve the following anatomic sites except:

    A. long bones and joints
    B. jaw
    C. chest
    D. abdomen
    E. none of the above

11. All of the following compounds may be given orally except:

    A. pentazocine (Talwin)
    B. hydromorphone (Dilaudid)
    C. nalbuphine (Nubain)
    D. methadone (Dolophine)

12. A true statement about the opioid antagonists naloxone and naltrexone is:

    A Both may be given parenterally.
    B. Both may be given orally.
    C. Naloxone may be given orally but naltrexone may be given parenterally.
    D. Naltrexone may be given orally but naloxone may be given parenterally.

13. A 50-year-old woman presents with easy bruisability and bleeding after minor trauma. She has been taking piroxicam (Feldene) 20 mg orally every day for the past three weeks for an arthritic condition. Physical exam shows several petechiae over her extremities and the abdomen. Lab data show normal coagulation profile except for prolonged bleeding time. She was advised to discontinue taking Feldene. The time required for restoration of normal hemostasis after discontinuation of piroxicam is:

    A. 1 day
    B. 3 days
    C. 5 days
    D. 7–10 days

14. All of the following medications may be given parenterally except:

    A. ketorolac (Toradol)
    B. diazepam (Valium)
    C. amitriptyline (Elavil)
    D. oxycodone

15. The μ(mu)-opioid receptors mediate all of the following except:

    A. supraspinal analgesia
    B. mydriasis
    C. euphoria
    D. respiratory depression

16. Convulsions can be caused by the administration of high doses of the following opioids except:

    A. meperidine
    B. morphine
    C. methadone
    D. none of the above

17. All of the following are inactive prodrugs that are converted to active analgesic metabolites in the liver except:

    A. codeine
    B. sulindac (Clinoril)
    C. salicyl salicylate (Disalicid)
    D. hydromorphone (Dilaudid)

18. One of the following compounds crosses the blood-brain barrier:

    A. ibuprofen (Motrin)
    B. indomethacin (Indocin)
    C. tolmetin (Tolectin)
    D. sulindac (Clinoril)

19. All of the following analgesics are contraindicated in renal failure except:

    A. hydromorphone (Dilaudid)
    B. ibuprofen (Motrin)
    C. meperidine (Demerol)
    D. morphine sulfate

QUESTIONS 20–22: A 37-year-old African American woman with history of sickle cell anemia presents to the emergency department with severe sharp pain of several hours duration involving her low back and legs. Past history is significant for frequent attacks of painful episodes that usually have been treated with parenteral or oral hydromorphone (Dilaudid). She consumes an average of 100 mg of hydromorphone per week. Physical exam is significant for moderate tenderness over the lumbosacral spine and tibiae. Her current painful episode was treated with 10 mg of nalbuphine (Nubain) intramuscularly (i.m.). About 30 minutes later she became agitated and complained of headache, abdominal cramps, sweating and running nose.

20. The most likely cause of these new signs and symptoms is:

    A. increase in the nociceptive activity of her original painful episode.
    B. onset of cerebrovascular accident complicating her disease.
    C. side effects of nalbuphine.
    D. withdrawal signs and symptoms precipitated by nalbuphine.

21. Diagnostic work-up of this patient at this point should include:

    A. CAT scan of the head
    B. ultrasonography of the abdomen
    C. immediate psychiatric evaluation
    D. none of the above

22. Appropriate treatment of this patient at this point includes:

    A. increase the dose of nalbuphine to 15 mg i.m.
    B. continue nalbuphine and add diphenhydramine (Benadryl) 25 mg i.m.
    C. discontinue nalbuphine and give hydromorphone (Dilaudid).
    D. continue nalbuphine and give acetaminophen for the headache.

23. The most common cause of hospitalization of patients with sickle cell anemia is:

    A. acute chest syndrome
    B. cerebrovascular accidents (strokes)
    C. acute musculoskeletal painful episodes (painful crises)
    D. leg ulcers

24. Acute chest syndrome that complicates sickle cell disease is characterized by all of the following except:

A. chest pain, fever, and leukocytosis
B. new pulmonary infiltrates on chest X-ray
C. tachypnea
D. normal arterial oxygen tension (PO_2)

25. The mechanism by which hydroxyurea exerts its beneficial effect by decreasing the frequency of acute sickle cell painful episodes is thought to be due to:

A. bone marrow suppression
B. induction of Hb F production
C. prolongation of red cell survival
D. induction of macrocytosis

QUESTIONS 26–27: A 33-year-old African American woman with known history of sickle cell anemia complains of sudden onset of pain in the right upper quadrant. She tells you that her pain is sharp, is somewhat different from that of her usual crisis pain, and gets worse with deep inspiration. She also noted that her eyes became yellow and her urine became tea colored. She complains of no tiredness, weakness, or easy fatigability. Physical exam was pertinent for icteric sclerae, hepatomegaly of 16 cm liver span, and diffuse tenderness in the right upper quadrant. Lab data showed Hb = 6.4 g% (her usual Hb in the steady state is 7.5 g%), reticulocyte count of 15%, total serum bilirubin of 16 mg% with direct bilirubin of 4.5 mg%, prothrombin time of 15" (N = 12") and liver enzymes (AST and ALT) increased to 2.5 times the upper level of normal values.

26. The most likely diagnosis of this clinical picture is:

A. acute sickle cell painful crisis
B. aplastic crisis
C. hepatic crisis
D. acute cholecystitis

27. The patient described above was admitted to the hospital, put on bed rest and was started on analgesic therapy for her pain. The most important second step in the management of this patient is:

A. continue conservative treatment and monitor serum bilirubin level and PT.
B. transfuse with two units of red blood cells immediately.
C. order ultrasonography of the abdomen to rule out cholelithiasis.
D. order serologic tests for hepatitis B and C.

QUESTIONS 28–67: MATCHING

Directions: The group of questions below consists of lettered headings followed by a list of numbered items. For each numbered item select the one lettered option that is most closely related to it. Each lettered option may be selected once, more than once, or not at all. In two cases the lettered options are incorporated in a table. Place letters on lines following numbered items.

QUESTIONS 28–37

    A. opioid agonist
    B. mixed opioid agonist-antagonist
    C. partial opioid agonist
    D. opioid antagonist
    E. none of the above

28. pentazocine ____
29. methadone ____
30. buprenorphine ____
31. naproxen ____
32. naltrexone ____
33. oxycodone ____
34. nalbuphine____
35. naloxone____
36. hydromorphone ____
37. ketorolac ____

QUESTIONS 38–42

Quantitative Hemoglobin Electrophoresis

	% HB F	% Hb A	% Hb S	% Hb A_2
A.	1.0	94	0	E5.0
B.	25.0	72	0	3.0
C.	6.0	0	91	3.0
D.	2.5	12.5	79	6.0
E.	1.0	56.5	40	2.5

38. Sickle cell anemia ____
39. hereditary persistence of fetal hemoglobin (HPFH) ____
40. β-thalassemia trait ____
41. Hb S-β^+-thalassemia (sickle-β^+-thalassemia) ____
42. sickle cell trait ____

QUESTIONS 43–52

    A. Schedule I substance
    B. Schedule II substance
    C. Schedule III substance
    D. Schedule IV substance
    E. Schedule V substance

43. codeine ____
44. codeine and acetaminophen (Tylenol #3) ____
45. an antitussive preparation containing codeine (such as Ryna C-liquid) ____
46. diazepam ____
47. heroin ____
48. fentanyl ____
49. marijuana ____
50. methylphenidate ____
51. lorazepam ____
52. meperidine ____

QUESTIONS 53–62

    A. osteomyelitis
    B. myoclonus and/or seizure disorder
    C. hematuria
    D. *E. coli* urinary tract infection
    E. staphylococcal pneumonia
    F. cerebrovascular accident (stroke)
    G. retinopathy
    H. aplastic crisis
    I. priapism
    J. megaloblastic crisis

53. This complication of sickle cell disease is most common in adult females and may be recurrent in nature. ____

54. Occurs most frequently in children with sickle cell anemia and its treatment requires chronic transfusion or exchange transfusion. ____

55. This complication may be seen in any carrier of the sickle gene such as sickle cell anemia, Hb SC disease, and sickle cell trait. ____

56. Occurs in some adults with sickle cell disease who are taking Meperidine (Demerol) on a long-term basis. ____

57. This complication is most frequently seen in patients with Hb SC disease. _____

58. This complication of sickle cell disease is prevented by treatment with folic acid on a chronic basis. _____

59. Occurs in sickle cell anemia typically after a viral infection and is characterized by worsening of the anemia and a marked decrease in the reticulocyte count. _____

60. If this complication persists for more than 24 hours, it may be associated with impotence. _____

61. This complication is one of the causes of the acute chest syndrome. _____

62. This complication is often caused by unusual pathogens such as salmonella species. _____

QUESTIONS 63–67: For each patient described below select the most likely hemoglobin electrophoresis profile (A–E):

	% HB A	% Hb S	% Hb A2	% Hb F
A.	56	42	2	0
B.	0	50	50	0
C.	0	95	2	3
D.	10	80	6	4
E.	0	75	2	23

63. A 35-year-old African American woman had a history of retinopathy that required laser therapy. Hb is 11.5 g/dl and the indices are microcytic and hyperchromic. One of her parents had Hb C trait. _____

64. A 25-year-old African American man with history of gross hematuria. Hb, Hct, and examination of the peripheral smear are normal. No history of painful episodes. His mother has normal hemoglobin electrophoresis profile. _____

65. A 24-year-old African American woman who has been taking 2500 mg of hydroxyurea orally daily for the last year. Her Hb at present is 9 g/dl and the MCV is 140 fl. She used to have frequent painful episodes before taking hydroxyurea. _____

66. A 30-year-old African American man with microcytic hypochromic indices on routine evaluation. Hb is 12 g% and the MCV 68 fl. No history of blood transfusion. Serum iron and ferritin were within normal. History of occasional mild painful episodes. _____

67. A 25-year-old African American man with history of 10–12 painful episodes per year. Hb is 8.5 g/dl, reticulocyte count 15%, and the MCV is 90 fl. Examination of the peripheral smear shows 10% irreversibly sickled cells. Past history includes cholecystectomy, avascular necrosis, and acute chest syndrome. ____

QUESTIONS 68–92: COMPARISON-MULTIPLE TRUE-FALSE

Directions: The set of lettered headings below is followed by a list of numbered items. For each item select (put letter on line after item):

A. If the item is associated with (A) only
B. If the item is associated with (B) only
C. If the item is associated with both (A) and (B)
D. If the item is associated with neither (A) nor (B)

QUESTIONS 68–72

A. sickle cell trait
B. sickle cell anemia
C. both
D. neither

68. hematuria ____
69. leg ulcers ____
70. massive splenomegaly in adults ____
71. confers resistance to infection by *Plasmodium falciparum* ____
72. hyposthenuria (difficulty in concentrating the urine) ____

QUESTIONS 73–77

A. morphine sulfate
B. meperidine (Demerol)
C. both
D. neither

73. Serum concentration of metabolites increases in the presence of renal failure. ____
74. available in controlled-release oral form. ____
75. May be given by any route: oral, intravenous, intramuscular, subcutaneous, or rectal ____

76. mixed agonist-antagonist ____
77. lipophilic ____

QUESTIONS 78–82

    A. cancer pain
    B. sickle pain
    C. both
    D. neither

78. Recurrent acute episodes of pain are a hallmark. ____
79. Deafferentation type of pain is relatively common. ____
80. May be somatic or visceral in nature. ____
81. Requires treatment with opioid analgesics. ____
82. Nonpharmacologic modalities of therapy alone are effective in achieving pain relief in most patients. ____

QUESTIONS 83–87

    A. μ-opioid receptors
    B. κ-opioid receptors
    C. both
    D. neither

83. mediate supraspinal analgesia ____
84. associated with miosis ____
85. associated with dysphoria ____
86. associated with sedation ____
87. associated with diuresis ____

QUESTIONS 88–92

    A. pure opioid agonists
    B. opioid agonists-antagonists
    C. both
    D. neither

88. have a ceiling effect ____
89. associated with psychotomimetic side effects often ____
90. high addictive potential ____
91. inhibit platelet function ____

92. mediate their effects via interaction with specific receptors in the central nervous system ____

QUESTIONS 93–120: TRUE OR FALSE

Directions: For each set of numbered items you are to respond either True (T) or False (F). Put letter on line at end of statement.

QUESTIONS 93–97: True statements bout sickle cell anemia include:

93. Sickle cell anemia manifests itself immediately after birth because genetic mutations are present in both the β and γ chains of the hemoglobin molecule. ____

94. Splenomegaly is a common finding in adult patients with sickle cell anemia. ____

95. The acute sickle cell painful crisis is the most common clinical manifestation of the disease in adults and is the usual reason for hospitalization. ____

96. Cholelithiasis is common in sickle cell anemia and is the result of the increased red cell destruction due to the sickle mutation. ____

97. Sickle cell trait is usually associated with mild anemia and decreased life span. ____

QUESTIONS 98–102: True statements about acute chest syndrome include:

98. The most important diagnostic finding of the syndrome is the presence of new pulmonary infiltrates on chest X-ray. ____

99. Streptococcal pneumonia is the most common underlying cause of the syndrome in adults. ____

100. Treatment may include blood transfusion or exchange transfusion. ____

101. The diagnosis of pulmonary fat embolism is best made by looking for fat inclusion bodies (oil-red stain) in bronchial washings obtained by bronchoscopy. ____

102. The presence of blister cells in peripheral blood is diagnostic of acute chest syndrome. ____

QUESTIONS 103–107: True statements about the treatment of sickle cell anemia with hydroxyurea include:

103. Hydroxyurea may cure sickle cell anemia. ____

104. Hydroxyurea exerts its beneficial effect by increasing the level of fetal hemoglobin. ____

105. Responders to hydroxyurea experience fewer episodes of acute chest syndrome than nontreated patients. ____

106. Hydroxyurea may be given to pregnant women with sickle cell anemia. ____

107. Myelosuppression is the most common toxic effect of hydroxyurea. ____

QUESTIONS 108–112: True statements about the treatment of sickle pain include:

108. Health care providers, in general, are well aware of the unique nature of sickle pain and demonstrate a positive attitude toward patients with sickle cell disease. ____

109. Opioid analgesics are the mainstay of management of sickle pain. ____

110. Most patients with sickle cell disease are addicted to opioids. ____

111. Antihistamines are the most commonly used adjuvants in treating sickle pain. ____

112. A multidisciplinary approach is most desirable in the management of sickle pain. ____

QUESTIONS 113–115: True statements about pain receptors include:

113. The C-polymodal receptors are responsive to chemical stimulation. ____

114. The Aδ-receptors and fibers are unmyelinated. ____

115. The C-polymodal receptors transmit stimuli at a relatively slow rate in the range of 2 m/sec. ____

QUESTIONS 116–120: Patients with sickle cell disease who do the following are most likely suffering from maladaptive and aberrant behavior suggestive of drug addiction:

116. Forge prescriptions written for opioid medications on more than one occasion. ____

117. Hoard opioid medications for later use to treat pain as needed. ____

118. Request specific opioids for their pain. ____

119. Report loss of prescription and/or medications on a recurrent basis. ____

120. Exhibit uncouth behavior and unkempt appearance. ____

Appendix B

Answers to Appendix A:
Sickle Cell Knowledge Self-assessment for Medical Personnel

1. C	31. E	61. E	91. D
2. D	32. D	62. A	92. C
3. D	33. A	63. B	93. F
4. C	34. B	64. A	94. F
5. D	35. D	65. E	95. T
6. D	36. A	66. D	96. T
7. D	37. E	67. C	97. F
8. D	38. C	68. C	98. T
9. A	39. B	69. B	99. F
10. E	40. A	70. D	100. T
11. C	41. D	71. A	101. T
12. D	42. E	72. C	102. F
13. D	43. B	73. C	103. F
14. D	44. C	74. A	104. T
15. B	45. E	75. B	105. T
16. D	46. D	76. D	106. F
17. D	47. A	77. B	107. T
18. B	48. B	78. B	108. F
19. A	49. A	79. A	109. T
20. D	50. B	80. C	110. F
21. D	51. D	81. C	111. T
22. C	52. B	82. D	112. T
23. C	53. D	83. A	113. T
24. D	54. F	84. C	114. F
25. B	55. C	85. D	115. T
26. C	56. B	86. C	116. T
27. A	57. G	87. B	117. F
28. B	58. J	88. B	118. F
29. A	59. H	89. B	119. T
30. C	60. I	90. A	120. F

Abbreviations and Acronyms

2,3-DPG	2,3-diphosphoglycerate
A	adenine
a-t-c	A prescription to take a medication at scheduled intervals, "around-the-clock" (not as-needed)
a.c.	ante cibos, before meals
AA	amino acid; also refers to the genotype of normal hemoglobin (β^A/β^A).
AHCPR	Agency for Health Care Policy and Research (U.S.)
AIDS	acquired immunodeficiency syndrome
ALT	alanine aminotransferase; same as SGPT
APAP	acetaminophen
ASA	aspirin
AST	aspartate aminotransferase; same as SGOT
ATP	adenosine triphosphate
b.i.d.	bis in die, twice a day
BAC	bovine adrenal chromaffin cells
BMT	bone marrow transplantation
C	cytosine
cDNA	complimentary DNA
CGRP	calcitonin gene-related peptide
CNS	central nervous system
CPK	creatinine phosphokinase
CRP	C-reactive protein
CSA	Controlled Substances Act
CSF	cerebrospinal fluid
CT scan	computed tomographic scan
CVA	cerebrovascular accident
DEA	Drug Enforcement Administration
DIC	disseminated intravascular coagulation
DNA	deoxyribonucleic acid
EMG	electromyography
EMLA	eutectic mixture of local anesthetic
EPO	erythropoietin
FDA	Food and Drug Administration
Fe	iron
fl	femtoliter, 10^{-15} liter

FPA	fibrinopeptide A
g	gram
G	guanine
G6PD	glucose-6-phosphate dehyrogenase
GABA	γ-aminobutyric acid
GI	gastrointestinal
Glu	glutamic acid
h.s.	hora somni, at bedtime
Hb	hemoglobin
Hb F	fetal hemoglobin
Hb S	sickle hemoglobin
Hct	Hematocrit
HDW	hemoglobin distribution width
HIV	human immunodeficiency virus
HU	hydroxyurea
i.m.	intramuscular
i.v.	intravascular
IASP	International Association for the Study of Pain
ICAM	intracellular adhesion molecule
IL	interleukin
ISC	irreversibly sickled cell
IVS	intervening sequence
kb	kilobase; 1000 base pairs of DNA or 1000 bases of RNA
kd	kilodalton
kg	kilogram, 10^3 g
LDH	lactate dehydrogenase
Lys	lysine
MAOI	monamine oxidase inhibitors
Mb	myoglobin
MCH	mean corpuscular hemoglobin
MCHC	mean corpuscular hemoglobin concentration
MCPP	multiple-copy prescription programs
MCV	mean corpuscular volume
mg	milligram, 10^{-3} g
microgram	one-millionth of a gram; abbreviated mg; 10^{-6} g.
ml	milliliter, 10^{-3} liter
MRI	magnetic resonance imaging
mRNA	messenger ribonucleic acid
ng	nanogram, 10^{-9} g
NRS	numerical rating scale
NSAID	nonsteroidal anti-inflammatory drug
OTC	over the counter
P50	oxygen pressure in torrs at which 50% of hemoglobin carries oxygen

p.c.	post cibum, after meals
PCA	patient-controlled analgesia
PCV	packed red cell volume, same as hematocrit
pg	picogram, 10^{-12} g
PICC	peripherally inserted central catheter
Plt	platelet
PNA	peripheral afferent nociceptor
p.o.	per os, orally
pr	an abbreviation used with prescriptions, meaning to take a medication, usually a suppository, through the rectum.
p.r.n.	pro re nata, as needed
q.d.	quaque die, daily
q.h.	quaque hora, every hour
q.i.d.	quater in die, four times a day
q2h	every two hours
q3h	every three hours
rRNA	ribosomal ribonucleic acid
RBC	red blood cell
RDW	red cell distribution width
RES	reticuloendothelial system
retic	reticulocyte count
RSC	reversibly sickled cell
s.c.	subcutaneous
SAA	serum amyloid A
SCD	sickle cell disease
SG	substantia gelatinosa
SGOT	serum glutamate-oxaloacetate transaminase
SGPT	serum glutamate-pyruvate transaminase
SP	substance P
SS	sickle cell anemia
SSRI	selective serotonin reuptake inhibitor
stat	statim, immediately
T	thymine
tRNA	transfer ribonucleic acid
t.i.d.	ter in die, three times a day
TENS	transcutaneous electrical nerve stimulation
TNF-α	tumor necrosis factor-α
U	uracil
Val	valine
VAS	visual analog scale
VCAM	vascular cell adhesion molecule
WBC	white blood cell
WHO	World Health Organization

Glossary

α-Thalassemia   A condition characterized by imbalanced globin chain synthesis due to decreased or absent synthesis of α-globin chains.

α-Thalassemia trait   A condition characterized by mild globin chain imbalance and microcytic anemia due to deletion of two α-globin genes. This deletion could be in *trans* (genotype: $-\alpha/-\alpha$), which is common in African Americans, or in *cis* (genotype: $--/\alpha\alpha$), which is common in Asians.

β-Thalassemia   A condition characterized by imbalanced globin chain synthesis due to decreased or absent synthesis of β-globin chains.

β^+-Thalassemia gene   A mutant β^{thal} gene that results in decreased synthesis of β globin.

β^0-Thalassemia gene   A mutant β^{thal} gene that does not result in the synthesis of any normal β globin.

β-Thalassemia intermedia   Moderate globin chain imbalance and moderate anemia due to inheritance of one or two β^{thal} genes. It is usually a clinical diagnosis.

β-Thalassemia major or Cooley's anemia   Profound globin chain imbalance and severe anemia due to inheritance of two β^{thal} genes. Transfusion dependent.

β-Thalassemia minor or trait (β-thal trait)   Minimal globin chain imbalance and anemia due to inheritance of a single β^{thal} gene.

δβ-Thalassemia   A condition characterized by decreased or absent synthesis of δ and β globin chains and an increased synthesis of γ globin chains, α/non-α (β + γ) chain synthesis is less imbalanced than β-thalassemia.

2,3-Diphosphoglycerate (2,3-DPG)   Intermediate product in the glycolytic pathway that functions as an important regulator in hemoglobin oxygen affinity.

Acetaminophen   An analgesic used to treat mild pain and reduce fever (for example, Tylenol).

Acupressure   A variation of acupuncture in which finger pressure is applied instead of needles.

Acupuncture   A therapeutic practice of Chinese origin involving of the introduction of fine needles at certain points in the skin along vital "lines of force," sometimes far removed from the site of pain.

Acute pain   A warning of a physical condition needing correction; biologically meaningful, useful, limited in time.

Addiction   Psychological craving for a drug; the need to obtain and use a drug for nonmedical reasons overwhelms and controls the addict's life, despite the risk of harm. Extremely rare in the cancer patient, but still feared by patient and doctor alike. Distinct from **Tolerance** and **Physical dependence.**

Adjuvant analgesic   A drug that is not a primary analgesic but that research shows has independent or additive analgesic properties.

Allele   One of several mutational forms of a specific gene.

Allodynia Pain due to a non-noxious stimulus to normal skin.

Amphetamine A group of stimulant drugs that stimulate nerve activity in the brain and increase wakefulness and alertness.

Analgesia Absence of pain on noxious stimulation.

Analgesics Medications that relieve pain.

Antiemetic Any drug that helps relieve vomiting and nausea.

Anticonvulsant Drug that reduces the frequency and severity of seizures.

Antidepressant A medicine used to treat depression.

Anxiolytic Medication used to reduce anxiety, agitation, or tension.

Arthralgia Pain in a joint, usually due to arthritis or arthropathy.

Autosomal dominant inheritance Inheritance of a gene that is located on a chromosome other than the sex (X or Y) chromosome, and which in single state may give rise to a phenotype that may be expressed through two or more generations.

Base pair (bp) A partnership of A with T or of C with G in a DNA double helix; in RNA, A pairs with U.

Basophilic stippling Granules of aggregated RNA forming inclusions in erythrocytes.

Behavioral techniques A coping strategy in which patients are taught to monitor and evaluate their own behavior and to modify their reactions to pain.

Bioavailability The degree to which a certain drug reaches its site of action or the fraction of the dose that reaches the systemic circulation following administration by any route.

Biofeedback A behavioral technique to control and modify emotional, nervous, and muscle responses by altering blood pressure and pulse. Must be taught by a professional.

Bolus An "escape" or "rescue" dose. An extra dose of medication to take as needed (p.r.n.) to relieve pain that breaks through despite medication that is given at regularly scheduled intervals.

Breakthrough pain A sudden flare-up of pain.

Ceiling dose A dose beyond which a drug will do no further good. Aspirin and acetaminophen, for example, have ceiling, or maximum, doses; morphine and other opioids do not.

Central pain Pain associated with a lesion of the central nervous system.

Chemotherapy Treatment of infections or malignant disease that acts selectively on the cause of the disorder.

Chiropractic A theory of healing that relies on manual manipulation and adjustment of the spine. It is based on the belief that disease results from lack of normal nerve function.

Chronic pain Prolonged pain, usually lasting for more than six months, for which the cause may or may not be known. Intensity may range from mild to severe.

Cis On the same side. *Cis*-mutations occur on the same side of a chromosome.

Codeine A weak opiate used for pain relief, often with other drugs in tablet or liquid mixtures.

Codon A triplet of nucleotides that specifies an amino acid or a termination signal.

Coping strategies   Varying methods patients use to deal with a particular disease or diagnosis.

Crisis   From the Greek *krisis;* meaning a turning point in the course of a disease with the development of new signs and symptoms.

Cryotherapy   The therapeutic use of cold to reduce discomfort, limit progression of tissue edema, or break a cycle of muscle spasm. Cryotherapy is a form of counterirritation.

Cutaneous pain   Pain generated from the skin.

Deafferentation pain   Pain due to loss of sensory input, or abnormal input, into the central nervous system (e.g., postherpetic neuralgia).

Deformability   The ability of a red cell to change its shape reversibly.

Deletion   Loss or removal of a sequence of DNA with the regions on either side being joined together.

Dependence   Also called physical dependence, a common and natural result of the body growing used to a medication, particularly an opioid such as morphine. If the drug were suddenly stopped, the patient would undergo physical problems associated with withdrawal (also called abstinence syndrome). It is easily avoided by reducing the dose of the drug gradually. Distinct from **Addiction** and **Tolerance.**

Distraction   A method to relieve pain by taking the sufferer's attention away from it.

Domain   A discrete continuous part of the amino acid sequence of a protein to which a particular function can be attributed.

Dominant   Allele that determines the phenotype displayed in a heterozygote, the other allele being recessive.

Dose   The amount of medication prescribed.

Drug receptors   Cell components that combine with a drug to alter the function of the cell. Morphine receptors are located primarily in specialized parts of the brain and spinal cord. Like a lock and key, the receptor recognizes only a specific type of drug.

Drug tolerance   The loss of effectiveness of an analgesic after repeated administration.

Dysesthesia   An unpleasant abnormal sensation, whether spontaneous or evoked.

Dysphoria   A mental state in which the patient experiences a general, unpleasant sense of not feeling like oneself; the opposite of euphoria.

Elimination half-life   The time required for the blood concentration of a certain drug to decrease by 50% of the original value.

Enhancer   A DNA sequence that increases the expression of a gene in *cis*-configuration. It can function in many locations, upstream or downstream, relative to the promoter.

Enhancers   Drugs that are given in combination with other drugs to increase their usefulness.

Enzymopathy   Any disturbance of enzyme function, especially inherited deficiencies of specific enzymes.

Epidural   Situated within the spinal canal, on or outside the dura mater (tough membrane surrounding the spinal cord); synonyms are "extradural" and "peridural."

Epidural anesthesia A method of pain relief in which a local anesthetic is injected into the epidural space in the middle and lower back to numb the nerves leading to the chest and lower half of the body.

Equianalgesic Having equal pain-killing effect; morphine sulfate, 10 mg intramuscularly, is generally used for opioid analgesic comparisons.

Etiology Study of the causes of disease, many of which are multifactorial in origin. Many diseases are of unknown etiology.

Exon A polynucleotide sequence in DNA that codes information for protein synthesis and that is copied and spliced together with other such sequences to form messenger RNA.

Faith/religious healing A method of trying to cure disease by prayer and religious faith.

Fentanyl An opioid analgesic used as a supplementary analgesic in anesthesia. Also used in the transdermal pain patch.

First-pass effect The biotransformation of a drug during its first passage through the portal circulation of the liver.

Gate control theory of pain An explanation of how electrical stimulation can sometimes block the sensation of pain.

Gene A unit of heredity whose main function is to determine the structure of peptide chains (sequence of amino acids) of proteins such as globin chains and enzymes.

Genotype The genetic constitution of an individual. With respect to a particular locus, the two genes present at that locus in that individual (for instance, β^A/β^S is the genotype, at the β-globin locus on chromosome 11 of a person with sickle cell trait).

Glucose-6-phosphate dehydrogenase (G6PD) An NADP-specific enzyme in the hexose monophosphate shunt catalyzing the dehydrogenation of glucose-6-phosphate to 6-phosphogluconate.

Guided imagery Therapy in which patients are encouraged to imagine a real or imaginary setting.

Haplotype The specific combination of alleles in a defined region of a chromosome.

Hb H disease A form of α-thalassemia characterized by mild to moderate microcytic anemia due to the deletion of three α-globin genes (genotype: $--/-\alpha$).

Heat therapy The use of heat to relieve pain in parts of the body.

Heinz bodies Inclusions of erythrocytes representing oxidized hemoglobin that has denatured and precipitated.

Hemoglobin A (Hb A) The major hemoglobin of adult human beings, it consists of a tetramer of two α chains and two β chains plus a heme moiety ($\alpha_2\beta_2$).

Hemoglobin A2 (Hb A2) The minor hemoglobin of adult human beings, it consists of a tetramer of two α chains and two δ chains plus a heme moiety ($\alpha_2\delta_2$).

Hemoglobin F (Hb F) The major hemoglobin during fetal life; decreases to less than 1% during adulthood. It consists of two α chains and two γ chains plus a heme moiety ($\gamma_2\gamma_2$).

Hemoglobin S (Hb S) An abnormal Hb where the sixth amino acid, glutamic acid, of the β chain is replaced by valine ($\beta^{Glu\rightarrow Val}$).

Hemolytic episode An event that results in the release of hemoglobin from erythrocytes.

Hereditary persistence of fetal hemoglobin (HPFH) A condition characterized by decreased or absent synthesis of δ and β globin chains and an increased synthesis of γ globin chains; α/non-α chain synthesis is balanced.

Heterozygous A patient with one or more pairs of dissimilar alleles is said to be heterozygous at that particular gene locus on homologous chromosomes.

Hexose monophosphate shunt Metabolic pathway primarily responsible for generating reducing power for cells in the form of NADPH.

Holistic medicine An alternative therapy aimed at treating the whole person, both body and mind.

Homozygous A patient with identical alleles at the same locus of homologous chromosomes is said to be homozygous.

Hybridization The pairing of complementary RNA or DNA strands to give an RNA-DNA hybrid or a DNA duplex.

Hydrops fetalis A severe form of α-thalassemia that is incompatible with life due to the deletion of all four α-globin genes (genotype: − −/− −).

Hyperalgesia Increased sensitivity to noxious stimulation.

Hypnosis State or condition that occurs when appropriate suggestions elicit distortions (revisions) of perception, memory, or mood.

Iatrogenic Induced inadvertently by the medical treatment or procedures of a physician.

Imagery A pain-relief technique that uses mental images produced by memory or imagination.

Informed consent A discussion between patient and physician that explains what procedure the physician will perform and its risks and benefits.

Intraspinal opioid therapy A technique, which may be epidural (or intrathecal or subarachnoid), in which morphine (or another opioid) is given directly near their receptors in the spine. Only tiny amounts are needed, and usually pain relief is potent but with few side effects. An invasive but efficient means of delivering medication.

Intron A segment of DNA that is transcribed, but is removed from within the primary transcript by splicing together the sequences (exons) on either side of it.

Ischemia A condition in which there is not enough blood getting to cell tissue and which often produces pain.

Lancinating Characterized by piercing or stabbing sensations.

Linkage The property of genes to be inherited together as a result of their neighboring location on the same chromosome; it is measured by percent recombination between loci.

Linkage disequilibrium A situation whereby two linked alleles are found in a population to be in *cis*, or in tandem to each other, more frequently than would be expected by chance. At least two explanations are possible: (1) the mutation giving rise to one of the alleles is rather recent (therefore recombination has not yet had the time to cause equilibration with other linked genes); (2) the arrangement in tandem of the two alleles is favored by selection.

Locus The position on a chromosome where a particular gene is located. In diploid organism, like humans, there are at each locus two genes (one on each of the two homologous chromosomes); with the only exception being most of the X chromosome in males, who are haploid for this region.

Lumbar puncture A procedure in which a needle is introduced between two bones of the spine to remove a small amount of spinal fluid for diagnostic purposes or to inject medication for anesthesia.

Meditation A technique using soothing thought, reflection, and contemplation to alleviate pain.

Metastasis The spread of cancer from one part of the body to another by way of the lymph system or bloodstream.

Methemoglobin Hemoglobin molecule with iron in the ferric (+3) state and thus not efficient in transporting oxygen.

Migraine A severe headache lasting from a few hours to a few days, accompanied by disturbances of vision and/or nausea and vomiting.

Missense mutation A change in a DNA base that results in a sequence of three base pairs that code for a different amino acid than the original code.

Mixed opioid agonist-antagonist A compound that has an affinity for two or more types of opioid receptors and blocks opioid effects on one receptor type while producing opioid effects on a second receptor type.

Morbidity The state of being diseased.

Morphine An opioid medication; the first drug of choice for severe cancer pain.

Mortality The death rate, or the number of deaths per 100,000 of the population per year.

Mucosal Referring to the mucous membranes that line the respiratory tract, alimentary canal, urinary and genital passages, and eyelids. The membranes secrete a fluid that contains mucus to keep them moist and lubricated.

Myofascial pain A large group of muscle disorders characterized by the presence of hypersensitive points, called trigger points, within one or more muscles or the investing connective tissue together with a syndrome of pain, muscle spasm, tenderness, stiffness, limitation of motion, weakness, and occasionally autonomic dysfunction.

NADP/NADPH Nicotinamide adenine dinucleotide phosphate and its reduced form (NADPH). Pyridine coenzymes that function in several oxidative-reductive reactions in cells.

Narcotic A drug derived from opium to opium-like compounds, with potent analgesic effects, and with the potential for physical dependence and tolerance after repeated administration. From the Greek *narki,* meaning numbness or stupor.

Neuralgia Pain in the distribution of a nerve or nerves.

Neuritis Inflammation of a nerve or nerves.

Neuron A nerve cell.

Neuropathic pain Pain that stems from a damaged nerve; it is usually burning, tingling, numbing, or itching in character.

Neuropathy A disturbance of function or pathological change in a nerve: in one nerve, mononeuropathy; in several nerves, mononeuropathy multiplex; symmetrical and bilateral, polyneuropathy.

Neuropeptide A neural secretion that transmits a chemical message from one neuron to another.

Nociception The process of pain transmission, usually relating to a receptive neuron for painful sensations.

Nociceptor A receptor preferentially sensitive to a noxious or potentially noxious stimulus.

Nonsense mutation Any change in DNA that results in a three-base-pair sequence that does not code for an amino acid, and thus terminates the protein sequence.

Noxious Harmful, causing injury to health or well-being.

Operant conditioning Use of environmental influences to reward or eliminate behaviors.

Opiate A naturally occurring alkaloid derived from opium. Morphine and codeine are examples.

Opiate receptor Opiate-binding sites found throughout primary afferents and the neuraxis.

Opioid A morphine-like drug that produces pain relief.

Opioid agonist Any morphine-like compound that produces bodily effects including pain relief, sedation, constipation, and respiratory depression.

Opioid partial agonist A compound that has an affinity for and stimulates physiologic activity at the same cell receptors as opioid agonists but that produces only a partial (i.e., submaximal) bodily response.

Opium The dried powdered mixture of alkaloids obtained from the unripe capsules of poppy seeds.

Oxymorphone A synthetic opioid with analgesic actions similar to those of morphine but more potent.

Pain An unpleasant sensory and emotional experience associated with actual or potential tissue damage or described in terms of such damage.

Pain assessment The determination of a patient's pain through one or more pre-determined modalities.

Pain behaviors Movements or verbal and nonverbal communications indicating that pain is being experienced.

Pain diary A daily journal used to chart a patient's pain.

Pain history Information taken by a provider from a patient about past pain treatments and medications.

Pain team A diverse group of health care providers in a hospital or other facility who work together to provide pain relief to patients.

Pain threshold The least stimulus intensity at which a subject perceives pain.

Pain tolerance The level of pain, intensity, or duration that a patient is able to endure.

Painful crisis The sudden and striking onset of severe pain in a patient with sickle cell anemia or other sickle cell syndrome. Same as **Painful episode.**

Painful episode See **Painful crisis.**

Paresthesia An abnormal sensation, whether spontaneous or evoked.

Patient's bill of rights A general statement of patient rights voluntarily adopted by most health care providers, covering matters such as access to care, patient dignity and confidentiality, personal safety, consent to treatment, and explanation of charges. Similar rights have been studied statutorily adopted in several states (cf. Minn. Stat. ξ 144.651) and by the federal government.

Patient education Provision of information to the patient on preoperative procedures and expected postoperative sensations, plus instruction to help decrease mobility-related discomfort.

Patient-controlled analgesia (PCA) Self-administration of an analgesic by a patient. PCA is available either from a programmed pump that delivers the drug through an intravenous line or taken orally.

Phantom limb pain The persistence of pain from a limb that was amputated.

Pharmacodynamics A branch of pharmacology that studies the mechanism of action of drugs and their biochemical and physiological effects.

Pharmacokinetics A branch of pharmacology that studies the factors affecting drug movement in the body.

Pharmacology A science that studies drugs.

Phenothiazines Drugs used to treat psychotic illness and also used as antihistamines and antiemetics.

Phenotype The physical appearance or makeup of an individual. In relation to a particular genetic character, the phenotype reflects the genotype conferring that character, plus the possible effects of the environment. In addition, the phenotype (what appears) depends on what we analyze (the way we look at it). Thus, while genotype is an absolute concept, phenotype is a relative concept.

Physical dependence An expected physical condition that results from the continued use of some medications, such as opioids. If medication were suddenly stopped, flu-like symptoms (withdrawal) would occur. Distinct from **Addiction** and **Tolerance.**

Physical medicine The use of physical agents in the management of disease/disorders. These include heat, cold, electricity, radiant, electromagnetic forces, traction, exercises, etc.

Physical modalities Therapeutic interventions that use physical methods, such as heat, cold, massage, or exercise, to relieve pain.

Physical therapy The health profession that treats pain in muscles, nerves, joints, and bones with exercise, electrical stimulation, hydrotherapy, and the use of massage, heat, cold, and electrical devices.

Poikilocytosis Presence in the blood of erythrocytes showing abnormal variation in shape.

Polychromasia Variation in the hemoglobin content of the erythrocytes of the blood.

Polymerase chain reaction (PCR) A technique for amplifying in vitro by a very large factor (10^5 or more) an individual DNA sequence. The reaction must be primed by using specific oligonucleotides, so prior sequence information is necessary.

Prodrug   A pharmacologically inactive compound that, after administration, is converted to an active drug.

Prognosis   A medical appraisal of the course of disease and the prospects for recovery.

Progressive muscle relaxation   A cognitive-behavioral strategy in which muscles are alternately and systematically tensed and then relaxed.

Promoter   A DNA sequence located upstream of the transcribed portion of a gene and essential for its transcription because it is the binding site for RNA polymerase.

Pruritus   A condition marked by excessive itching.

Pseudo-addiction   A drug-seeking behavior that is often construed as a psychological craving for a medication, usually an opioid such as morphine, but in fact is the result of undermedication and the desire for pain relief.

Psychological dependence (addiction)   Pattern of compulsive drug use characterized by a continued craving for an opioid and the need to use the opioid for effects other than pain relief.

Pyrimidine 5′ nucleotidase   Enzyme important in degrading pyrimidine nucleotides.

Recessive   An allele that is obscured in the phenotype of a heterozygote by the dominant allele, often due to inactivity or absence of the product of the recessive allele.

Recombinant DNA   Any DNA molecule constructed artificially by bringing together DNA segments of different origin. The impact of the respective technology has been so great that the phrase "recombinant DNA revolution" has been coined.

Referred pain   Pain that is generated from one area but felt in another.

Rehabilitation   A treatment process that integrates medical, physical, social, psychologic, emotional, and vocational aspects to help patients with impairments maximize function and resume their usual roles.

Relaxation   A variety of techniques used to decrease anxiety and muscle tension, such as imagery, distraction, and progressive muscle relaxation.

Restriction enzymes   Recognize specific short sequences (mostly four or six bases) of DNA and cleave the duplex wherever those sequences are found. These sequences are called restriction sites.

RFLP (restriction fragment length polymorphism)   Genetic variation in the size of a DNA fragment detectable, after digestion with a particular restriction enzyme, by a particular probe. RFLP results from a point mutation in a restriction site, or from a shift in its position due to a deletion or to a duplication.

Sedation   The use of a drug to reduce excessive anxiety, often as premedication to produce relaxation before an uncomfortable procedure.

Sedative   A drug used to produce calmness. Sedatives include sleep medications, antianxiety drugs, antipsychotic drugs, and antidepressant drugs.

Self-statement   Involves instructing patients to substitute positive thoughts for such negative ones as "I can't stand this" or "How much longer will this go on?"

Serotonin   A neurotransmitter released by the brain that is thought to be involved in controlling states of consciousness and mood.

Sickle cell anemia   A hereditary disease characterized by abnormally shaped red blood cells that result in a very severe form of anemia.

Sickle-α-Thalassemia   Genotype: $-\alpha/-\alpha$; β^s/β^s. Occurs in about 5% of patients with sickle cell anemia. Clinically characterized by mild anemia, increased incidence of retinopathy and avascular necrosis, and decreased incidence of leg ulcers and stroke.

Sicklemia   Sickle cell trait. An obsolete term that was used in the 1940s and 1950s but rarely used after that.

Silent carrier α-thalassemia   A condition characterized by deletion of one α-globin gene (genotype: $-\alpha/\alpha\alpha$) that causes minimal globin chain imbalance and, typically, no anemia.

Somatic   Derived from Greek word for "body." Somatosensory input refers to sensory signals from all tissues of the body including skin, viscera, muscles, and joints, but usually refers to input for body tissue other than viscera.

Somatic pain   Pain associated with the body.

Southern blotting   The procedure for transferring denatured DNA from an agarose gel to a nitrocellulose filter, where it can be recognized by an appropriate probe.

Spherocytosis   Presence in the blood of small, globular, hemoglobinated erythrocytes without the usual central pallor.

Splicing   Describes the removal of introns from an RNA primary transcript and joining of the exons; thus introns are spliced out, while exons are spliced together.

Stop codon   A three-base-pair sequence in DNA that does not code for an amino acid, and thus results in termination of the protein sequence.

Substantia gelatinosa   Lamina II of the dorsal horn of the spinal cord where C fibers terminate.

Suffering   A state of severe distress associated with events that threaten the intactness of the person.

Tactile strategies   Techniques that provide comfort through the sense of touch, such as stroking or massage.

Termination codon   This is one of three triplet sequences (UAG, UAA, or UGA) that cause termination of protein synthesis; also called stop codons or nonsense codons.

Thromboembolism   The blockage of a blood vessel by a fragment that has broken off and been carried from a blood clot elsewhere in the circulatory system.

Titration   An adjustment in which a patient will need larger doses of a drug over time to receive the same relief. It is an expected effect of using opioids and is unrelated to addiction. Distinct from **Physical dependence** and **Addiction.**

Tolerance   A common physiologic result of chronic opioid use in which a larger dose of opioid is required to maintain the same level of analgesia.

Topical anesthesia   An anesthetic applied locally on the skin to produce temporary numbness.

Torr   A measure of partial pressure of oxygen or other gases in calculated mmHg.

Trans   Configuration of two sites is called *trans* when their location is on two different chromosomes.

Transcription   Synthesis of RNA on a DNA template.

Transgenic   Animals produced by introducing new DNA sequences into the germ line by microinjection into the egg or into the blastocyst.

Translation   Synthesis of protein on an mRNA template.

Trigger point   A hypersensitive area or site in muscle or connective tissue, usually associated with myofascial pain syndromes.

Ultrasound   The use of high-frequency sound waves as a diagnostic tool to detect abnormalities in the body. The procedure is considered painless and safe, and is particularly useful for examining fluid-filled organs and soft organs.

Vector   A DNA molecule capable of replication and specially engineered to facilitate cloning of another DNA molecule of interest. The vector is usually a plasmid, a phage, or a YAC (see below), but may also be an animal virus, such as a retrovirus.

Visceral pain   Pain associated with the abdominal cavity.

Visual analog scale   A pain assessment tool in which the patient rates his or her pain on a scale of zero (no pain) to 10 (severe pain).

Yeast artificial chromosome (YAC)   Eukaryocyte vector suitable for cloning large pieces of DNA up to 2000 kb.

References

Abel SR. Tramadol: an alternative analgesic to traditional opioids and NSAids. J Pharm Care Pain Symptom Control 1995; 3:5–29.

Abildgaard CF, Simone JV, Schulman I. Factor VIII (antihaemorphilic factor) activity in sickle cell anemia. Br J Haematol 1967; 13:19–27.

Abrams MR, Phillips G Jr, Whitworth E. Adaptation and coping: a look at a sickle cell patient population over age 30—an integral phase of the life long developmental process. In: Nash KB (Ed). Psychosocial Aspects of Sickle Cell Disease. New York: The Haworth Press, 1994, pp 141–160.

Achord JL. Gastroenterologic and hepatobiliary manifestations. In: Embury SH, Hebbel RP, Mohandas N, Steinberg MH (Eds). Sickle Cell Disease: Basic Principles and Clinical Practice. New York: Raven Press, 1994, pp 665–666.

Adams PC, Speechley M. The effect of arthritis on the quality of life in hereditary hemochromatosis. J Rheumatol 1996; 23:707–710.

Adams RJ. Neurological complications. In: Embury SH, Hebbel RP, Mohandas N, Steinberg MH (Eds). Sickle Cell Disease: Basic Principles and Clinical Practice. New York: Raven Press, 1994, pp 599–621.

Adams-Graves P, Kedar A, Koshy M, et al. RheothRx (poloxamer 188) injection for the acute painful episode of sickle cell disease: a pilot study. Blood 1997; 90:2041–2046.

Addae SK. Mechanism for the high incidence of sickle cell crisis in the tropical cool season. Lancet 1971; 2:1256.

Adedeji MO. Complications of sickle cell disease in Benin City, Nigeria. East Afr Med J 1988; 65:3–7.

Adeyokunnu AA, Hendrickse RG. Salmonella osteomyelitis in childhood. Arch Dis Child 1980; 55:175–184.

Adragna NC, Fonseca P, Lauf PK. Hydroxyurea affects cell morphology, cation transport, and red blood cell adhesion in cultured vascular endothelial cells. Blood 1994; 83:553–560.

Agrawal NM, Roth S, Graham DY, et al. Misoprostol compared with sucralfate in the prevention of nonsteroidal anti-inflammatory drug-induced gastric ulcer: a randomized, controlled trial. Ann Intern Med 1991; 115:195–200.

Akenzua GI, Amiegheme OR. Inhibitor of in vitro neutrophil migration in sera of children with homozygous sickle cell gene during painful crisis. Br J Haematol 1981; 47:345–352.

Akinola NO, Stevens SME, Franklin IM, Nash GB, Stuart J. Rheological changes in the prodromal and established phases of sickle cell vaso-occlusive crisis. Br J Haematol 1992; 81:598–602.

Akinyanju O, Akinsete I. Leg ulceration in sickle cell disease in Nigeria. Trop Geogr Med 1979; 31:87–91.

Al-Khatti A, Veith RW, Papayannopoulou T, et al. Stimulation of fetal hemoglobin synthesis by erythropoietin in baboons. N Engl J Med 1987; 317:415–420.

Al-Momen AK. Recombinant human erythropoietin induced rapid healing of a chronic leg ulcer in a patient with sickle cell disease. Acta Haematol 1991; 86:46–48.

Al-Rashid R. Orbital apex syndrome secondary to sickle cell anemia. J Pediatr 1979; 95:426–427.

Ali M, McDonald JW. Reversible and irreversible inhibition of platelet cyclooxygenase and serotonin release by nonsteroidal anti-inflammatory drugs. Thromb Res 1978; 13:1057–1065.

Alkjaersig N, Fletcher A, Joist H, Chaplin H Jr. Hemostatic alterations accompanying sickle cell pain crises. J Lab Clin Med 1976; 88:440–449.

Alleyne SI, Wint E, Serjeant GR. Social effects of leg ulceration in sickle cell anemia. South Med J 1977; 70:213–214.

Allison AC. Protection afforded by sickle cell trait against subtertian malarial infection. Br Med J 1954; 1:290–294.

Allison AC. Malaria in carriers of the sickle cell trait and in newborn children. Exper Parasitol 1957; 6:418–447.

Altman KL, Watman RN, Solomon K. Surgically induced splenogenic anemia in the rabbit. Nature 1951; 168:827.

American Pain Society. Principles of Analgesic Use in the Treatment of Acute Pain and Cancer Pain, 3rd ed. Skokie, IL: American Pain Society, 1993.

American Psychiatric Association staff. Diagnostic and Statistical Manual of Mental Disorders: DSM-IV, 4th ed. Washington, DC: American Psychiatric Association, 1994.

Amjad H. Bannerman RM, Judisch JM. Sickling pain and season. Br Med J 1974; 1:54.

Anderson D, Hauser SD, McGarity KL, et al. Selective inhibition of cyclooxygenase (COX)-2 reverses inflammation and expression of COX-2 and interleukin-6 in rat adjuvant arthritis. J Clin Invest 1996; 97: 2672–2679.

Anderson MF, Went LN, Mac Iver JE, Dixon HG. Sickle cell disease in pregnancy. Lancet 1960; 2:516–521.

Angarola RT, Joranson DE. More federal drug control initiatives: Are they warranted? Will they consider the patient? American Pain Society Bulletin 1993; 3:1–2, 8–9.

Ankra-Badu GA. Sickle cell leg ulcers in Ghana. East Afr Med J 1992; 69:366–369.

Anku VD, Haris JW. Peripheral neuropathy and lead poisoning in a child with sickle cell anemia. J Pediatr 1974; 85:337–340.

Antonarakis SE, Boehm CD, Giardina PV, Kazazian HH. Nonrandom association of polymorphic restriction sites in the β-globin gene cluster. Proc Natl Acad Sci USA 1982; 79:137–141.

Archibald RMCL, Kemp HBS, Marks LH, Wynn Parry CB. Orthopaedics. In: Edwards FC, McCallum RI, Taylor PH (Eds). Fitness for Work: The Medical Aspects. Oxford: Oxford University Press, 1990, pp 126–141.

Armaly MF. Ocular manifestations in sickle cell disease. Arch Intern Med 1974; 133:670–679.

Armstrong PJ, Bersten A. Normeperidine toxicity. Anesth Analg 1986; 65:536–538.

Ashcroft MT, Serjeant GR. Growth, morbidity and mortality in a cohort of Jamaican adolescents with homozygous sickle cell disease. West Indian Med J 1981; 30:197–201.

Asher R. Munchausen's syndrome. Lancet 1951; 1:339–341.

Asher SW. Multiple cranial neuropathies, trigeminal neuralgia, and vascular headaches in sickle cell disease: a possible common mechanism. Neurology 1980; 30:210–211.

Athanasou NA, Hatton C, McGee JO'D, Weatherall DJ. Vascular occlusion and infarction in sickle cell crisis and the sickle chest syndrome. J Clin Pathol 1985; 38:659–664.

Bailey S, Higgs DR, Morris DR, Serjeant GR. Is the painful crisis of sickle cell disease due to sickling? [letter] Lancet 1991; 337:735.

Baker DH. Roentgen manifestations of Cooley's anemia. Ann N Y Acad Sci 1964; 119:641–661.

Balkaran B, Char G, Morris JS, et al. Stroke in a cohort of patients with homozygous sickle cell disease. J Pediatr 1992; 120:360–366.

Ballas SK. Disorders of the red cell membrane: a reclassification of hemolytic anemias. Am J Med Sci 1978; 276:4–22.

Ballas SK. The pathophysiology of hemolytic anemias. Transfus Med Rev 1990a; 4:236–256.

Ballas SK. Treatment of pain in adults with sickle cell disease. Am J Hematol 1990b; 34:49–54.

Ballas SK. Sickle cell anemia with few painful crises is characterized by decreased red cell deformability and increased number of dense cells. Am J Hematol 1991; 36:122–130.

Ballas SK. Bone-marrow transplantation in sickle-cell anemia: Why so few so late? Lancet 1992a; 340:1226.

Ballas SK. Munchausen sickle cell painful crisis. Ann Clin Lab Sci 1992b; 22:226–228.

Ballas SK. Management of sickle cell disease. Hospital Physician 1993; 29:12–15, 29–35.

Ballas SK. A cautionary note regarding the use of controlled release agonists (oral and/or transdermal in acute sickle cell painful episodes [abstract #2196]). Blood 1994a; 84(Suppl. 1): 553a.

Ballas SK. Neurobiology and treatment of pain. In: Embury SH, Hebbel RP, Mohandas N, Steinberg MH (Eds). Sickle Cell Disease: Basic Principles and Clinical Practice. New York: Raven Press Ltd., 1994b, pp 745–772.

Ballas SK. Sickle cell disease. In: Rakel RE (Ed). Conn's Current Therapy. Philadelphia: WB Saunders, 1995a; pp 318–327.

Ballas SK. The sickle cell painful crisis in adults: phases and objective signs. Hemoglobin 1995b; 19:323–333.

Ballas SK. Attitudes toward adult patients with sickle cell disease: silent prejudice or benign neglect. J Assoc Acad Minor Phys, 1996a; 7:62.

Ballas SK. Sickle cell pain [comment]. Pain Digest 1996b; 6:317.

Ballas SK. Factitious sickle cell painful episodes: a secondary type of Munchausen syndrome. Am J Hematol 1996c; 53:254–258.

Ballas SK, Delengowski A. Pain measurement in hospitalized adults with sickle cell painful episodes. Ann Clin Lab Sci 1993; 23:358–361.

Ballas SK, Kocher W. Erythrocytes in Hb SC disease are microcytic and hyperchromic. Am J Hematol 1988; 28:37–39.

Ballas SK, Park CH. Severe hypoxemia secondary to acute sternal infarction in sickle cell anemia. J Nuclear Med 1991; 32:1617–1618.

Ballas SK, Reyes PF. Peripheral neuropathy in adults with sickle cell disease. American Journal of Pain Management 1997; 7:53–58.

Ballas SK, Riddick GS. Clinical profile of the adult "problem" patient with sickle cell anemia. In: Book of Abstracts, 20th Meeting of the National Sickle Cell Disease Program, Boston, MA, March 18–21,1995, p 73.

Ballas SK, Smith ED. Red cell changes during the evolution of the sickle cell painful crisis. Blood 1992; 79:2154–2163.

Ballas SK, Lewis CN, Noone AM, et al. Clinical, hematologic, and biochemical features of Hb SC disease. Am J Hematol 1982; 13:37–51.

Ballas SK, Larner J, Smith ED, et al. The xerocytosis of Hb SC disease. Blood 1987; 69:124–130.

Ballas SK, Larner J, Smith ED, Schwartz E, Rappaport EF. Rheological predictors of the severity of the painful sickle cell crisis. Blood 1988; 72:1216–1223.

Ballas SK, Dover GJ, Charache S. The effect of hydroxyurea on the rheological properties of sickle erythrocytes in vivo. Am J Hematol 1989a; 32:104–111.

Ballas SK, Talacki CA, Rao VM, Steiner RM. The prevalence of avascular necrosis in sickle cell anemia: correlation with α-thalassemia. Hemoglobin 1989b; 13:649–655.

Ballas SK, Talacki CA, Adachi K, et al. The XmnI site $(-158, C \rightarrow T)$ 5′ to the Gγ gene: correlation with the Senegalese haplotype and Gγ globin expression. Hemoglobin 1991; 15:393–405.

Ballas SK, Rubin RN, Gabuzda TC. Treating sickle cell pain like cancer pain [letter]. Ann Intern Med 1992; 117:263.

Ballas SK, Barton F, Castro, Bellevue R. Narcotic analgesic use among adult patients with sickle cell anemia [abstract #2554]. Blood 1995a; 86(Suppl. 1):642a.

Ballas SK, Park CH, Jacobs SR. The spectrum of painful episodes in adult sickle cell disease. Pain Digest 1995b; 5:73–89.

Ballas SK, Carlos TM, Dampier C. Guideline for Standard of Care of Acute Painful Episodes in Patients With Sickle Cell Disease. Philadelphia: Thomas Jefferson University, 1996.

Ballas SK, Gay RN, Chehab FF. Is Hb A2 elevated in adults with sickle-α-thalassemia (β^S/β^S; $-\alpha/-\alpha$)? Hemoglobin 1997; 21:405–420.

Barabino GA, McIntire LV, Eskin SG, Sears DA, Udden M. Rheological studies of erythrocyte-endothelial cell interactions in sickle cell disease. Prog Clin Biol Res 1987; 240:113–127.

Barltrop D. Lead poisoning. Arch Dis Child 1971; 46:233–235.

Barnhart MI, Henry RL, Lusher JM. Sickle Cell, 2nd ed. Kalamazoo: The Upjohn Company, 1976, pp 15–35.

Baron M, Leiter E. The management of priapism in sickle cell anemia. J Urol 1978; 119:610–611.

Barreras L, Diggs LW. Bicarbonates, pH, and percentage of sickle cells in venous blood in patients with sickle cells crisis. Am J Med Sci 1964; 247:710–718.

Barrett-Connor E. Sickle cell disease and viral hepatitis. Ann Intern Med 1968; 69:517–527.

Barrett-Connor E. Acute pulmonary disease and sickle cell anemia. Am Rev Respir Dis 1971a; 104:159–165.

Barrett-Connor E. Bacterial infection and sickle cell anemia; an analysis of 250 infections in 106 patients and a review of the literature. Medicine 1971b; 50:97–112.

Barrett-Connor E. Pneumonia and pulmonary infarction in sickle cell anemia. JAMA 1973; 224:997–1000.

Barton AJ, Gallegos X. Relaxation and biofeedback. In: Wall PD, Melzack R (Eds). Textbook of Pain, 3rd ed. Edinburgh: Churchill Livingstone 1994, pp 1321–1336.

Basbaum AI. The generation and control of pain. In: Rosenberg RN, Grossman RG, Schochet SS Jr, Heinz ER, Willis WD (Eds). The Clinical Neurosciences, Neurobiology. New York: Churchill Livingstone, 1983, pp V301–V324.

Basbaum AI, Fields HL. Endogenous pain control systems: brainstem spinal pathways and endorphin circuitry. Annu Rev Neurosci 1984; 7:309–338.

Basford JR. Physical agents and biofeedback. In: Delisa JA (Ed). Rehabilitation Medicine: Principles and Practice. Philadelphia: JB Lippincott, 1988, pp 257–275.

Bauer J. Sickle cell nomenclature [letter]. Arch Intern Med 1974; 134:388.

Bauer J, Fisher LJ. Sickle cell disease. Arch Surg 1943; 47:553–563.

Baum K, Dunn DT, Maude GH, Serjeant GR. The painful crisis of homozygous sickle cell disease: a study of risk factors. Arch Intern Med 1987; 147:1231–1234.

Beaver W. Combination analgesics. Am J Med 1984; 77:38–53.

Beaver WT. Impact of non-narcotic oral analgesics on pain management. Am J Med 1988; 84:3–15.

Beaver WT, Feise GA. A comparison of the analgesic effect of oxymorphone by rectal suppository and intramuscular injection in patients with postoperative pain. J Clin Pharmacol 1977; 17:276–291.

Beaver WT, Wallenstein SL, Houde RW, Rogers A. A comparison of the analgesic effect of methotrimeprazine and morphine in patients with cancer. Clin Pharmacol Ther 1966; 7:436–446.

Beaver WT, Wallenstein SL, Houde RW, Rogers A. Comparisons of the analgesic effects of oral and intramuscular oxymorphone and of intramuscular oxymorphone and morphine in patients with cancer. J Clin Pharmacol 1977; 17:186–198.

Beckett AH, Casey AF. Synthetic analgesics, stereochemical considerations. J Pharm Pharmacol 1954; 6:986–991.

Becton DL, Raymond L, Thompson C, Berry DH. Acute phase reactants in sickle cell disease. J Pediatr 1989; 115:99–102.

Beet EA. Primary splenic abscess and sickle cell disease. East Afr Med J 1949; 22:180–186.

Beinhauer LG, Gruhn JG. Dermatologic aspects of congenital spherocytic anemia. Arch Dermatol 1957; 75:642–646.

Bell MA, Weddell AGM. A descriptive study of the blood vessels of the sciatic nerve in the rat, man and other mammals. Brain 1984a; 107:871–898.

Bell MA, Weddell AGM. A morphometric study of intrafascicular vessels of mammalian sciatic nerve. Muscle Nerve 1984b; 7:524–534.

Bellet PS, Kalinyak KA, Shukla R, Gelfand MJ, Rucknagel DL. Incentive spirometry to prevent acute pulmonary complications in sickle cell disease. N Engl J Med 1995; 333:699–703.

Benedetti C, Butler SH. Systemic analgesics. In: Bonica JJ (Ed). The Management of Pain, 2nd ed. 1990, pp 1640–1675.

Benjamin LJ. Biochemical and cellular alterations in sickle cell anemia: Crisis markers and therapeutic monitors. In: Beuzard Y, Charache S, Galacteros F (Eds). Approaches to the Therapy of Sickle Cell Anemia. Paris: Les Editions INSERM, 1986, pp 451–454.

Benjamin LJ. Pain in sickle cell disease. In: Foley KM, Payne RM (Eds). Current Therapy of Pain. Toronto: BC Decker, 1989, pp 90–104.

Benjamin LJ, Nagel RL. The comprehensive sickle cell center day hospital: an alternative to the emergency room for management of acute sickle pain. In: Program of the 16th Annual Meeting of the National Sickle Cell Centers, Mobile, AL, March 24–26, 1991, p 14.

Benjamin LJ, Jones RL, Peterson CM, Zellars R, Harpel P. Hemostatic alterations in sickle cell anemia: objective markers of vaso-occlusive crisis. Blood 1985; 66(Suppl. 1):318a.

Benjamin LJ, Berkowitz LR, Orringer E, et al. A collaborative, double-blind randomized trial of cetiedil citrate in sickle cell crisis. Blood 1986; 67:1442–1447.

Bennett OM, Namnyak SS. Bone and joint manifestations of sickle cell anemia. J Bone Joint Surg 1990; 72B:494–499.

Bentz C, Ballas SK. Neurobehavioral features of sickle cell disease. Neuropsychiatry, Neuropsychology and Behavioral Neurology 1994; 7:36–40.

Benz EJ Jr. Synthesis, structure, and function of hemoglobin. In: Kelly WN, DeVita VT (Eds). Textbook of Internal Medicine, Vol 1. Philadelphia: JB Lippincott, 1989, p 236.

Bertrand Y, Lefrene JJ, Leverger G, et al. Autoimmune haemolytic anaemia revealed by human parvovirus linked erythroblastopenia. Lancet 1985; 2:382–383.

Beurling-Harbury C, Schade SG. Platelet activation during pain crisis in sickle cell anemia patients. Am J Hematol 1989; 31:237–241.

Billet HH, Kim K, Fabry ME, Nagel RL. The percentage of dense cells does not predict incidence of sickle cell painful crisis. Blood 1986; 68:301–303.

Billet HH, Fabry ME, Nagel RL. Hemoglobin distribution width: a rapid assessment of dense red cells in the steady state and during painful crisis in sickle cell anemia. J Lab Clin Med 1988a; 112:339–344.

Billet HH, Nagel RL, Fabry ME. Evolution of laboratory parameters during sickle cell painful crisis: evidence compatible with dense red cell sequestration without thrombosis. Am J Med Sci 1988b; 296:293–298.

Billet HH, Patel Y, Rivers SP. Venous insufficiency is not the cause of leg ulcers in sickle cell disease. Am J Hematol 1991; 37:133–134.

Blau CA, Constantoulakis P, Shaw CM, Stamatoyannopoulos G. Fetal hemoglobin induction with butyric acid: efficacy and toxicity. Blood 1993; 81:259.

Blei F, Guarini L, Carriero D. Elevated levels of circulating intercellular adhesion molecule-1 (ICAM-1) in sickle cell disease. In: Book of Abstracts, 18th Annual Meeting of the National Sickle Cell Disease Program, Philadelphia, PA, May 22–25, 1993, p 77a.

Boctor AM, Eickholt M, Puglsley TA. Meclofenamate sodium is an inhibitor of both the 5-lipooxygenase and cyclooxygenase pathways of the arachidonic acid cascade in vitro. Prostaglandins Leukotrienes Med 1986; 23:229–238.

Bohrer SP (Ed). Bone Ischemia and Infarction in Sickle Cell Disease. St Louis: Warren H Green, 1981.

Bohrer S. Bone changes in the extremities in sickle cell anemia. Semin Radiol 1987; 22:176–185.

Boivie J. Central pain. In: Wall PD, Melzack R (Eds). Textbook of Pain, 3rd ed. Edinburgh: Churchill Livingstone, 1994, pp 871–902.

Bonica JJ. Neurophysiologic and pathologic aspects of acute and chronic pain. Arch Surg 1977; 112:750–761.

Bonica JJ. Definitions and taxonomy of pain. In: The Management of Pain, 2nd ed. Philadelphia: Lea & Febiger 1990a; pp 18–27.

Bonica JJ. Postoperative pain. In: JJ Bonica (Ed). The Management of Pain, 2nd ed. Philadelphia: Lea & Febiger, 1990b, pp 461–480.

Bonica JJ, Ventafridda V, Twycross RG. Cancer Pain. In: Bonica JJ (Ed). The Management of Pain, 2nd ed. Philadelphia: Lea & Febiger, 1990, pp 400–460.

Boros L, Thomas C, Weiner WJ. Large cerebral vessel disease in sickle cell anemia. J Neurol Neurosurg Psychiatry 1976; 39:1236–1239.

Bouvier CA, Gaynor E, Clintron JR, Bernhardt B, Spaet TH. Circulating endothelium as an indication of vascular injury. Thromb Diath Hemorrh 1970; 40:163–168.

Brandon W. Sickle cell disease and the adult patient. Minority Nurse Newsl 1995; 2:1.

Bray MA. Leukotrienes in inflammation. Agents Actions 1986; 19:87–99.

Breda MA, Drinkwater DC, Laks H, et al. Prevention of reperfusion injury in the neonatal heart with leukocyte-depleted blood. J Thorac Cadiovasc Surg 1989; 7:654–665.

Breitbart W, Holland J. Psychiatric aspects of cancer pain. In: Foley KM, Bonica JJ, Ventafridda V (Eds). Advances in Pain Research and Therapy, Vol 16. New York: Raven Press, 1990, p 73.

Brena SF, Chapman SC. Chronic Pain: Management Principles. Clinics in Anesthesiology. Philadelphia: WB Saunders, 1985.

Briehl RW. Gelation of sickle cell hemoglobin IV. Phase transitions in hemoglobin S gels: separate measures of aggregation and solution-gel equilibrium. J Mol Biol 1978; 123:521–538.

Briehl RW, Ewert S. Effects of pH, 2,3–diphosphoglycerate and salts on gelation of sickle cell deoxyhemoglobin. J Mol Biol 1973; 80:445–458.

Bromberg PA. Pulmonary aspects of sickle cell disease. Arch Intern Med 1974; 133:652–657.

Brookoff D, Polomano R. Treating sickle cell pain like cancer pain. Ann Int Med 1992; 116:364–368.

Brooks PM, Day RO. Nonsteroidal antiinflammatory drugs: differences and similarities. N Engl J Med 1991; 324:1716–1725.

Brozovic M, Anionwu E. Sickle cell disease in Britain. J Clin Pathol 1984; 37:1321–1326.

Brozovic M, Davies SC, Yardumian A, et al. Pain relief in sickle cell crises [letter]. Lancet 1986; 2:624–625.

Brozovic M, Davies SC, Brownell AI. Acute admissions of patients with sickle cell disease who live in Britain. Br Med J 1987; 294:1206–1208.

Bruera E, Chadwich S, Brenneis C, et al. Methyl-phenidate associated with narcotics for the treatment of cancer pain. Cancer Treat Rep 1987; 71:67–70.

Brugnara C, Gee B, Armsby CC, et al. Therapy with oral clotrimazole induces inhibition of the Gardos Channel and reduction of erythrocyte dehydration in patients with sickle cell disease. J Clin Invest 1996; 97:1227–1234.

Brugsch HG, Gill D. Polyarthritis in sickle cell anemia. N Engl J Med 1944; 231:291–292.

Brusilow SW, Horwich A. Urea cycle enzymes. In: Scriver C, Beaudet A, Sly W, Valle D (Eds). The Metabolic Basis of Inherited Disease, 6th ed. New York: McGraw-Hill, 1989, p 629.

Buchanan GR. Infection. In: Embury SH, Hebbel RP, Mohandas N, Steinberg MH (Eds). Sickle Cell Disease: Basic Principles and Clinical Practice, New York: Raven Press, 1994, pp 567–587.

Buchanan GR, Glader BE. Benign course of extreme hyperbilirubinemia in sickle cell anemia: analysis of six cases. J Pediatr 1977; 91:21–24.

Buchanan GR, Glader BE. Leukocyte counts in children with sickle cell disease: comparative values in the steady state, vaso-occlusive crisis, and bacterial infection. Am J Dis Child 1978; 132:396–398.

Buchanan WP, Ungaro PC, Ranney JE. Objective laboratory parameters in the diagnosis of sickle cell pain crisis. North Carolina Med J 1988; 49:583–584.

Budd K. Chronic pain: challenge and response. Drugs 1994; 47(suppl. 1):33–38.

Bullingham RES, McQuay HJ, Moore A, Bennett MRD. Buprenorphine kinetics. Clin Phamacol Ther 1980; 28:667–672.

Bullingham RE, McQuay HJ, Porter EJ, Allen MC, Moore RA. Sublingual buprenorphine used postoperatively: ten hour plasma drug concentration analysis. Br J Clin Pharmacol 1982; 13:665–673.

Bunn HF, Forget BG (Eds). Hemoglobin: Molecular, Genetic and Clinical Aspects. Philadelphia: WB Saunders, 1986.

Bunting H. Sedimentation rates of sickled and non-sickled cells from patients with sickle cell anemia. Am J Med Sci 1939; 198:191–193.

Burch JW, Standford N, Majerus PW. Inhibition of platelet prostaglandin synthetase by oral aspirin. J Clin Invest 1978; 61:314–319.

Burghardt-Fitzgerald DC. Pain-behavior contracts: effective management of the adolescent in sickle cell crisis. J Pediatr Nurs 1989; 4:320–324.

Burns JJ, Berger BL, Lief PA, et al. The physiological disposition and fate of meperidine (Demerol) in man and a method for its estimation in plasma. J Pharmacol Exp Ther 1979; 16:667–672.

Butler DJ, Beltran LR. Functions of an adult sickle cell group: education, task orientation, and support. Health Soc Work 1993; 18:49–56.

Byrne JG, Appleyard RF, Lee CC, et al. Controlled reperfusion of the regionally ischemic myocardium with leukocyte-depleted blood reduces stunning, the no-reflow phenomenon, and infarct size. J Thorac Cardiovasc Surg 1992; 103:66–72.

Cacciola E, Giustolisi R, Musso R, Longo A. Antithrombin III concentrate for treatment of chronic leg ulcers in sickle cell beta-thalassemia: a pilot study. Ann Int Med 1989; 111:534–536.

Calis KA, Kohler DR, Corso DM. Transdermally administered fentanyl for pain management. Clin Pharmacol 1992; 11:22–36.

Campos VM, Solis EL. The analgesic and hypothermic effects of nefopam, morphine, aspirin, diphenhydramine and placebo. J Clin Pharmacol 1980; 20:42–49.

Cantees K, Dunwoody C, Carlos T, Stacey B. Promoting active patient participation in management of painful crisis utilizing patient controlled analgesia (PCA). In: Book of Abstracts, 20th Meeting of the National Sickle Cell Disease Program, Boston, MA, March 18–21, 1995, p 140.

Cantello R, Aguggia M, Gilli M, et al. Analgesic action of methylphenidate on parkinsonian sensory symptoms: mechanism and other physiological implications. Arch Neurol 1988:45:973–976.

Carr DB, Jacox AK, Chapman CR, et al. Acute Pain Management: Operative or Medical Procedures and Trauma. Clinical Practice Guideline no. 1, AHCPR Publication No. 92-0032. Rockville, MD: U.S. Department of Health and Human Services, Public Health Service, Agency for Health Care Policy and Research, 1992.

Casey JR, Kinney TR, Ware RE. Acute splenic sequestration in the absence of palpable splenomegaly. Am J Pediatr Hematol/Oncol 1994; 16:181–182.

Casey KL, Minoshima S, Berger KL, Koeppe RA, et al. Positron emission tomographic analysis of cerebral structures activated specifically by repetitive noxious heat stimuli. J Neurophysiol 1994; 71:802–807.

Castro O, Brambilla DJ, Thorington B, et al. The cooperative study of sickle cell disease. The acute chest syndrome in sickle cell disease: incidence and risk factors. Blood 1994; 84:643–649.

Cavenagh JD, Joseph AEA, Dills S, Bevan DH. Splenic sepsis in sickle cell disease. Br J Haematol 1994; 86:182–189.

Chabal C, Russell LC, Burchiel KJ. The effect of intravenous lidocaine, tocainide and mexiletine on spontaneously active fibers originating in rat sciatic neuromas. Pain 1989; 38:333–338.

Charache S. Treatment of sickle cell anemia. Annu Rev Med 1981; 32:195–206.

Charache S. Pharmacological modification of hemoglobin F expression in sickle cell anemia: an update on hydroxyurea studies. Experientia 1993; 49:126–132.

Charache S, Walker WG. Failure of desmopressin to lower serum sodium or prevent crisis in patients with sickle cell anemia. Blood 1981; 58:892–896.

Charache S, Duffy TP, Morrell RM. Toxic-therapeutic ratio of sodium cyanate (NaNCO) in sickle cell anemia. Clin Res 1974; 22:560a.

Charache S, Dover GJ, Moore RD, et al. Hydroxyurea: effects on hemoglobin F production in patients with sickle cell anemia. Blood 1992; 79:2555–2565.

Charache S, Terrin ML, Moore RD, et al. Effect of hydroxyurea on frequency of painful crises in sickle cell anemia. N Engl J Med 1995; 332:1317–1322.

Charache S, Barton FB, Moore RD, et al. Fetal hemoglobin, hydroxyurea, and sickle cell anemia: clinical utility of a hemoglobin "switching" agent. Medicine 1996; 75:300–326.

Cheetham RC, Heuhns ER, Rosemeyer MA. Participation of haemoglobins A, F, A$_2$, and C in polymerization of hemoglobin S. J Mol Biol 1979; 129:45–61.

Chernoff AI, Shapleigh JB, Moore CV. Therapy of chronic ulceration of the legs associated with sickle cell anemia. JAMA 1954; 155:1487–1491.

Cheskin LJ, Chami TN, Johnson RE, Jaffe JH. Assessment of nalmefene glucuronide as a selective gut opioid antagonist. Drug Alcohol Depend 1995; 39:151–154.

Christensen ML, Wang WC, Harris S, Eades SK, Williams JA. Transdermal fentanyl administration in children and adolescents with sickle cell pain crisis. J Pediatr Hematol/Oncol 1996; 18:372–376.

Chuang E, Ruchelli E, Mulberg AE. Autoimmune liver disease and sickle cell anemia in children: a report of three cases. J Pediatr Hematol Oncol 1997; 19:159–162.

Chun CH, Raff MJ, Contreras L, et al. Splenic abscess. Medicine 1980; 59:50–65.

Chung SMK, Ralston EL. Necrosis of the femoral head associated with sickle-cell anemia and its genetic variants. J Bone Joint Surg 1969; 51:33–58.

Ciabattoni G, Cinotti GA, Pierucci A, et al. Effects of sulindac and ibuprofen in patents with chronic glomerular disease: evidence for the dependence of renal function on prostacyclin. N Engl J Med 1984; 310:279–283.

Ciabattoni G, Boss AH, Patrignani P, et al. Effects of sulindac on renal and extrarenal eicosanoid synthesis. Clin Pharmacol Ther 1987; 41:380–383.

Clark LJ, Chan LS, Powars DR, Baker RF. Negative charge distribution and density on the surface of oxygenated normal and sickle red cells. Blood 1981; 57:675–678.

Clark MK, Mohandas N, Embury SH, Lubin BH. A simple laboratory alternative to irreversibly sickled cell (ISC) count. Blood 1982; 16:569–662.

Clarke HJ, Jinnah RH, Brooker AF, Michaelson JD. Total replacement of the hip for avascular necrosis in sickle cell disease. J Bone Joint Surg 1989; 71B:465–470.

Clive DM, Stoff JS. Renal syndromes associated with nonsteroidal anti-inflammatory drugs. N Engl J Med 1984; 310:563–572.

Co LL, Schmitz TH, Havdala H, Reyes A, Westerman MP. Acupuncture: an evaluation of the painful crises of sickle cell anaemia. Pain 1979; 7:181–185.

Code of Federal Regulations. Food and Drugs, 21 Parts 1300 to end. Washington, DC: Office of the Federal Register, National Archives and Records Administration, April 1, 1996, pp 82–186.

Cole TB, Sprinkle RH, Smith SJ, Buchanan GR. Intravenous narcotic therapy for children with severe sickle cell pain crisis. Am J Dis Child 1986; 140:1255–1259.

Cole-Strauss A, Yoon K, Xing Y, et al. Correction of the mutation responsible for sickle cell anemia by an RNA-DNA oligonucleotide. Science 1996; 273:1386–1389.

Collins AF, Dover GJ, Luban NLC. Increased fetal hemoglobin production in patients receiving valproic acid for epilepsy. Blood 1994; 84:1690–1691.

Conroy MC, Randinitis EJ, Turner JL. Pharmacology, pharmaconkinetics, and therapeutic use of meclofenamate sodium. Clin J Pain 1991; 7(Suppl. 1):S44–S48.

Constantoulakis P, Knitter G, Stamatoyannopoulos G. On the induction of fetal hemoglobin by butyrates: in vivo and in vitro studies with sodium butyrate and comparison of combination treatments with 5-azaC and araC. Blood 1989; 74:1963–1971.

Conti C, Tso E, Browne E. Oral morphine protocol for sickle cell crisis pain. Md Med J 1996; 15:43–47.

Conyard S, Krishnamurthy M, Dosik H. Psychological aspects of sickle cell anemia in adolescents. Health Soc Work 1980; 5:20–26.

Cook JE, Meyer J. Severe anemia with remarkable elongated and sickle-shaped red blood cells and chronic leg ulcers. Arch Intern Med 1915; 16:644–651.

Cooper SA, Beaver WT. A model to evaluate mild analgesics in oral surgery outpatients. Clin Pharmacol Ther 1976; 20:241–250.

Corvelli AI, Binder RA, Kales A. Disseminated intravascular coagulation in sickle cell crisis. South Med J 1979; 72:505–506.

Cousins MJ. Acute pain and the injury response: immediate and prolonged effects. Reg Anesth 1989; 14:162–179.

Cousins MJ. Acute post operative pain. In: Wall PD, Melzack R (Eds). Text book of Pain, 3rd ed. New York: Churchill Livingstone, 1994, pp 357–385.

Cozzi L, Tryon WW, Sedlacek K. The effectiveness of biofeedback-assisted relaxation in modifying sickle cell crises. Biofeedback Self Regul 1987; 12:51–61.

Crepeau RH, Edelstein SJ, Szalay M, et al. Sickle cell hemoglobin fiber structure altered by α-chain mutation. Proc Natl Acad Sci USA 1981; 78:1406–1410.

Cresta M. Energy expenditure in sicklemia [letter]. JAMA 1974; 228:287.

Crosby WH. The metabolism of hemoglobin and bile pigment in hemolytic disease. Am J Med 1995; 18:112–122.

Cummer CL, LaRocco CG. Ulcers of the legs in sickle cell anemia. Arch Dematol Syphilol 1940; 42:1015–1039.

David R, Barron BJ, Madewell JE. Osteomyelitis, acute and chronic. Radiol Clin North Am 1987; 25:1171–1201.

Davies SC. The hospital management of patients with sickle cell disease. Hematologica 1990; 75:96–106.

Davies SC, Bevan DH. Sickle cell pain crisis. Lancet 1996; 347:263.

Davies SC, Brozovic M. The presentation, management and prophylaxis of sickle cell disease. Blood Rev 1989; 3:29–44.

Davies SC, Luce PJH, Winn AA, et al. Acute chest syndrome in sickle cell disease. Lancet 1984; 1:36–38.

Davis H, Moore RM Jr., Gergen PJ. Cost of hospitalizations associated with sickle cell disease in the United States. Public Health Reports 1997; 112:40–43.

Dayhoff M (Ed). Atlas of Protein Sequence and Structure, Vol 5. Washington DC: Georgetown University Medical Center, 1972.

De Castro J, Van de Water A, Wouters L, et al. Comparative study of cardiovascular, neurologic and metabolic side effects of eight narcotics in dogs. Acta Anaesthesiol Belg 1979; 30:5–54.

De Ceulaer K, Higgs DR, Weatherall DJ, et al. α-Thalassemia reduces the hemolytic rate in homozygous sickle-cell disease. N Engl J Med 1983; 309:189–190.

De Ceulaer K, Forbes M, Roper D. Serjeant GR. Non-gouty arthritis in sickle cell disease: report of 37 consecutive crises. Ann Rheum Dis 1984; 43:599–603.

de Jong RH. Defining pain terms. JAMA 1980; 244:143.

Delhotal-Landes B, Flouvat B, Liote F, et al. Pharmacokinetic interactions between NSAIDS (Indomethicin or sulindac) and H2-receptor antagonists (cimetidine or ranitidine) in human volunteers. Clin Pharmacol Ther 1988; 44:442–452.

Devine DV, Kinney TR, Thomas PF, Rosse WF, Greenberg CS. Fragment D-dimer levers: an objective marker of vaso-occlusive crisis and other complications of sickle cell disease. Blood 1986; 68:317–319.

Diamond HS, Meisel A, Sharon I, Holden D, Cacatian A. Hyperuricosuria and increased tubular secretion of urate in sickle cell anemia. Am J Med 1975; 59:796–802.

Diamond HS, Meisel AD, Holden D. The natural history of urate over production in sickle cell anemia. Ann Intern Med 1979; 90:752–757.

Diggs LW. The blood picture in sickle cell anemia. South Med J 1932; 25:615–620.

Diggs LW. The crisis in sickle cell anemia. Hematologic Studies. Am J Clin Pathol 1956, 26:1109–1118.

Diggs LW. Sickle cell crisis. Am J Clin Pathol 1965; 44:1–19.

Diggs LW. Bone and joint lesions in sickle cell disease. Clin Orthop 1967; 52:119–143.

Diggs LW. Anatomic lesions in sickle cell anemia. In: Abramson H, Bertles JF, Wethers DL

(Eds). Sickle Cell Disease, Diagnosis, Management, Education, and Research. St Louis: CV Mosby, 1973, pp 189–229.

Diggs LW, Ching RE. Pathology of sickle cell anemia. South Med J 1934; 27:839–844.

Diggs LW, Flowers E. Sickle cell anemia in the home environment. Clin Pediatr 1971; 10:697–700.

Diggs LW, Vorder-Bruegge CF. Vascular occlusive mechanisms in sickle cell disease. J Natl Med Assoc 1954; 46:46–49.

Diggs LW, Pulliam HN, King JC. The bone changes in sickle cell anemia. South Med J 1937; 30:249–259.

DiPalma JR, DiGregorio GJ. Basic Pharmacology in Medicine, 3rd ed. New York: McGraw-Hill, 1990.

Dixon R, Crews T, Inturrisi CE, Foley K. Levorphanol: pharmacokinetics and steady-state plasma concentrations in patients with pain. Res Commun Chem Pathol Pharmacol 1983; 41:3–17.

Dorn L. Priapism. In: Symposium on Sickle Cell Disease. Nurs Clin North Am 1983; 18:149–151.

Dorwart BB, Gabuzda TG. Symmetric myositis and fasciitis: a complication of sickle cell anemia during vasoocclusion. J Rheumatol 1985; 12:590–595.

Dover GJ, Brusilow S, Samid D. Increased fetal hemoglobin in patients receiving sodium 4-phenylbutyrate. N Engl J Med 1992; 327:569–570.

Dover GJ, Brusilow S, Charache S. Induction of fetal hemoglobin production in subjects with sickle cell anemia by oral sodium phenylbutyrate. Blood 1994; 84:339–343.

Drug Facts and Comparisons, 51st ed. St. Louis: Facts and Comparison, 1997.

Drug Information for the Health Care Professional, 12th ed. Rockville, MD: USP DI, 1992.

Dubner R. Topical capsaicin therapy for neuropathic pain. Pain 1991; 47:247–248.

Dunn MJ, Hood VL. Prostaglandins and the kidney. Am J Physiol 1977; 233:169–184.

Durosinmi MA, Gevao SM, Esan GJ. Chronic leg ulcers in sickle cell disease: experience in Ibadan, Nigeria. Afr J Med Med Sci 1991; 20:11–14.

Durward A. The blood supply of nerves. Postgrad Med J 1948; 24:11–14.

Dykes GW, Crepeau RH, Edelstein SJ. Three-dimensional reconstruction of the 14-filament fibers of hemoglobin S. J Mol Biol 1979; 130:451–472.

Eaton JW. Malaria and the selection of the sickle gene. In: Embury SH, Hebbel RP, Mohandas N, Steinberg MH (Eds). Sickle Cell Disease: Basic Principles and Clinical Practice. New York: Raven Press, 1994, pp 13–18.

Eaton WA, Hofrichter J. Hemoglobin S gelation and sickle cell disease. Blood 1987; 70:1245–1266.

Ebong WW. Acute osteomyelitis in Nigerians with sickle cell disease. Ann Rheum Dis 1986; 45:911–915.

Eddy NB, Lee LE. The analgesic equivalence and relative side action liability of oxymorphone. J Pharmacol Exp Ther 1959; 125:116–121.

Edelstein SJ. Molecular topology in crystals and fibers of hemoglobin S. J Mol Biol 1981; 50:557–575.

Edelstein SJ, Stevenson I. Sickle cell anaemia and reincarnation beliefs in Nigeria. Lancet 1983; II:1140.

Eisele JH Jr, Grigsby EJ, Dea G. Clonazepam treatment of myoclonic contractions associated with high-dose opioids: case report. Pain 1991; 49:231–232.

Eisendrath SJ, Goldman B, Douglas J, Dimatteo L, Van Dyke C. Meperidine-induced delirium. Am J Psychiatry 1987; 144:1062–1065.

Elander J, Midence K. A review of evidence about factors affecting quality of pain management in sickle cell disease. Clin J Pain 1996; 12:180–193.

Emblen J, Halstead L. Spiritual needs and interventions: comparing the views of patients, nurses and chaplains. Clinical Nurse Specialist 1993; 7:175–182.

Embury SH, Hebbel RP, Mohandas N, Steinberg MH (Eds). Sickle Cell Disease, Basic Principles and Clinical Practice. New York: Raven Press, 1994a.

Embury SH, Hebbel RP, Steinberg MH, Mohandas N. Pathogenesis of vasoocclusion. In:

Embury SH, Hebbel RP, Mohandas N, Steinberg MH (Eds). Sickle Cell Disease: Basic Principles and Clinical Picture. New York: Raven Press Ltd, 1994b; pp 311–326.

Embury SM, Dozy AM, Miller J, et al. Concurrent sickle-cell anemia and α-thalassemia: effect on severity of anemia. N Engl J Med 1982; 306:270–274.

Emond AM, Holman R, Hayes RJ, et al. Priapism and impotence in homozygous sickle cell disease. Arch Intern Med 1980; 140:1434–1437.

Emond AM, Collis R, Darvill D, et al. Acute splenic sequestration in homozygous sickle cell disease: natural history and management. J Pediatr 1985; 107:201–206.

Engler R, Covell JW. Granulocytes cause reperfusion ventricular dysfunction after 15-minute ischemia in the dog. Circ Res 1987; 61:20–28.

Ennis JT, Serjeant GR, Middlemiss JH. Homozygous sickle cell disease in Jamaica. Br J Radiol 1973; 46:943–950.

Epps CH Jr., Bryant DD, Coles MJM, Castro O. Osteomyelitis in patients who have sickle cell disease. J Bone Joint Surg 1991; 73A:1281–1294.

Erenberg G, Rinsler SS, Fish BG. Lead neuropathy and sickle cell disease. Pediatrics 1974; 54:438–441.

Ernst AA, Weiss SJ, Lyons L, Johnson WD. Presentation and pain management with ketorolac in acute sickle cell disease related pain crises [abstract]. Clinical Research 1993; 41:363a.

Espinosa G. Hand-foot roentgen findings in sickle cell anemia. JAMA 1979; 71(2):171–173.

Espinoza LR, Spilberg I, Osterland CK. Joint manifestations of sickle cell disease. Medicine 1974; 53:295–305.

Evans GR. Haemoglobin disorders and their occupational implications. Occup Med 1994; 44:29–33.

Evans PV, Symmes AT. Bone marrow infarction with fat embolism and nephrosis in sickle cell disease. J Indiana State Med Assoc 1975; 50:1101–1105.

Fabry ME, Benjamin L, Lawrence C, Nagel RL. An objective sign in painful crisis in sickle cell anemia: the concomitant reduction of high density red cells. Blood 1984; 64:559–563.

Falk RJ, Jeannette JC. Renal disease. In: Embury SH, Hebbel RP, Mohandas N, Steinberg MH (Eds). Sickle Cell Disease: Basic Principles and Clinical Practice. New York: Raven Press, 1994, pp 673–680.

Farber MD, Koshy M, Kinney TR. Cooperative study of sickle cell disease: demographic and socioeconomic characteristics of patients and families with sickle cell disease. J Chron Dis 1985; 38:495–505.

Fenichel RL, Watson J, Eirich F. Electrophoretic studies of the plasma and serum proteins in sickle cell anemia. J Clin Invest 1950; 29:1620–1624.

Ferrante MF. Nonsteroidal anti-inflammatory drugs. In: Ferrante MF, Vade Bancoeur TR (Eds). Post Operative Pain Management. New York: Churchill Livingstone, 1993a, pp 133–143.

Ferrante MF. Opioids. In: Ferrante MF, Vade Boncoeur R (Eds). Postoperative Pain Management. New York: Churchill Livingstone, 1993b, pp 145–209.

Ferrer-Brechner T, Ganz P. Combination therapy with ibuprofen and methadone for chronic cancer pain. Am J Med 1984; 77:78–83.

Ferrone FA, Hofrichter J, Eaton WA. Kinetics of sickle hemoglobin polymerization: II. A double nucleation mechanism. J Mol Biol 1985; 183:611–631.

Ferster A, Vermylen C, Cornu G, et al. Hydroxyurea for treatment of severe sickle cell anemia: a pediatric clinical trial. Blood 1996; 88:1960–1964.

Fibach E, Prasanna P, Rodgers GP, Samid D. Enhanced fetal hemoglobin production by phenylacetate and 4-phenylbutyrate in erythroid precursors derived from normal donors and patients with sickle cell disease. Blood 1993; 82:2203–2206.

Fibach E, Schechter AN, Noguchi CT, Rodgers GP. Reducing erythropoietin in cultures of human erythroid precursors elevates the proportion of fetal haemoglobin. Br J Haematol 1994; 88:39–45.

Ficat RP. Treatment of avascular necrosis of the femoral head. In: Hungerford DS (Ed). The Hip. St Louis: Mosby, 1983; pp 279–295.

Ficat RP. Idiopathic bone necrosis of the femoral head. J Bone Joint Surg [Br] 1985; 67-B:3–9.

Fields HL. Pain. New York: McGraw-Hill, 1987.

Fine PG, Marcus M, DeBoer AJ, Vanderoord B. An open label study of oral transmucosal fentanyl citrate (OTFC) for the treatment of breakthrough cancer pain. Pain 1991; 45:149–155.

Fisher B. Hemoglobin Munchausen. JAMA 1974; 229:1044–1045.

Fishman B, Lascalzo M. Cognitive-behavioral interventions in management of cancer pain: principles and applications. Med Clin North Am 1987; 71:271–288.

Flacke JW, Flacke WE, Williams GD. Acute pulmonary edema following naloxone reversal high-dose morphine anesthesia. Anesthesiology 1977; 47:376–378.

Flegel KM, Cole CH. Inappropriate antidiuresis during carbamazepine treatment. Ann Intern Med 1977: 87:722–723.

Fleming AF, Storey J, Molineaux L, Iroko EA, Attai ED. Abnormal haemoglobins in the Sudan savanna of Nigeria: prevalence of hemoglobins and relationships between sickle cell trait, malaria and survival. Ann Trop Med Parasitol 1979; 73:161–172.

Foley KM. The practical use of narcotic analgesics. Med Clin North Am 1982; 66:1091–1103.

Foley KM. The treatment of cancer pain. N Engl J Med 1985; 313:84–95.

Foley KM. Pain syndromes in patients with cancer. Med Clin North Am 1987; 71:169–184.

Foley KM, Portenoy RK. Treatment of pain in sickle cell crisis [letter]. N Engl J Med 1994; 331:334.

Forbes K, Hanks GW, Justins DM, Cherry DA. Sickle cell pain crises. Lancet 1996; 347:262.

Forget BG. Gene therapy. In: Embury SH, Hebbel RP, Mohandas N, Steinberg MH (Eds). Sickle Cell Disease: Basic Principles and Clinical Practice. New York: Raven Press, 1994, pp 853–860.

Forrest WH, Brown BW, Brown CR. Dextroamphetamine with morphine for the treatment of postoperative pain. N Engl J Med 1977; 296:712–715.

Fowler MG, Whitt JK, Lallinger RR, et al. Neuropsychologic and academic functioning of children with sickle cell anemia. Dev Behav Pediatr 1988; 9:213–220.

Francis RB. Protein S-deficiency in sickle cell anemia. J Lab Clin Med 1988; 111:571–576.

Francis RB. Elevated fibrin D-dimer fragment in sickle cell anemia: evidence for activation of coagulation during the steady state as well as in painful crisis. Haemostasis 1989; 19:105–111.

Francis RB, Johnson CS. Vascular occlusion in sickle cell disease: current concepts and unanswered questions. Blood 1991; 77:1405–1404.

Franklin IM, Atkin K. Employment of persons with sickle-cell disease and sickle-cell trait. J Soc Occup Med 1986; 36:76–79.

Frempong KO. Stroke in sickle cell disease: demographic, clinical and therapeutic considerations. Semin Hematol 1991; 28:213–219.

Freye E. Cardiovascular effects of high doses of fentanyl, meperidine and naloxone in dogs. Anesth Analg 1974; 53:40–47.

Friedman EW, Webber AB, Osborn HH, Schwartz S. Oral analgesia for treatment of painful crises in sickle cell anemia. Ann Emerg Med 1986; 15:43–47.

Fromm GH. Trigeminal neuralgia and related disorders. In: Portenoy RK (Ed). Pain: Mechanisms and Syndromes. Philadelphia: WB Saunders Co, 1989; 7:305–319.

Fromm GH. Terrance CF, Chattha AS. Baclofen in the treatment of trigeminal neuralgia: double blind study and long term follow-up. Ann Neurol 1984; 15:240–244.

Fruchtman SM, Kaplan ME, Peterson P, et al. Acute leukemia (AL), hydroxyurea (HU) and polycythemia vera (PV): an analysis of risk and the Polycythemia Vera Study Group [abstract]. Blood 1994; 84(Suppl. 1):518a.

Fultz JM, Senay BC. Guidelines for the management of hospitalized narcotic addicts. Ann Inter Med 1975; 82:815–818.

Gage TP, Gagner JM. Ischemic colitis complicating sickle cell crisis. Gastroenterology 1983; 84:171–174.

Gal TJ. Naloxone reversal of buprenorphine-induced respiratory depression. Clin Pharmacol Ther 1989; 45:66–71.

Galloway SJ, Harwood-Nuss AL. Sickle cell anemia: a review. J Emerg Med 1988; 6:213–226.

Garty I, Koren A, Katzuni E. Uncommon sites of bone infarction in a sickle cell anemia patient. Eur J Nucl Med 1983; 8:367–368.

Garty I, Koren A, Garzozi H. Frontal and orbital bone infarctions causing periorbital swelling in patients with sickle cell anemia. Arch Ophthalmol 1984; 102:1486–1488.

Gaston MH, Verter JI, Woods G, et al. Prophylaxis with oral penicillin in children with sickle cell anaemia. N Engl J Med 1986; 314:1593–1599.

Gerber N, Apseloff G. Death from a morphine infusion during a sickle cell crisis. J Pediatr 1993; 123:322–325.

Giacomini KM, Giacomini JC, Gibson TP, Levy G. Propoxyphene and norpropoxyphene plasma concentrations after oral propoxyphene in cirrhotic patients with and without surgically constructed portacaval shunt. Clin Pharmacol Ther 1980; 28:417–424.

Gil KM. Coping with sickle cell disease pain. Ann Behav Med 1989; 11:49–57.

Gil KM, Abrams MR, Phillips G, Keefe FJ. Sickle cell disease pain: relation of coping strategies to adjustment. J Consult Clin Psychol 1989; 57:725–731.

Gil KM, Phillips G, Edens J, Martin NJ, Abrams M. Observation of pain behaviors during episodes of sickle cell disease pain. Clin J Pain 1994; 10:128–132.

Gilbert PE, Martin WR. The effects of morphine- and nalorphine-like drugs in the nondependent and morphine-dependent chronic spinal dog. J Pharmacol Exp Ther 1976; 198:66–82.

Gill FM, Sleeper LA, Weiner SJ, et al. Clinical events in the first decade in a cohort of infants with sickle cell disease. Blood 1995; 86:776–783.

Gill SJ, Spoe R, Benedict RC, Fall L, Wyman J. Ligand-linked phase equilibria of sickle cell hemoglobin. J Mol Biol 1980; 140:299–312.

Gilman JG, Huisman THJ. DNA sequence variation associated with elevated fetal $^{G}\gamma$-globin production. Blood 1985; 66:783–787.

Givner LB, Luddy RE, Schwartz AD. Etiology of osteomyelitis in patients with major sickle hemoglobinopathies. J Pediatr 1981; 99:411–413.

Glader BE, Propper RD, Buchanan GR. Microcytosis associated with sickle cell anemia. Am J Clin Pathol 1975; 72:63–64.

Gluckman E, Rocha V, Boyer-Chammard A, et al. Outcome of cord-blood transplantation from related and unrelated donors. N Engl J Med 1997; 337:373–381.

Goldberg MF. Treatment of proliferative sickle retinopathy. Trans Am Acad Ophthalmol Otolaryngol 1972; 75:532–536.

Goldberg MA, Husson MA, Bunn HF. The participation of hemoglobins A and F in the polymerization of sickle hemoglobin. J Biol Chem 1977; 252:3414–3421.

Golding JSR. The bone changes in sickle cell anemia. Ann Roy Coll Surg Eng 1956; 19:296–315.

Golino P, Piscione F, Willerson JT, et al. Divergent effects of serotonin on coronary artery dimensions and blood flow in patients with coronary atherosclerosis and control subjects. N Engl J Med 1991; 324:641–648.

Gonzalez ER, Ornato JP, Ware D, Bull D, Evens RP. Comparison of intramuscular analgesic activity of butorphanol and morphine in patients with SCD. Ann Emerg Med 1988; 17:788–791.

Gonzalez ER, Bahal N, Hansen LA, et al. Intermittent injection versus patient-controlled analgesia for sickle-cell crisis pain: comparison of patients in the emergency department. Arch Intern Med 1991; 151:1373–1378.

Gordon PA, Breeze GR, Mann JR, Stuart J. Coagulation fibrinolysis in sickle cell disease. J Clin Pathol 1974; 27:485–489.

Gornick ME, Eggers PW, Reilly TW, et al. Effects of race and income on mortality and use of services among Medicare beneficiaries. N Engl J Med 1996; 335:791–799.

Gourlay GK, Kowalski SR, Plummer JL, et al. The efficacy of transdermal fentanyl in the treatment of postoperative pain: a double-blind comparison of fentanyl and placebo systems. Pain 1990; 40:21–28.

Gourrier E, Karoubi P, El Hanache A, et al. Use of EMLA® cream in a department of neonatology. Pain 1996; 68:431–434.

Gradisek RE. Priapism in sickle cell disease. Ann Emerg Med 1983; 12:510–512.

Graham DY, Agrawal N, Roth SH. Prevention of NSAID-induced gastric ulcer with misoprostol: multicentre, double-blind, placebo-controlled trial. Lancet 1988; ii:1277–1280.

Green D, Scott JP. Is sickle cell crisis a thrombotic event? Am J Hematol 1986; 23:317–321.

Green D. Kwaan HC, Ruiz G. Impair fibrinolysis in sickle cell disease-relation to crisis and infection. Thromb Diath Haemorrh 1970; 24:10–16.

Greer M, Schotland D. Abnormal hemoglobin as a cause of neurologic disease. Neurology 1962; 12:114–123.

Griffin TC, McIntire D, Buchanan GR. High-dose intravenous methylprednisolone therapy for pain in children and adolescents with sickle cell disease. N Engl J Med 1994; 330:733–737.

Grundy R, Howard R, Evans J. Practical management of pain in sickling disorders. Arch Dis Child 1993; 69:1151–1153.

Hagen NA, Foley KM, Cerbones DJ, Portenoy RK, Inturrisi CE. Chronic nausea and morphine-6-glucuronide. J Pain Symptom Manage 1991; 6:125–128.

Hagger D, Wolff S, Owen J, Samson D. Changes in coagulation and fibrinolysis in patients with sickle cell disease compared with healthy black controls. Blood Coagul Fibrinolysis 1995; 6:93–99.

Hall H, Ciarucci K, Berman B. Self-regulation and assessment approaches for vaso-occlusive pain management for pediatric sickle cell anemia patients. Int J Psychosom 1992; 39:28–33.

Hallen B, Carlsson P, Uppfeldt A. A clinical study of lignocaine prilocaine cream to relief the pain of venipuncture. Br J Anaesth 1985; 57:326–328.

Handelsman E, Voulalas D. Albuterol inhalations in acute chest syndrome. Am J Dis Children 1991; 145:603–604.

Hanker GJ, Amstutz HC. Osteonecrosis of the hip in the sickle-cell diseases. J Bone Joint Surg 1988; 70A:499–506.

Hanna MH, Peat SJ, Woodham M, Knibb A, Fung C. Analgesic efficacy and CSF pharmacokinetics of intrathecal morphine-6-glucuronide: comparison with morphine. Br J Anaesth 1990; 64:547–550.

Hansen J, Ginman C, Hartvig P, et al. Clinical evaluation of oral methadone in treatment of cancer pain. Acta Anesthesiol Scand 1982; 74(Suppl.):124–127.

Harkness DR, Roth S. Clinical evaluation of cyanate in sickle cell anemia. In: Brown EB (Ed). Progress in Hematology, Vol. 9. New York: Grune and Stratton, 1975, pp 157–184.

Hart RG, Easton JD. Carbamazepine and hematological monitoring. Ann Neurol 1982; 11:309–312.

Hartrick CT, Pither CE. Tutorial 17: How to manage a difficult pain patient. Pain Digest 1995; 5:93–97.

Hatton CSR, Bunch C, Weatherall DJ. Hepatic sequestration in sickle cell anemia. Br Med J 1985; 290:744–745.

Hattori Y, Kutlar F, Kutlar A, McKie VC, Huisman THJ. Haplotypes of β^S chromosomes among patients with sickle cell anemia from Georgia. Hemoglobin 1986; 10:623–642.

Haut MJ, Cowan DH, Harris JW. Platelet function and survival in sickle cell disease. J Lab Clin Med 1973; 82:44–53.

Hawkey CJ. Non-steroidal anti-inflammatory drugs and peptic ulcers. Br Med J 1990; 300:278–284.

Haynes J, Allison RC. Pulmonary edema; Complication in the management of sickle cell pain crisis. Am J Med 1986; 80:833–840.

Hebbel RP. Beyond hemoglobin polymerization. The red blood cell membrane and sickle disease pathophysiology. Blood 1991; 77:214–237.

Hebbel RP, Boogaerts MAB, Eaton JW, Steinberg MH. Erythrocyte adherence to endothelium in sickle-cell anemia. N Engl J Med 1980a; 302:992–995.

Hebbel RP, Yamada O, Moldow CF, et al. Abnormal adherence of sickle erythrocytes to cultured vascular endothelium: possible mechanism for microvascular occlusion in sickle cell disease. J Clin Invest 1980b; 65:154–160.

Hebbel RP, Moldow CF, Steinberg MH. Modulation of erythrocyte-endothelial interactions and the vaso-occlusive severity of sickling disorders. Blood 1981; 58:947–952.

Hebbel RP, Visser MR, Goodman JL, Jacob HS, Vercellotti GM. Potentiated adherence of sickle erythrocyte to endothelium infected by virus. J Clin Invest 1987; 80:1503–1506.

Heckler FR, Dibbell DG, McCraw JB. Successful use of muscle flaps or myocutaneous flaps in patients with sickle cell disease. Plast Reconstr Surg 1977; 60:902–908.

Heel RC, Brogden RN, Speight TM, Avery GS. Buprenorphine: a review of its pharmacological properties and therapeutic efficacy. Drugs 1979; 17:81–110.

Hendrickse JP de V, Harrison KA, Watson-Williams EJ, Luzzatto L, Ajcbor LN. Pregnancy in homozygous sickle cell anemia. J Obstet Gynecol Br Comm 1972; 79:396–409.

Heng MC. Local hyperbaric oxygen administration for leg ulcers [editorial]. Br J Dermatol 1983; 109:232–234.

Heng MC, Pilgrim JP, Beck FW. A simplified hyperbaric oxygen technique for leg ulcers. Arch Dermatol 1984; 120:640–645.

Herbert B. Hidden agenda. The New York Times 1996; July 15:p A13.

Hermens JM, Hanifin JM, Hirschman CA. Comparison of histamine release in human skin mast cells by morphine, fentanyl and oxymorphone. Anesthesiology 1985; 62:124–129.

Hernanz A, DeMiguel E, Romera N, et al. Calcitonin gene-related peptide II, Substance P and vasoactive intestinal peptide in plasma and synovial fluid from patients with inflammatory joint disease. Br J Rheumatol 1993; 32:31–35.

Hernigou P, Galacteros F, Bachir D, Goutallier D. Deformities of the hip in adults who have sickle-cell disease and had avascular necrosis in childhood. J Bone Joint Surg [Am] 1991; 73-A:81–92.

Hernigou P, Bachir D, Galacteros F. Avascular necrosis of the femoral head in sickle cell disease. Treatment of collapse by the injection of acrylic cement. J Bone Joint Surg (Br) 1993; 75-B:875–880.

Herrick JB. Peculiar elongated and sickle-shaped red blood corpuscles in a case of severe anemia. Arch Intern Med 1910; 6:517–521.

Herz A, Teschemacher HJ. Activities and sites of antinociceptive action of morphine-like analgesics and kinetics of distribution following intravenous intracerebral and intraventricular application. Adv Drug Res 1971; 6:79.

Higgs DR, Aldridge BE, Lamb J, et al. The interaction of alpha-thalassemia and homozygous sickle-cell disease. N Engl J Med 1982; 306:1441–1446.

Higgs DR, Vickers MA, Wilkie AOM, et al. A review of the molecular genetics of the human alpha globin gene cluster. Blood 1989; 73:1081–1104.

Hill CS. The negative influence of licensing and disciplinary boards and drug enforcement agencies on pain treatment with opioid analgesics. J Pharmaceutical Care in Pain and Symptom Control 1993; 1:43–62.

Hill MC, Oh KS, Bowerman JW, Siegelman SS, James AE. Abnormal epiphyses in sickling disorders. Am J Roentgenol 1975; 124:34–43.

Hodenpyl E. A case of apparent absence of the spleen, with general compensatory lymphatic hyperplasia. Med Record 1898; 54:695–698.

Hofrichter J, Ross PD, Eaton WA. A physical description of hemoglobin S gelation. In: Hercules JI, Cottan GL, Waterman MR, Schecter AN (Eds). Proceedings of the Symposium on Molecular and Cellular Aspects of Sickle Cell Disease, DHEW Publication no (NIH) 76-1007. Bethesda, MD: U.S. Department of Health, Education and Welfare, 1976, p 185.

Holbrook CT. Patient-controlled analgesia pain management for children with sickle cell disease. J Assoc Acad Minor Phys 1990; 1:93–96.

Holley FO, Van-Steennis C. Postoperative analgesia with fentanyl: pharmacokinetics and pharmacodynamics of constant-rate I.V. and transdermal delivery. Br J Anaesth 1988; 60:608–613

Homi J, Reynolds J, Skinner A, Hanna W, Serjeant GR. General anaesthesia in sickle-cell disease. Br Med J 1979; 1599–1601.

Horton JAB. The Diseases of Tropical Climates and Their Treatment. London: Churchill, 1874.

Hoskin PJ, Hanks GW. Opioid agonist-antagonist drug in acute and chronic pain states. Drugs 1991; 41:326–344.

Houck CS, Sullivan LJ, Wilder RT, Rusy LM, Burrows FJ. Pharmacokinetics of a higher dose of rectal acetaminophen in children [abstract]. Anesthesia 1995; 83:A1126.

Houde RW. Analgesic effectiveness of narcotic agonist-antagonists. Br J Clin Pharmacol 1979; 7:297–308.

Houde RW, Wallenstein SL, Beaver WT. Clinical measurement of pain. In: de Stevens G (Ed). Analgesics. New York: Academic, 1975, pp 75–81.

Howard R. Preoperative and postoperative pain control. Arch Dis Child 1993; 69:699–703.

Huang JC, Gay R, Khella SL. Sickling crisis, fat embolism, and coma after steroids. Lancet 1994; 344:951–952.

Hughes JG, Diggs LW, Gillespie CE. Involvement of the nervous system in sickle cell anemia. J Pediatr 1940; 17:166–184.

Huisman THJ, Carver MFH, Efremov GD. A syllabus of human hemoglobin variants. Augusta, GA: The Sickle Cell Anemia Foundation, 1996.

Huisman THJ, Carver MFH, Boysal E. A Syllabus of Thalassemia Mutations. Augusta, GA: The Sickle Cell Anemia Foundation, 1997.

Hull DH. Other important medical conditions. In: Ernsting J, King P (Eds). Aviation Medicine. London: Butterworths, 1988, p 616.

Hunter RL, Papadea C, Gallagher CJ, Finlayson DC, Check IJ. Increased whole blood viscosity during coronary artery bypass surgery. Studies to evaluate the effects of soluble fibrin and poloxamer 188. Thromb Haemost 1990; 63:6–12.

Hupert C, Yacoub M, Turgeon LR: Effect of hydroxyzine on morphine analgesia for the treatment of postoperative pain. Anesth Analg 1980; 59:690–696.

Ibrahim AS. Relationship between meteorological changes and occurrence of painful sickle cell crises in Kuwait. Trans R Soc Trop Med Hyg 1980; 74:159–161.

Ingram VM. A specific chemical difference between the globins of normal human and sickle-cell anemia haemoglobin. Nature 1956; 178:792–794.

Insel PA. Analgesic antipyretic and antiinflammatory agents and drugs employed in the treatment of gout. In: Hardman JG, Limbird LE, Malinoff PB, Ruddon RW, Gilman AG (Eds). Goodman and Gilman's The Pharmacological Basis of Therapeutics, 9th ed. New York: McGraw-Hill, 1996, pp 617–657.

International Association for the Study of Pain. Pain terms: list with definitions and notes on usage. Pain 1979; 6:249–252.

International Association for the Study of Pain. Pain terms: a list with definitions and notes on usage. Pain 1982; 14:205–206.

Inturrisi CE, Umans JG. Meperidine biotransformation and central nervous system toxicity in animals and humans. In: Foley KM, Inturrisi CE (Eds). Opioid Analgesics in the Management of Clinical Pain. Advances in Pain Research and Therapy, Vol 8. New York: Raven Press, 1986, pp 143–154.

Inturrisi CE, Colburn WN, Verebey K, et al. Propoxyphene and norpropoxyphene kinetics after single and repeated doses of propoxyphene. Clin Pharmacol Ther 1982; 31:157–167.

Isichei E. A history of the Igbo people. London: Macmillan, 1976, pp 26–27.

Ittyerah R, Alkjaersig N, Fletcher A, Chaplin H. Coagulation Factor XIII concentration in sickle cell disease. J Lab Clin Med 1976; 88:546–554.

Itzchak Y, Glickman MG, Gottschalk A, Lange R, Downing E. Hemodynamic and morphologic evaluation of the spleen after splenic vein ligation in the dog. Invest Radiol 1978; 13:155–160.

Ives TJ, Guerra MF. Constant morphine infusion for severe sickle cell crisis. Drug Intelligence and Clinical Pharmacy 1987; 21:625–626.

Iwegbu CG, Fleming AF. Avascular necrosis of the femoral head in sickle-cell disease: a series from the Guinea Savannah of Nigeria. J Bone Joint Surg 1985; 67-B(1):29–32.

Izzo V, Pagnoni B, Rigoli M. Recent acquisitions in pain therapy: meclofenamic acid. Clin J Pain 1991; 7(Suppl. 1):S49–S53.

Jackson JF, Odom JL, Bell WN. Amelioration of sickle cell disease by persistent fetal hemoglobin. JAMA 1961; 177:867–869.

Jacox AK, Carr DB, Payne R, et al. Management of Cancer Pain. Clinical Practice Guideline no. 9, AHCPR Publication no. 94-0592. Rockville, MD: U.S. Department of Health and Human Services, Public Health Service, Agency for Health Care Policy and Research, 1994.

Jaffe JH, Martin WR. Opioid analgesics and antagonists. In: Gilman AG, Goodman LS, Rall TW, Murad F (Eds). The Pharmacological Basis of Therapeutics, 7th ed. New York: Macmillan, 1985, p 491.

Jaffe JH, Martin WR. Opioid analgesics and antagonists. In: Goodman LS, Gilman A, Rall TW, Nies AS, Taylor B (Eds). Goodman and Gilman's The Pharmacological Basis of Therapeutics, 8th ed. New York: Pergamon Press, 1990, pp 485–521.

Jandle JH, Jacob HS, Daland CA. Hypersplenism due to infection: a study of 5 cases manifesting hemolytic anemia. N Engl J Med 1961; 264:1063–1071.

Jänig W. Can reflex sympathetic dystrophy be reduced to an alpha-adrenoreceptor disease? APS J 1992; 1:16–22.

Janis MG. Leukocyte alkaline phosphatase in sickle cell disease. N Engl J Med 1976; 294:163.

Jennings RB, Sommers HM, Smuth GA, Flack HA, Linn G. Myocardial necrosis induced by temporary occlusion of a coronary artery in the dog. Arch Pathol Lab Med 1960; 70:82–92.

Jensen WW, Lessin LS. Membrane alterations associated with hemoglobinopathies. Semin Hematol 1970; 4:409–426.

Jessel TM, Dodd J. Functional chemistry of primary afferent neurons. In: Wall PD, Melzack R (Eds). Textbook of Pain, 2nd ed. Edinburgh: Churchill Livingstone 1989, pp 82–99.

Jiak H, Miettinen OS, Shapiro S, et al. Comprehensive drug surveillance. JAMA 1970; 213:1455–1460.

Johnson CS, Verdegem TD. Pulmonary complications of sickle cell disease. Semin Respir Med 1988; 9(3):287–295.

Johnson CS, Omata M, Tong MJ, et al. Liver involvement in sickle cell disease. Medicine 1985; 64:349–356.

Johnson FL, Mentzer WC, Kalinyak KA, Sullivan KM, Abboud MR. Bone marrow transplantation for sickle cell disease: the United States experience. Am J Pediatr Hematol Oncol 1994; 16:22–26.

Joiner CH. Cation transport and volume regulation in sickle red blood cells. Am J Physiol 1993; 264 (Cell Physiol 33):C251–C270.

Jones SR, Binder RA, Donowho EM Jr. Sudden death in sickle cell trait. N Engl J Med 1970; 282:323–325.

Joyce TH, Skjonsky BS, Taylor B, Morrow DH, Hess KR. Dermal analgesia in children using a eutectic mixture of lidocaine and prilocaine. Anesth Analg 1990; 70:S184.

Kaiko RF. Discussion. In: Foley K, Inturrisi CE (Eds). Opioid Analgesics in the Management of Clinical Pain. Advances in Pain Research and Therapy, Vol 8., New York: Raven Press, 1986, pp 235–240.

Kaiko RF, Foley KM, Grabinski PV, et al. Central nervous system excitatory effects of meperidine in cancer patients. Ann Neurol 1983; 13:180–185.

Kalinyak KA, Morris C, Ball WS, et al. Bone marrow transplantation in a young child with sickle cell anemia. Am J Hematol 1995; 48:256–261.

Kalso E, Vainio A. Morphine and oxycodone hydrochloride in the management of cancer pain. Clin Pharmacol Ther 1990; 47:639–646.

Kan YW, Dozy AM. Polymorphism of DNA sequence adjacent to human β-globin structural gene: relationship to sickle mutation. Proc Natl Acad Sci USA 1978; 65:5631–5635.

Kanver RM, Foley RM. Patterns of narcotic drug use in a cancer pain clinic. Ann NY Acad Sci 1981; 362:161–172.

Kapelushni J, Koren G, Solh H, Greenberg M, DeVeber L. Evaluating the efficacy of EMLA in alleviating pain associated with lumbar puncture: comparison of open and double-blinded protocols in children. Pain 1990; 42:31–34.

Kaplan SS, Nardi M. Impairment of leukocyte function during sickle cell crisis. J Reticuloendothelia Soc 1977; 22:499–506.

Karayalcin G, Lanzkowsky P. Plasma protein C levels in children with sickle cell disease. Am J Pediatr Hematol/Oncol 1989; 11:320–323.

Karayalcin G, Imran M, Rosner F. Blister cells: association with pregnancy, sickle cell disease, and pulmonary infarction. JAMA 1972; 219:1727–1729.

Karayalcin G, Lanzkowsky P, Kari AB. Serum-α-hydroxybutyrate dehydrogenase levels in children with sickle cell disease. Am J Pediatr Hematol Oncol 1981; 3:169–171.

Kastanis E, Hsu E, Luke KH, McKee JA. Systemic lupus erythematosus and sickle hemoglobinopathies: a report of two cases and review of the literature. Am J Hematol 1987; 25:211–214.

Katz J, Kavanagh BP, Sandler AN, et al. Preemptive analgesia: clinical evidence of neuroplasticity contributing to post operative pain. Anesthesiology 1992; 77:439–446.

Katz N, Ferrante FM. Nociception. In: Ferrante FM, VadeBoncoeur TR (Eds). Post Operative Pain Management. New York: Churchill Livingstone 1993; pp 17–67.

Kaul DK, Fabry ME, Nagel RL. Microvascular sites and characteristics of sickle cell adhesion to vascular endothelium in shear flow conditions: pathophysiological implications. Proc Natl Acad Sci USA 1989; 86:3356–3360.

Kaul DK, Fabry ME, Nagel RL. The pathophysiology of vascular obstruction in the sickle syndromes. Blood Rev 1996; 10:29–44.

Keeley K, Buchanan GR. Acute infarction of the long bones in children with sickle cell anemia. J Pediatr 1982; 101:170–175.

Kenny MW, George AJ, Stuart J. Platelet hyperactivity in sickle cell disease: a consequence of hyposplenism. J Clin Pathol 1980; 33:622–625.

Kenny MW, Meakin M, Worthington DJ, Stuart J. Erythrocyte deformability of oxygenated sickle erythrocytes in the asymptomatic state and in painful crisis. Br J Haematol 1985; 59:363–368.

Keynon J. Acupressure Techniques: A Self-Help Guide. Rochester: Healing Arts Press, 1988.

Khojasteh A, Evans W, Reynolds RD, Thomas G, Saivarese JJ. Controlled release morphine in the treatment of cancer pain with pharmacokinetic correlation. J Clin Oncol 1987; 5:956–961.

Khouri RK, Upton J. Bilateral lower limb salvage with free flaps in a patient with sickle cell ulcers. Ann Plast Surg 1991; 27:574–576.

Kincaid-Smith P. Effects of non-narcotic analgesics on the kidney. Drugs 1986; 32(Suppl. 4):109–128.

Kirpatrick DV, Barrios NJ, Hambert JH. Bone marrow transplantation for sickle cell anemia. Semin Hematol 1991; 28:240–243.

Kirson LE, Tomaro AJ. Mental nerve paresthesis secondary to sickle cell crisis. Oral Surg 1979; 48:509–512.

Kitahata LM, Collins JG, Robinson CJ. Narcotic effects on the nervous system. In: Kitahata LM, Collins JG (Eds). Narcotic Analgesics in Anesthesiology. Baltimore: Williams & Wilkins, 1982, p 57.

Kitchen EA, Dawson W, Rainsford KD, Cawston T. Inflammation and possible modes of action of anti-inflammatory drugs. In: Rainsford KD (Ed). Anti-inflammatory and anti-rheumatic drugs. Vol. 1., Inflammation Mechanisms and Actions of Traditional Drugs. Boca Raton, FL: CRC Press, 1985, pp 21–87.

Klug PP, Kaye N, Jensen WN. Endothelial cell and vascular damage in the sickle cell disorders. Blood Cells 1982; 8:175–184.

Konotey-Ahulu FID. Hereditary qualitative and quantitative erythrocyte defects in Ghana: an historical and geographical survey. Ghana Med J 1968; 7:118–119.

Konotey-Ahulu FID. Patterns of Clinical Haemoglobinopathy. East Afr Med J 1969; 46:149–156.

Konotey-Ahulu FID. Mental nerve neuropathy: a complication of sickle cell crisis. Lancet 1972; 2:388.

Konotey-Ahulu FID. The sickle cell diseases. Arch Int Med 1974; 133:611–619.

Konotey-Ahulu FID. The sickle cell disease: clinical manifestations including the "sickle crisis." Arch Intern Med 1979; 133:611–619.

Konotey-Ahulu FID. The Sickle Cell Disease Patient. London: Macmillan, 1991.

Koren G. Management of childhood pain: new approaches to procedure-related pain: use of eutectic mixture of local anesthetics in young children for procedure-related pain. J Pediatr 1993; 122:S30–S35.

Koren A, Fedchteyn S, Katzuni E. Early diagnosis of bone infarction in children with sickle cell anemia by using MDP 99m Tc scanning. Harefuah 1982; 102:182–185.

Koren A, Garty I, Katzuni E. Bone infarction in children with sickle cell disease: Early diagnosis and differentiation from osteomyelitis. Eur J Pediatr 1984; 142:93–97.

Koshy M, Enstuah R, Koranda A, et al. Leg ulcers in patients with sickle cell disease. Blood 1989; 74:1403–1408.

Kosterlitz WH. Opiate actions in guinea pig ileum and mouse vas deferens. Neurosci Res Bull 1975; 13:68–70.

Kripke BJ, Finck AJ, Shah N, Snow JC. Naloxone antagonism after narcotic supplemented anesthesia. Anesth Analg 1976; 55:800–805.

Kumar A, Posner G, Marsh F, Bellvue R, Dosik H. Acute pancreatitis in sickle cell crisis. J Natl Med Assoc 1989; 81:91–92.

Kumar S, Powars D, Allen J, Haywood LJ. Anxiety, self-concept, and personal and social adjustments in children with sickle cell anemia. J Pediatr 1976; 88:859–863.

Kwaan HC, Green D. The inhibitors of fibrinolysis in sickle cell disease. Thromb Diath Haemorrh 1973; 53(Suppl):263–270.

Labie D, Pagnier J, Lapoumeroulie C, et al. Common haplotype dependency of high $^{G}\gamma$-globin gene expression and high HbF levels in β-thalassemia and sickle cell anemia patients. Proc Natl Acad Sci USA 1985; 82:2111–2114.

Lachant NA, Oseas RS. Case report: vaso-Occlusive crisis-associated neutrophil dysfunction in patients with sickle cell disease. Am J Med Sci 1987; 30:253–257.

Lande WM, Andrews DL, Clark MR, et al. The incidence of painful crisis in homozygous sickle cell disease: correlation with red cell deformability. Blood 1988; 72:2056–2059.

Langman MJS. Treating ulcers in patients receiving anti-arthritic drugs [editorial]. QJM 1989; 73:1089–1091.

Lasagna L, Beecher HK. The optimal dose of morphine. JAMA 1954; 156:230–234.

Lasagna RG, DeKornfeldt TJ. Methotrimeprazine: a new phenothiazine derivative with analgesic properties. JAMA 1961; 178:887.

Laska EM, Sunshine A, Mueller F, et al. Caffeine as an analgesic adjuvant. JAMA 1984; 251:1711–1718.

Latasch L, Probst S, Dudziak R. Reversal by nalbuphine of respiratory depression caused by fentanyl. Anesth Analg 1984; 63:814–816.

Lawrence C, Fabry ME. Erythrocyte sedimentation rate during steady state and painful crisis in sickle cell anemia. Am J Med 1986; 81:801–808.

Lawrence C, Fabry ME, Nagel RL. Red cell distribution width parallels dense red cell disappearance during painful crises in sickle cell anemia. J Lab Clin Med 1985; 105:706–710.

Lebby R. Case of absence of the spleen. South J Med Pharm 1846; 1:481–483.

Lee G, DeMaria AN, Amsterdam EA, et al. Comparative effects of morphine, meperidine and pentazocine on cardiocirculatory dynamics in patients with acute myocardial infarction. Am J Med 1976; 60:949–955.

Lee J, Forrester P. EMLA for postoperative analgesia for day case circumcision in children: a comparison with dorsal nerve of penis block. Anesthesia 1992; 47:1081–1083.

Lee RE, Golding JS, Serjeant GR. The radiological features of avascular necrosis of the femoral head in homozygous sickle cell disease. Clin Radiol 1981; 32:205–214.

Lee RC, McTavish D, Sorkin EM. Tramadol: a preliminary review of its pharmacodynamic and pharmacokinetic properties, and therapeutic potential in acute and chronic pain states. Drugs 1993; 46:313–340.

Leff RD, Aldo-Benson MA, Spitz-Fife R. Tophaceous gout in a patient with sickle cell-thalassemia: case report and review of the literature. Arthitis Rheum 1983; 26:928–929.

Lehmann JF, de Lateur BF. Diathermy and superficial heat and cold therapy. In: Kottke FJ, Stillwell GK, Lehmann JF (Eds). Krusen's Handbook of Physical Medicine and Rehabilitation, 3rd ed. Philadelphia: WB Saunders, 1982, pp 275–350.

Lehmann JF, de Lateur BF. Ultrasound, shortwave, microwave, superficial heat and cold in the treatment of pain. In: Wall PD, Melzack R (Eds). Textbook of Pain, 2nd ed. Edinburgh: Churchill Livingstone, 1989, pp 932–941.

Leichtman DA, Brewer GJ. Elevated plasma levels of fibrinopeptide A during sickle cell anemia pain crisis: evidence for intravascular coagulation. Am J Hematol 1978; 5:183–190.

Leivy FE, Schnabel TG. Abdominal crisis in sickle anemia. Am J Med Sci 1932; 183:381–391.

Levin J, Taiwo Y. Inflammatory pain. In: Wall PD, Melzack R (Eds). Textbook of Pain. 3rd ed. New York: Churchill Livingstone, 1994, pp 45–56.

Levine J. Pain and analgesia: the outlook for more rational treatment. Ann Intern Med 1984; 100:269–276.

Levy M. Pharmacokinetics of metamizol metabolites. In: Burne K (Ed). 100 years of pyrazolone drugs. Basel: Birkhauser Verlag, 1986, pp 199–204.

Levy M. Adverse reactions to OTC analgesics: an epidemiological evaluation. In: Brune K (Ed). Agents and Actions. Supplement 25: Non-opioid (OTC) Analgesics: Risks/Benefits in Perspective. Basel: Birkhauser Verlag, 1988, pp 21–31.

Lew Vl, Freemen CJ, Ortiz OE, Bookchin RM. A mathematical model of the volume, pH, and ion content regulation in reticulocytes: application to the pathophysiology of sickle cell dehydration. J Clin Invest 1991; 87:100–112.

Leysen JE, Gommeren W, Niemegeers CJ. [^{3}H] Sufentanil, superior ligand for μ opiate receptors: binding properties and regional distribution in rat brain and spinal cord. Eur J Pharmacol 1983; 87:209–225.

Lindenbaum J. Hemoglobin Munchausen. JAMA 1974; 228:498.

Lipowsky HH, Sheikh NU, Katz DM. Intravital microscopy of capillary hemodynamics in sickle cell disease. J Clin Invest 1987; 80:117–127.

Lippman SM, Ginzton LE, Thigpen T, Tanaka KR, Laks MM. Mitral valve prolapse in sickle cell disease. Arch Intern Med 1985; 145:435–438.

Liu JE, Gzesh DJ, Ballas SK. The spectrum of epilepsy in sickle cell anemia. J Neuro Sci 1994; 123:6–10.

Livingstone FB. Anthropological implications of sickle cell gene distribution in West Africa. Am Anthropology 1958; 60:533–562.

Livingstone FB. Malaria and human polymorphisms. Ann Rev Genet 1971; 5:33–64.

Longnecker DE, Grazis PA, Eggers GWN. Naloxone for antagonism of morphine induced respiratory depression. Anesth Analg 1973; 52:447–453.

Lubin B, Vichinsky E. Sickle cell disease. In: Hoffman R, Benz EJ, Shattil SJ, et al. (Eds). Hematology: Basic Principles and Practice. New York: Churchill Livingstone, 1991, pp 450–471.

Lucas GS, Caldwell NM, Stuart J. Fluctuating deformability of oxygenated sickle erythrocytes in the asymptomatic state and in painful crisis. Br J Haematol 1985; 59:363–368.

Lukens JN. Sickle cell disease. Dis Mon 1981; 27:1–56.

Lutzker LG, Alavi A. Bone and marrow imaging in sickle cell disease: diagnosis of infarction. Semin Nucl Med 1976; 6:83–93.

Luzzato L, Nwachuku-Jarrett ES, Reddy S. Increased sickling of parasitized erythrocytes as mechanisms of resistance against malaria in the sickle cell trait. Lancet 1970; 1:319–322

Lycka BA. EMLA, a new and effective topical anesthetic. J Dermatol Surg Oncol 1992; 18:859–862.

Maccarrone C, West RJ, Broomhead AF, Hudson GP. Single dose pharmacokinetics of Kapanol™ a new oral sustained-release formulation. Clinical Drug Investigation 1994; 7:262–274.

Mackie I, Bull H, Brozovic M. Altered Factor VIII complexes in sickle cell disease. Br J Haematol 1980; 46:499–502.

Magdoff-Fairchild B, Poillon WN, Li TI, Bertles JF. Thermodynamic studies of polymerization of deoxygenated sickle cell hemoglobin. Proc Natl Acad Sci USA 1976; 73:990–994.

Mahmood A. Fibrinolytic activity and sickle cell crises. Br Med J 1969; 1:52–53.

Mahmood A, Macintosh DM, Shaper AG. Fibrinolytic activity in the clinical crisis of sickle cell anemia. Br Med J 1967; 3:653–654.

Mallory TB. Sickle cell anemia: case records of the Massachusetts General Hospital. N Engl J Med 1941; 225:626–630.

Malloy J, Wade A, Ballas SK. Managing conflict between nursing staff and hospitalized patients with sickle cell disease [abstract 180a]. In: Book of Abstracts, 18th Meeting of the National Sickle Cell Disease Program, Philadelphia, PA, May 22–25, 1993.

Mallouh AA. Subperiosteal bleeding with acute bone infarcts in children with sickle cell disease. Am J Dis Children 1987; 141:1251.

Mallouh AA, Talab Y. Bone and joint infection in patients with sickle cell disease. J Pediatr Orthop 1985; 5:158–162.

Malmberg AB, Yaksh TL. Pharmacology of spinal action of ketorolac, morphine, ST-91, U50488H, and L-PIA on the formalin test and isobolographic analysis of the NSAID interaction. Anesthesiology 1993; 79:270–281.

Manci EA, Maisel DA, Conrad ME. Systemic necrotizing vasculitis in sickle cell disease. Am J Hematol 1987; 26:93–96.

Mankin HJ. Nontraumatic necrosis of bone (osteonecrosis). N Engl J Med 1992; 326:1473–1479.

Mann JR. Sickle cell haemoglobinopathies in England. Arch Dis Child 1981; 56:676.

Margolies MP. Sickle Cell Anemia: a composite study and survey. Medicine 1951; 30:357–443.

Marino C, McDonald E. Rheumatoid arthritis in a patient with sickle cell disease. J Rhematol 1990; 17:970–972.

Marks RM, Sachar EJ. Undertreatment of medical inpatients with narcotic analgesics. Ann Intern Med 1973; 78:173–181.

Marsten PD, Shah KK. Artificially induced edema in sickle cell anemia. J Trop Med Hyg 1964; 67:31–34.

Martin CR, Cobb C, Tatter D, Johnson C, Haywood J. Acute myocardial infarction in sickle cell anemia. Arch Intern Med 1983; 143:830–831.

Martin WR, Jasiaki DR, Mansky PA. Naltrexone, an antagonist for the treatment of heroin dependence. Arch Gen Psychiatry 1973; 28:784–791.

Martin WR, Eades CG, Thompson JA, Huppler RE, Gilbert PE. The effects of morphine-and nalorphine-like drugs in the nondependent and morphine-dependent cyclazocine-dependent spinal dog. J Pharmacol Exp Ther 1976; 197:517–532.

Maruta T, Swanson DW, Finlayson RE. Drug abuse and dependency in patients with chronic pain. Mayo Clin Proc 1979; 54:241–244.

Mason VR. Sickle cell anemia. JAMA 1922; 79:1318–1320.

Mather LE, Denson DD. Pharmacokinetics of systemic opioids for the management of pain. In: Sinatra et al. (Eds). Acute Pain Mechanism and Management. St. Louis, MO: Mosby–Year Book, 1992.

Mather LE, Gourlay GK. Biotransformation of opioids: significance for pain therapy. In: Nimmo WS, Smith G (Eds). Opioid Agonist/Antagonist Drugs in Clinical Practice. Amsterdam: Excerpta Medica, 1984, p 31.

Mather LE, Denson DD, Raj PP. Tutorial 22: Pharmacokinetics and pharmacodynamics of analgesic agents. Pain Digest 1996; 6:34–41.

Maze M. Clinical implications of membrane receptor function in anesthesia. Anesthesiology 1980; 55:160–171.

McCall IW, Desai P, Serjeant BE, Serjeant GR. Cholelithiasis in Jamaican patients with homozygous sickle cell disease. Am J Hematol 1977; 3:15–21.

McDonald CR, Eichner ER. Concurrent primary pneumococcemia, disseminated intravascular coagulation, and sickle cell anemia. South Med J 1978; 71:858–860.

McDonaugh KT, Nienhuis AW. Induction of the human γ-globin gene promoter in K562 cells by sodium butyrate: reversal of repression by CCAAT displacement protein [abstract]. Blood 1991; 78(Suppl.):255a.

McFadden EP, Clarke JG, Davies GJ, et al. Effect of intracoronary serotonin on coronary vessels in patients with stable angina and patients with variant angina. N Engl J Med 1991; 324:648–654.

McGivney WT, Crooks GM. The care of patients with severe chronic pain in terminal illness. JAMA 1984; 251:1182–1188.

McGrath PA (Ed). Pain in Children: Nature, Assessment, Treatment. New York: Guilford Press, 1990.

McKusick VA. Molecular Genetics. Bethesda, MD: Foundation for Advanced Education in the Sciences, Inc, 1987.

McPherson E, Perlin E, Finke H, Castro O, Pittman J. Patient-controlled analgesia in patients with sickle cell vaso-occlusive crisis. Am J Med Sci 1990; 299:10–12.

McQuay HJ. Pre-emptive analgesia. Br J Anaesth 1992; 69:1–3.

McQuay HJ, Bullingham RE, Bennett MR, Moore RA. Delayed respiratory depression: a case report and a new hypothesis. Acta Anaesthesiol Belg 1979; 30(Suppl.):245–247.

Meltzer BA. Sickle cell pain crisis. Lancet 1996; 347:262.

Melzack R. The tragedy of needless pain. Sci Am 1990; 262:27–33.

Melzack R, Wall PD. Pain mechanisms: a new theory. Science 1965; 150:971–979.

Melzack R, Stillwell DM, Fox EJ. Trigger points and acupuncture points for pain: correlations and implications. Pain 1977; 3:3–23.

Meradante S. Opioids and akathisia. J Pain Symptom Manage 1995; 10:415.

Merskey H (Ed). Classification of chronic pain: description of chronic pain syndromes and definitions of pain terms. Pain 1986; (Suppl. 3):S216–S221.

Merskey H. Development of a universal language of pain syndromes. In: Bonica JJ, Lindblom U, Iggo A (Eds). Advances in Pain Research and Therapy. Vol 5., New York: Raven Press, 1983, pp 37–52.

Mian E, Mian M, Beghe F. Lyophilized Type-1 collagen and chronic leg ulcers. Int J Tissue React 1991; 13:257–269.

Michaelis LL, Hickey PR, Clark TA, Dixon WM. Ventricular irritability associated with the use of naloxone. Ann Thorac Surg 1974; 18:608–614.

Middlemiss JH, Raper AB. Skeletal changes in the hemoglobinopathies. J Bone Joint Surg 1966; 48B:693–702.

Midence K, Elander J. Adjustment and coping in adults with sickle cell disease: an assessment of research evidence. Br J Health Psychol 1996; 1:95–111.

Miller RL, Webster ME, Melmon KL. Interaction of leukocytes and endotoxin with the plasmin and kinin systems. Eur J Pharmacol 1975; 33:53–60.

Miller RP, Roberts RJ, Fischer LJ. Acetaminophen elimination kinetics in neonates, children and adults. Clin Pharmacol Ther 1976; 19:284–294.

Miller RR, Jick H. Clinical effects of meperidine in hospitalized medical patients. J Clin Pharmacol 1978; 18:180–189.

Milner PF, Squires JE. Post-transfusion crisis in sickle cell anemia. In: Nagel RL (Ed). Pathophysiological Aspects of Sickle Cell Vasoocclusion. New York: Alan R. Liss, 1987, pp 351–359.

Milner PF, Kraus AP, Sebes JI, et al. Sickle cell disease as a cause of osteonecrosis of the femoral head. N Engl J Med 1991; 325:1476–1481.

Milner PF, Kraus AP, Sebes JI, et al. Osteonecrosis of the humeral head in sickle cell disease. Clin Orthop Related Res 1993; 289:136–143.

Miser AW, Narang PK, Dothage JA, et al. Transdermal fentanyl for pain control in patients with cancer. Pain 1989; 37:15–21.

Misra AL. Metabolism of opiates. In: Adler ML, Manara L, Samanin R (Eds). Factors Affecting the Action of Narcotics. New York: Raven Press, 1978, p 297.

Mitchell A, Fisher AP, Brunner M, Ware RG, Hanna M. Pethidine for painful crisis in sickle cell disease. Br Med J 1991; 303:249.

Mohandas N, Evans E. Adherence of sickle erythrocytes to vascular endothelial cells: requirement for both cell membrane changes and plasma factors. Blood 1984; 64:232–287.

Mohandas N, Clark MR, Jacobs MS, Shohet SB. Analysis of factors regulating erythrocyte deformability. J Clin Invest 1980; 66:563–573.

Moldenhauer CC, Roach GW, Finlayson DC, et al. Nalbuphine antagonism of ventilatory depression following high-dose fentanyl anesthesia. Anesthesiology 1985; 62:647–650.

Moncada S, Vane JR. Arachidonic and acid metabolites and the interactions between platelets and blood-vessel walls. N Engl J Med 1979; 300:1142–1147.

Monplaisir N, Merault G, Poyart C, et al. A variant with lower solubility than hemoglobin S and producing sickle cell disease in heterozygotes. Proc Natl Acad Sci USA 1986; 83:9363–9367.

Montgomery CJ, McCormack JP, Reichert CC, Marsland CP. Plasma concentrations after high dose (45 mg/kg) rectal acetaminophen in children. Can J Anaesth 1995; 42:982–986.

Montilla E, Frederick WS, Cass LJ. Analgesic effects of methotrimeprazine and morphine. Arch Intern Med 1963; 111:725–728.

Morgan AG, Venner AM. Immunity and leg ulcers in homozygous sickle cell disease. J Clin Lab Immunol 1981; 6:51–55.

Morrison RS. Update on sickle cell disease: incidence of addiction and choice of opioid in pain management. Pediatr Nurs 1991; 17:503.

Moulin DE, Kreeft JH, Murray PN, Murray-Parsons N, Bouquillon AI. Comparison of continuous subcutaneous and intravenous hydromorphone infusions for management of cancer pain. Lancet 1991; 337:465–468.

Mukherjee MB, Colah KB, Ghosh K, Mohanty D, Krishnamoorthy R. Milder clinical course of sickle cell disease in patients with α-thalassemia in the Indian subcontinent [letter]. Blood 1997; 89:732

Munetz MR, Cornes CL. Distinguishing akathisia from tardive dyskinesia: a review of the literature. J Clin Psychopharmacol 1983; 3:343–350.

Murphy MR, Hug CC Jr. Pharmacokinetics of intravenous morphine in patients anesthetized with enflurane-nitrous oxide. Anesthesiology 1981; 54:187–192.

Murray M, May A. Painful crises in sickle cell disease; patients' perspectives. Br Med J 1988; 297:452–454.

Nadel C, Portadin G. Sickle cell crisis: psychological factors associated with onset. NY State J Med 1977; 77:1075–1078.

Nadelson T. The Munchausen spectrum: borderline character features. Gen Hosp Psychiat 1979; 1:11–17.

Nadvi S, Sarnaik S, Ravindranath Y. Association of seizures with meperidine in sickle cell diseases. In: Book of Abstracts, 20th Meeting of the National Sickle Cell Disease Program, Boston, MA, March 18–21, 1995, p 210.

Nagel RL. The origin of the hemoglobin S gene. Einstein Quart J Biol Med 1984; 2:53–62.

Nagel RL, Bookchin RM, Johnson J, et al. Structural basis of the inhibitory effects of hemoglobin F and hemoglobin A_2 on the polymerization of Hb S. Proc Natl Acad Sci USA 1979; 76:670–674.

Nagel RL, Fabry ME, Pagnier J, et al. Hematologically and genetically distinct forms of sickle cell anemia in Africa: the Senegal type and the Benin type. N Engl J Med 1985; 312:880–884.

Nagel RL, Rao SK, Dunda-Belkhodja O, et al. The hematologic characteristics of sickle cell anemia bearing the Bantu haplotype: the relationship between Ggamma and Hb F level. Blood 1987; 69:1026–1030.

Nagel RL, Erlingsson S, Fabry ME, et al. The Senegal DNA haplotype is associated with the amelioration of anemia in African American sickle cell anemia patients. Blood 1991; 77:1371–1375.

Nagel RL, Vichinsky E, Shah M, et al. F reticulocyte response in sickle cell anemia treated with recombinant human erythropoietin: a double-blind study. Blood 1993; 81:9–14.

Nash K. Family counseling in sickle cell anemia. Urban Health 1977; September, 44–47.

Nash KB, Kramer KD, Hughes M, Powell A, Telfair J. Sickle cell mutual help groups. A five year study: information, findings and resources. Chapel Hill, NC: Psychosocial Research Division of Duke University/University of North Carolina, 1992.

Neel JV. The inheritance of the sickling phenomenon with particular reference to sickle cell disease. Blood 1951; 6:389–412.

Neely CL, Wajima T, Kraus AP, Diggs LW, Barreras L. Lactic acid dehydrogenase activity and plasma hemoglobin elevations in sickle cell disease. Am J Clin Pathol 1969; 52:167–169.

Neumann HN, Diggs LW, Schlenker FS, Barreras L. Increased urinary porphyrin excretion in sickle cell crises. Proc Soc Exp Biol Med 1966; 123:1–4.

Newman RG. The need to redefine "addiction." N Engl J Med 1983; 308:1096–1098.

Nibu K, Adachi K. Effect of FS ($\alpha_2\gamma\beta^S$) hybrid hemoglobin on Hb S nucleation and aggregation. Biochim Biophys Acta 1985; 829:97–102.

Nishimura SL, Rect LD, Pasternak GW. Biochemical characterization of high affinity ^{3}H-binding: further evidence for μ1 sites. Mol Pharmacol 1984; 25:29–37.

Nguyen TV, Margolis DJ. Hydroxyurea and lower leg ulcers. Cutis 1993; 52:217.

Noguchi CT, Schechter AN. The intracellular polymerization of sickle hemoglobin and its relevance to sickle cell disease. Blood 1981; 58:1057–1068.

Nossel H. Radioimmunoassay of fibrinopeptides in relation to intravascular coagulation and thrombosis. N Engl J Med 1976; 295:428–432.

O'Brien CP, McLellan AT. Myths about the treatment of addiction. Lancet 1996; 347:237–240.

O'Brien WM, Bagby GF. Rare adverse reactions to nonsteroidal anti-inflammatory drugs. J Rheumatol 1985; 12:13-200, 347–353, 562–567, 785–790.

Ofosu MD, Castro O, Alarif L. Sickle cell leg ulcers are associated with HLA-B35 and -Cw4. Arch Dermatol 1987; 123:482–484.

Ohaeri JU, Shokunbi WA, Akinlade KS, Dare LO. The psychosocial problems of sickle cell disease sufferers and their methods of coping. Soc Sci Med 1995; 40:955–960.

O'Hara AE. Roentgenographic osseous manifestations of the anemias and the leukemias. Clin Orthop 1967; 52:63–82.

Ohnishi A, Peterson CM, Dyck PJ. Axonal degeneration in sodium cyanate induced neuropathy. Arch Neurol 1975; 32:530–534.

Oliver OJ. The use of methotrimeprazine in terminal care. Br J Clin Pract 1985; 39:339–340.

O'Neill WM, Sherrard JS. Pain in human immunodeficiency virus disease: a review. Pain 1993; 54:3–14.

Onwubalili JK. Sickle cell anaemia, an explanation for the ancient myth of reincarnation in Nigeria. Lancet 1983; II(Aug 27):503–505.

Orkin SH, Kazaian HH Jr, Antonarakis SE, et al. Linkage of β-thalassemia mutations and β-globin gene polymorphisms with DNA polymorphisms in the human β-globin gene cluster. Nature 1982; 296:627–631.

Osborne RJ, Joel SP, Slevin ML. Morphine intoxication in renal failure: the role of morphine-6-glucuronide. Br J Med 1986; 292:1548–1549.

O'Shea B, McGennis AM, Cahil M, Folvey J. Munchausen syndrome. Br J Hosp Med 1984; 31:269–274.

Pagnier J, Mears JG, Dunda-Beklhodja O, et al. Evidence for the multicenter origin of the sickle cell hemoglobin gene in Africa. Proc Natl Acad Sci USA 1984; 81:1771–1773.

Palmer J, Broderick KA, Niaman JL. Acute lung syndrome during painful sickle cell crisis: relation to site of pain and narcotic requirement. Blood 1983; 62:5,59a.

Parris WCV. Alternative pain medicine: current modalities and principles. Current Review Pain 1997; 1:54–60.

Pasternak GW. Multiple morphine and enkephalin receptors and the relief of pain. JAMA 1988; 259:1362–1367.

Pasternak GW, Wood PJ. Multiple μ opiate receptors. Life Sci 1986; 38:1889–1898.

Pasternak GW, Childers SR, Snyder SH. Opiate analgesia: evidence for mediation by a sub-population of opiate receptors. Science 1980; 208:514–516.

Pasternak GW, Bodnar RJ, Clarke JA, Inturrisi CE. Morphine-6-glucuronide, a potent mu agonist. Life Sci 1987; 41:2845–2849.

Paszty C, Brion CM, Manci E, et al. Transgenic knockout mice with exclusively human sickle hemoglobin and sickle cell disease. Science 1997; 278:876–878.

Paterson JCS, Sprague CC. Observation on the genesis of crises in sickle cell anemia. Ann Intern Med 1959; 50:1500–1507.

Patient's Bill of Rights. In: Weiner RS (Ed). Innovations in Pain Management: A Practical Guide for Clinicians, Vol. 2, Appendix F. Orlando: Paul M Deutsch Press, 1993.

Patrono C, Dunn MJ. The clinical significance of inhibition of renal prostaglandin synthesis. Kidney Int 1987; 32:1–12.

Patterson RH, Wilson H, Diggs LW. Sickle cell anemia: a surgical problem. Surgery 1950; 28:393–403.

Paul D, Standifer KM, Intrurrisi CE, et al. Pharmacological characterization of morphine-6 beta-glucuronide, a very potent morphine metabolite. J Pharmacol Exp Ther 1989; 251:477–483.

Pauling L, Itano H, Singer SJ, Wells IC. Sickle cell anemia: a molecular disease. Science 1949; 110:543–548.

Payne R. Anatomy, physiology and neuropathology of cancer pain. Med Clin North Am 1987; 71:153–167.

Payne RM. Pain in the drug abuser. In: Foley KM, Payne RM (Eds). Current Therapy of Pain. Toronto: BC Decker, 1989a, pp 46–54.

Payne R. Pain management in sickle cell disease: rationale and techniques. Annals NY Acad Sci 1989b; 565:189–206.

Payne R. Transdermal fentanyl: suggested recommendations for clinical use. J Pain Symptom Manage 1992; 7(Suppl.):S40–S44.

Payne R. Pain management in sickle cell anemia. Anesth Clin N Am 1997; 15:306–318.

Pegelow CH. Survey of pain management therapy for children with sickle cell disease. Clin Pediatr 1992; 31:211–214.

Perlin E, Finke H, Castro O, et al. Treatment of sickle cell pain crises: a clinical trial of diflunisal (Dolobid). Clin Trials J 1988; 25:254–264.

Perlin E, Finke H, Castro O, et al. Infusional/patient-controlled analgesia in sickle-cell vaso-occlusive crises. Pain Clin 1993; 6:113–119.

Perlin E, Finke H, Castro O, et al. Enhancement of pain control with ketorolac tromethamine in patients with sickle cell vaso-occlusive crisis. Am J Hematol 1994; 46:43–47.

Perlman SL. Modern techniques of pain management. West J Med 1988; 148:54–6l.

Perrine RP, Brown MJ, Clegg JB, Weatherall DJ, May A. Benign sickle cell anemia. Lancet 1972; 2:1163–1167.

Perrine RP, Pembrey ME, John P, Perrine S, Shoup F. Natural history of sickle anemia in Saudi Arabs: a study of 270 subjects. Ann Intern Med 1978; 88:1–6.

Perrine SP, Greene MF, Faller DV. Delay in the fetal globin switch in infants of diabetic mothers. N Engl J Med 1985; 312:334–338.

Perrine SP, Rudolph A, Faller DV, et al. Butyrate infusions in the ovine fetus delay the biologic clock for globin gene switching. Proc Natl Acad Sci USA 1988; 85:8540–8542.

Perrine SP, Faller DV, Swerdlow P, et al. Pharmacologic prevention and reversal of globin gene switching. In: Stamatoyannopoulos G, Nienhuis AW (Eds). The Regulation of Hemoglobin Switching: Proceedings of the Seventh Conference on Hemoglobin Switching, Airlie, VA, September 8–11, 1990. Baltimore: Johns Hopkins University Press, 1991, pp 425–436.

Perrine SP, Ginder GD, Faller DV, et al. A short-term trial of butyrate to stimulate fetal-globin-gene expression in the beta-globin disorders. N Engl J Med 1993; 328:81–86.

Perutz MF. Structure and mechanism of haemoglobin. Br Med Bull 1976; 32:195–208.

Perutz MF, Mitchison JM. State of haemoglobin in sickle cell anaemia. Nature 1950; 166:677–679.

Pescor MJ. The Kolb classification of drug addicts. Public Health Rep 1939; 155(Suppl.).

Peters M, Plaat BE, ten Cate H, et al. Enhanced thrombin generation in children with sickle cell disease. Thromb Haemost 1994; 71:169–172.

Peterson CM, Tsairis P, Ohnishi A, et al. Sodium cyanate induced polyneuropathy in patients with sickle-cell disease. Ann Intern Med 1974; 81:152–158.

Phillips G, Slingluff C, Hartman J, Thomas P, Akwari O. Totally implantable intravenous catheters in the management of sickle cell anemia. Am J Hematol 1988; 29:134–138.

Phillips G Jr, Coffey B, Tran-Son-Tay R, et al. Relationship of clinical severity to packed red rheology in sickle cell anemia. Blood 1991; 78:2735–2739.

Phillips G Jr, Eckman JR, Hebbel RP. Leg ulcers and myofascial syndromes. In: Embury SH, Hebbel RP, Mohandas N, Steinberg MH (Eds). Sickle Cell Disease: Basic Principles and Clinical Practice. New York: Raven Press Ltd, 1994, pp 681–688.

Pieters RC, Rojer RA, Saleh AW, Saleh AEC, Duits AJ. Molgramostim to treat SS-sickle cell leg ulcers. Lancet 1995; 345:528.

Piletta P, Porchet HC, Dayer P. Central analgesic effect of acetaminophen but not of aspirin. Clin Pharmacol Ther 1991; 49:350–354.

Pillans PI, O'Conner N. Tissue necrosis and necrotizing fasciitis after intramuscular administration of diclofenac. Ann Pharm Ther 1995; 29:264–266.

Platt A, Eckman J. The Georgia Sickle Cell Center, a comprehensive emergency clinic model. In: Program of the 15th Annual Meeting of the National Sickle Cell Centers, Pathobiology and Clinical Management of Sickle Cell Disease: Recent Advances. Berkeley, CA, May 16–18, 1990, p 100.

Platt OS, Guinan EC. Bone marrow transplantation in sickle cell anemia: the dilemma of choice. N Engl J Med 1996; 335:426–427.

Platt OS, Thorington BD, Brambilla DJ, et al. Pain in sickle cell disease: rates and risk factors. N Engl J Med 1991; 325:11–16.

Platt OS, Brambilla DJ, Rosse WF, et al. Mortality in sickle cell disease: life expectancy and risk factors for early death. N Engl J Med 1994; 330:1639–1644.

Poillon WN, Bertles JF. Deoxygenated sickle hemoglobin: effects of lyotropic salts on its solubility. J Biol Chem 1979; 254:3462–3467.

Pollack CV, Sanders DY, Severance HW. Emergency department analgesia without narcotics for adults with acute sickle cell pain crisis: case reports and review of crisis management. J Emerg Med 1991; 9:445–452.

Poncz M, Kane E, Gill FM. Acute chest syndrome in sickle cell disease: etiology and clinical correlate. J Pediatr 1985; 107:861–866.

Pond SM, Tong T, Benowitz NL, Jacob P, Rigod J. Presystemic metabolism of meperidine to normeperidine in normal and cirrhotic subjects. Clin Pharmacol Ther 1981; 30:183–188.

Portenoy RK. Adjuvant analgesics. In: Doyle D, Hanks GW, McDonald N (Eds). Oxford Textbook of Palliative Medicine. Oxford: Oxford University Press, 1993, pp 187–203.

Portenoy RK. Opioid therapy for chronic nonmalignant pain: a review of the clinical issues. J Pain Symptom Manage 1996; 11:203–217.

Portenoy RK, Foley M. Chronic use of opioid analgesics in non-malignant pain: report of 38 cases. Pain 1986; 25:171–186.

Portenoy RK, Moulin DE, Rogers A, Inturrisi CE, Foley KM. I.V. infusion of opioids for cancer pain: clinical review and guidelines for use. Cancer Treat Rep 1986; 70:575–581.

Portenoy RK, Foley KM, Stulman J, et al. Plasma morphine and morphine-6-glucuronide during chronic morphine therapy for cancer pain: plasma profiles, steady state concentrations and the consequences of renal failure. Pain 1991; 47:13–19.

Portenoy RK, Thaler HT, Inturrisi CE, Friedlander-Klar H, Foley KM. The metabolite, morphine-6-glucuronide, contributes to the analgesia produced by morphine infusion in pain patients with normal renal function. Clin Pharm Ther 1992; 51:422–431.

Portnoy BA, Herion JC. Neurological manifestations in sickle cell disease. Ann Intern Med 1972; 76:643–652.

Powars D. Natural history of sickle cell disease: the first ten years. Semin Hematol 1976; 12:267–285.

Powars DR. Sickle cell anemia and major organ failure. Hemoglobin 1990; 14:573–598.

Powars DR, Johnson CS. Priapism. In: Sickle Cell Disease. Hematol Oncol Clin North Am 1996; 10:1353–1372.

Powars D, Wilson B, Imbus C, Pegelow C, Allen J. The natural history of stroke in sickle cell disease. Am J Med 1978; 65:461–471.

Powars DR, Weiss JN, Chan LS, Schroeder WA. Is there a threshold level of fetal hemoglobin that ameliorates morbidity in sickle cell anemia? Blood 1984; 63:921–926.

Powars D, Weidman JA, Odom-Maryon T, Niland JC, Johnson C. Sickle cell lung disease: prior morbidity and the risk of pulmonary failure. Medicine 1988; 67:66–76.

Powars DR, Chan L, Schroeder WA. β^S-Gene-cluster haplotypes in sickle cell anemia: clinical implications. Am J Pediatr Hematol Oncol 1990a; 12:367–374.

Powars DR, Chan L, Schroeder WA. The variable expression of sickle cell disease is genetically determined. Semin Hematol 1990b; 27:360–376.

Powars DR, Elliott-Mills DD, Chan L, et al. Chronic renal failure in sickle cell disease: risk factors, clinical course, and mortality. Ann Intern Med 1991; 115:614–620.

Powers RD. Management protocol for sickle cell disease patients with acute pain: impact on emergency department and narcotic use. Am J Emerg Med 1986; 4:267–268.

Poyhia R, Olkkola KT, Seppala T, Kalso E. The pharmacokinetics of oxycodone after intravenous injection in adults. Br J Clin Pharmacol 1991; 32:516–518.

Pryle BJ, Grech H, Stoddart PA, et al. Toxicity of norpethidine in sickle cell crisis. Br Med J 1992; 304:1478–1479.

Quan DB, Wandres DL. Clonidine in pain management. Ann Pharmacother 1993; 27:313–315.

Quintero E, Gines P, Arroyo V, et al. Sulindac reduces the urinary excretion of prostaglandins and impairs renal function in cirrhosis with ascites. Nephron 1986; 42:298–303.

Radnay PA, Brodman E, Mankikar D, Duncalf D. The effect of equi-analgesic doses of fentanyl, morphine, meperidine and pentazocine on common bile duct pressure. Anaesthetist 1980; 29:26–29.

Ragusa A, Lombardo M, Sortino G, et al. Beta^S gene in Sicily is in linkage disequilibrium with the Benin haplotype: implications for gene flow. Am J Hematol 1988; 27:139–141.

Ramsay RE, Wilder BJ, Berger JR, et al. A double-blind study comparing carbamazepine and phenytoin as initial seizure therapy in adults. Neurology 1983; 33:904–910.

Ravina A, Minuchin O, Kehrmann H. A simple disposable hyperbaric oxygen device for the treatment of wounds. Isr J Med Sci 1983; 19:845–847.

Rees DC, Chrvi P, Grimwade D, et al. The metabolites of nitricoxide in sickle-cell disease. Br J Haematol 1995; 9:834–837.

Reid CD, Charache S, Lubin B, et al. Management and Therapy of Sickle Cell Disease, 3rd ed. NIH Publication no. 95-2117. Bethesda, MD: National Heart, Lung, and Blood Institute, National Institutes of Health, 1995.

Reindorf CA, Walker-Jones D, Adekile AD, Lawal O, Oluwole SF. Rapid healing of sickle cell leg ulcers treated with collagen dressing. J Natl Med Assoc 1989; 81:866–868.

Reisine T, Pasternak G. Opioid analgesics and antagonists. In: Hardman JG, Limbird LE, Molinoff PB, Ruddon RW, Gilman AG (Eds). Goodman & Gilman's The Pharmacological Basis of Therapeutics, 9th ed. New York: McGraw-Hill, 1996, pp 521–555.

Reynolds J. The skull and spine. Semin Radiol 1987; 22:168–175.

Reynolds MD. Gout and hyperuricemia associated with sickle cell anemia. Semin Arthritis Rheum 1983; 12:404–413.

Richardson SGN, Matthews KB, Stuart J, Geddes AM, Wilcox RM. Serial changes in coagulation and viscosity during sickle cell crisis. Br J Haematol 1979; 41:95–103.

Rieber EE, Veliz G, Pollack S. Red cells in sickle cell crisis: observations on the pathophysiology of crisis. Blood 1977; 49:967–969.

Rieder RF, Safaya S, Gillette P, et al. Effect of β-globin gene cluster haplotype on the hematological and clinical features of sickle cell anemia. Am J Hematol 1991; 36:184–189.

Roberts DG, Gerber JG, Barnes JS, Zerbe GO, Nies AS. Sulindac is not renal sparing in man. Clin Pharmacol Ther 1985; 38:258–265.

Robieux IC, Kellner JD, Coppes MJ, et al. Analgesia in children with sickle cell crisis: comparison of intermittent opioids vs. continuous infusion of morphine and placebo controlled study of oxygen inhalation. Pediatr Hematol Oncol 1992; 9:317–326.

Rodgers GP, Dover GJ, Uyesada N, et al. Augmentation by erythropoietin of the fetal hemoglobin response to hydroxyurea in sickle cell disease. N Engl J Med 1993; 328:73–80.

Rooks WH II, Tomolonis AJ, Maloney PJ, Wallach MB, Schuler ME. The analgesic and anti-inflammatory profile of (±)-5-benzoyl-1,2-dihydro-3H pyrrolo [1,2a] pyrrole-1-carboxylic acid (RS-37619). Agents Actions 1982; 12:684–690.

Rooks WH II, Maloney PJ, Shott LD, et al. The analgesic and anti-inflammatory profile of ketorolac and its tromethamine salt. Drugs Exp Clin Res 1985; 11:479–492.

Ropper AH. The Guillain-Barré syndrome. N Engl J Med 1992; 326:1130–1136.

Rosa RM, Bierer BE, Thomas R, et al. A study of induced hyponatremia in the prevention and treatment of sickle cell crisis. N Engl J Med 1980; 303:1138–1143.

Rosen L. Videophotometric skin capillaroscopy for assessment of microvascular disturbances. Journal of the Oslo City Hospitals 1989; 39:107–121.

Rosner F, Karayalain G. Decreased leukocyte alkaline phosphatase activity in sickle cell anemia. Ann Intern Med; 80:668–669.

Ross E. Pharmacokinetics: the dynamics of drug absorption, distribution, and elimination. In: Hardman TA, Lombard LE, Molinoff PB, Ruddon RW, Gilman AG (Eds). Goodman & Gilman's The Pharmacological Basis of Therapeutics, Edition G. New York: McGraw-Hill, 1996a, pp 3–27.

Ross E. Pharmacodynamics: mechanism of drug action and the relationship between drug concentration and effect. In: Hardman TA, Lombard LE, Molinoff PB, Ruddon RW, Gilman AG (Eds). Goodman & Gilman's The Pharmacological Basis of Therapeutics, Edition G. New York: McGraw-Hill, 1996b, pp 29–41.

Ross PD, Hofrichter J, Eaton WA. Calorimetric and optical characterization of sickle cell hemoglobin gelation. J Mol Biol 1975; 96:239–256.

Ross PD, Hofrichter J, Eaton WA. Thermodynamics of gelation of sickly deoxyhemoglobin. J Mol Biol 1977; 115:111–134.

Roth EF, Friedman M, Ueda Y, et al. Sickling rates of human AS red cells infected in vitro with Plasmodium falciparum malaria. Science 1978; 202:650–652.

Roth EF, Bardfeld PA, Goldsmith SJ, Radel E, Williams JC. Sickle cell crisis as evaluated from measurements of hydroxybutyrate dehydrogenase and myoglobin in plasma. Clin Chem 1981; 27:314–316.

Roth HJ. Pharmacokinetics and biotransformation of pyrazolones. In: Brune K (Ed). Agents and Actions. Supplement 19: 100 Years of Pyrazolone Drugs. Basel: Birkhauser Verlag, 1986, pp 205–221.

Roth SH, Bennett RE. Non-steroidal anti-inflammatory drug gastropathy. Recognition and response. Arch Intern Med 1987; 147:2093–2100.

Roth SH. Nonsteroidal anti-inflammatory drugs: gastropathy, deaths, and medical practice. Ann Intern Med 1988; 109:353–354.

Roth S, Agrawal N, Mahowald M, et al. Misoprostol heals gastroduodenal injury in patients with rheumatoid arthritis receiving aspirin. Arch Intern Med 1989; 149:775–779.

Rothman SM, Nelson JS. Spinal cord infarction in a patient with sickle cell anemia. Neurology 1980; 30:1072–1076.

Rothschild BM, Sienknecht CW, Kaplan SB, Spindler JS. Sickle cell disease associated with uric acid deposition disease. Ann Rheum Dis 1980; 39:392–395.

Routledge PA, Shand DG. Presystemic drug elimination. Annu Rev Pharmacol Toxicol 1979; 19:447–468.

Rowbotham DJ, Wyld R, Peacock JE, Duthie DJR, Nimmo WS. Transdermal fentanyl for the relief of pain after upper abdominal surgery. Br J Anaesthesiol 1989; 63:56–59.

Royal JE, Harris VJ, Sansi PK. Facial bone infarcts in sickle living organism syndromes. Radiology 1988; 169:529–531.

Rozenberg MC, Holmsen H. Adenine nucleotide metabolism of blood platelets. IV. Platelet aggregation response to exogenous ATP and ADP. Biochim Biophys Acta 1968; 157:280–288.

Rucknagel DL, Kalinyak KA, Gelfan MJ. Rib infarcts and acute chest syndrome in sickle cell diseases. Lancet 1991; 337:831–833.

Rumack BH, Peterson RG. Acetaminophen overdose: incidence, diagnosis, and management in 416 patients. Pediatrics 1978; 62(suppl):898–903.

Russell MO, Goldberg HI, Hodson A, et al. Effect of transfusion therapy on arteriographic abnormalities and on recurrence of stroke in sickle cell disease. Blood 1984; 63:162–169.

Ryan TM, Ciavatta DJ, Townes TM. Knockout-transgenic mouse model of sickle cell disease. Science 1997; 278:873–876.

Saarinen UM, Chorba TL, Tattersall P, et al. Human parvovirus B19-induced epidemic acute red cell aplasia in patients with hereditary hemolytic anemia. Blood 1986; 67:1411–1417.

Sabbagh R, Kedar A. Increased prolactin level and pituitary adenoma as a cause of headache in two patients with sickle cell disease. Pediatr Hematol Oncol 1996; 13:101–105.

Sadat-Ali M, Sankaran-Kutty M, Kutty K. Recent observations on osteomyelitis in sickle cell disease. Int Orthop 1985; 9:97–99.

Sadat-Ali M, Ammar A, Corea JR, Ibrahim AW. The spine in sickle cell disease. Int Orthop 1993; 18:154–156.

Sagen J, Kemmler JE, Wang H. Adrenal medullary transplants increase spinal cerebrospinal fluid catecholamine levels and reduce pain sensitivity. J Neurochem 1991; 56:623–627.

Saito S, Saito M, Nishina T, et al. Long term rests of total hip arthroplasty for osteonecrosis of the femoral head: a comparison with osteoarthritis. Clin Orthop 1989; 244:198–207.

Saleh AW, van Goethem A, Jansen R, et al. Isobutyramide therapy in patients with sickle cell anemia. Am J Hematol 1995; 49:244–246.

Samuel RE, Salmon ED, Briehl RW. Nucleation and growth of fibers and gel formation in sickle cell haemoglobin. Nature 1990; 345:833–835.

Samuels-Reid J, Scott RB. Painful crises and menstruation in sickle cell disease. South Med J 1985; 78:384–385.

Sanders DY, Severance HW, Pollack CV. Sickle cell vaso-occlusive pain crisis in adults: alternative strategies for management in the emergency department. South Med J 1992; 85:808–811.

Saper JR, Silberstein S, Gordon CD, Hamel RL. Pine JW Jr (Eds). Handbook of Headache Management: A Practical Guide to Diagnosis and Treatment of Head, Neck, and Facial Pain. Baltimore: Williams & Wilkins, 1993.

Sarnaik SA, Lusher JM. Neurological complications of sickle cell anemia. Am J Pediatr Hematol/ Oncol 1982; 4:386–394.

Sartori PCE, Gordon GJ, Darbyshire PJ. Continuous papaveretum infusion for the control of pain in painful sickling crisis. Arch Dis Child 1990; 65:1151–1153.

Saunders CM. The management of terminal illness. London: Edward Arnold, 1967.

Savitt TH, Goldberg MF. Herrick's 1910 case report of sickle cell anemia. JAMA 1989; 261:266–271.

Sawe J, Dahlstrom B, Paalzow L, Rane A. Morphine kinetics in cancer patients. Clin Pharmacol Ther 1981; 30:629–635.

Sawe J, Svensson JO, Rane A. Morphine metabolism in cancer patients on increasing oral doses— no evidence for autoinduction or dose dependence. J Clin Pharmacol 1983; 16:85–93.

Schafer AI, Miller B, Lester EP, Bowers TK, Jacob HS. Monoclonal gammopathy in hereditary spherocytosis: possible pathogenetic relation. Ann Intern Med 1978; 88:45–46.

Scharf MB, Lobel JS, Caldwell E, et al. Nocturnal oxygen desaturation in patients with sickle cell anemia. JAMA 1983; 249:1753–1755.

Schechter AN, Noguchi CT, Rodgers GP. Sickle cell disease. In: Stamatoyannopoulos G, Nienhuis AW, Leder P, Majerus PW (Eds). The Molecular Basis of Blood Diseases. Philadelphia: WB Saunders, 1987:179–218.

Schecter NL, Berrien FB, Katz SM. The use of patient-controlled analgesia in adolescents with sickle cell pain crisis: a preliminary report. J Pain Symptom Manage 1988; 3:109–113.

Schmucker P, VanAckern K, Franke N, et al. Hemodynamic and respiratory effects of pentazocine: studies on surgical cardiac patients. Anaesthetist 1980; 29:475–480.

Schraeder BD, Ballas SK, Capaldi E, et al. Demographic and social characteristics of adults with sickle cell disease who require frequent and lengthy hospitalizations [abstract 178a]. In: Book of Abstracts, 18th Meeting of the National Sickle Cell Disease Program, Philadelphia, PA, May 22–25, 1993.

Schug SA, Merry AF, Acland RH. Treatment principles for the use of opioids in pain of nonmalignant origin. Drugs 1991; 42:228–239.

Schumacher HR. Rheumatological manifestations of sickle cell disease and other haemoglobinopathies. Clin Rheum Dis 1975; 1:37–52.

Schumacher HR, Andrews R, McLaughlin G. Arthropathy in sickle cell disease. Ann Intern Med 1973; 78:203–211.

Schumacher HR. Murray WM, Dalinka MK. Acute muscle injury complicating sickle cell crisis. Semin Arthritis Rheum 1990; 19:234–237.

Schwartz E, McElfresh AE. Treatment of painful crises of sickle cell disease: a double blind study. J Pediatr 1964; 64:132–133.

Schwartzman RJ. Reflex sympathetic dystrophy and causalgia. Neurol Clin 1992; 10:953–973.

Schwartzman RJ, McLellan TL. Reflex sympathetic dystrophy: a review. Arch Neurol 1987; 44:555–561.

Scott JP, Hillery CA, Brown ER, Misiewicz V, Labotka KJ. Hydroxyurea therapy in children severely affected with sickle cell disease. J Pediatr 1996; 128:820–828.

Sears DA. The morbidity of sickle cell trait: a review of the literature. Am J Med 1978; 64:1021–1036.

Sears DA. Sickle cell trait. In: Embury SH, Hebbel RP, Mohandas N, Steinberg MH (Eds). Sickle Cell Disease: Basic Principles and Clinical Practice. New York: Raven Press, 1994, pp 381–394.

Sebes JI, Kraus AP. Avascular necrosis of the hip in the sickle cell hemoglobinopathies. J Can Assoc Radiol 1983; 34:136–139.

Seeff LB, Cuccherini BA, Zimmerman HI, Adler E, Benjamin SB. Acetaminophen hepatotoxicity in alcoholics. Ann Intern Med 1986; 104:399–404.

Seeler RA. Intensive transfusion therapy for priapism in boys with sickle cell anemia. J Urol 1973a; 110:360–361.

Seeler RA. Non-seasonability of sickle cell crisis. Lancet 1973b; 2:743.

Seigel MI, McConnell RT, Cuatrecasas P. Aspirin-like drugs interfere with arachidonate metabolism by inhibition of the 12-hydroperoxy-5,8,10,14-eicosatetraenoic acid peroxidase activity of the lipoxygenase pathway. Proc Natl Acad Sci USA 1979; 76:3774–3778.

Sekar M, Mimpriss TJ. Buprenorphine, benzodiazepines and prolonged respiratory depression [letter]. Anaesthesia 1987; 42:567–568.

Semble EL, Wu C. Anti-inflammatory drugs and gastric mucosal damage. Semin Arthritis Rheum 1987; 16:271–286.

Serjeant GR. Leg ulceration in sickle cell anemia. Arch Intern Med 1974; 133:690–694.

Serjeant GR. Fetal haemoglobin in homozygous sickle cell disease. Clin Haematol 1975; 4:109–122.

Serjeant GR. Stilboestrol and stuttering priapism in homozygous sickle cell disease. Lancet 1985; ii:1274–1276.

Serjeant GR. Sickle Cell Disease, 2nd ed. Oxford: Oxford University Press, 1992.

Serjeant GR, Chalmers RM. Is the painful crisis of sickle cell disease 'a steal syndrome'? J Clin Pathol 1990; 43:789–791.

Serjeant GR, Serjeant BE, Desai P, et al. The determinants of irreversibly sickled cells in homozygous sickle cell disease. Br J Haematol 1978; 40:431–438.

Serjeant GR, De Ceulaer C, Lethbridge R, et al. The painful crisis of homozygous sickle cell disease: clinical features. Br J Haematol 1994; 87:586–591.

Seto SSY, Freeman JM. Lead neuropathy in children. Am J Dis Child 1964; 107:337–342.

Sevelius H, McCoy JF, Colmore JP. Dose response to codeine in patients with chronic cough. Clin Pharmacol Ther 1971; 12:449–455.

Shapiro BS. The management of pain in sickle cell disease. Pediatr Clin North Am 1989; 36:1029–1045.

Shapiro B. Sickle cell disease related pain. IASP Newsletter. Seattle: International Association for the Study of Pain, Jan/Feb 1991, pp 2–4.

Shapiro B. Management of painful episodes in sickle cell disease. In: Scheaffer NL, Berde CB, Yaster M (Eds). Pain in Infants, Children, and Adolescents. Baltimore: Williams & Wilkins, 1993, pp 385–410.

Shapiro BS. Pain in sickle cell disease. Pain Clinical Updates 1997, 5(2):1–4, newsletter, Seattle: IASP.

Shapiro BS, Dinges DF, Orne EC, Ohene-Frempong K, Orne MT. Recording of crisis pain in sickle cell disease. In: Tyler DC, Krane EJ (Eds). Advances in Pain Research Therapy, Vol. 15. New York: Raven Press, 1990, pp 313–321.

Shapiro BS, Cohen DE, Howe CJ. Patient-controlled analgesia for sickle-cell-related pain. J Pain Symptom Manage 1993; 8:22–28.

Shapiro BS, Dinges DF, Orne EC, et al. Home management of sickle cell-related pain in children and adolescents: natural history and impact on school attendance. Pain 1995; 61:139–144.

Shapiro BS, Benjamin LJ, Payne R, Heidrich G. Sickle cell-related pain: perceptions of medical practitioners. J Pain Symptom Manage 1997; 14:168–174.

Sharpsteen JR Jr, Powars D, Johnson C, et al. Multisystem damage associated with tricorporal priapism in sickle cell disease. Am J Med 1993; 94:289–295.

Shealy CN. Opioids and controlled substances in chronic benign pain: a survey of state medical boards. Am J Pain Med 1997; 7:10–14.

Sheehan AG, Machida H, Butzner JD. Acute pancreatitis in a child with sickle cell anemia. J Natl Med Assoc 1993; 85:70–72.

Sheehy T. Sickle cell hepatopathy. South Med J 1977; 70:533–538.

Sheehy T, Law DE, Wade BH. Exchange transfusion for sickle cell intrahepatic cholestasis. Arch Intern Med 1980; 140:1364–1366.

Sheline YI, Freedland KE, Carney RM. How safe are serotonin reuptake inhibitors for depression in patients with coronary heart disease? Am J Med 1997; 102:54–59.

Sher GD, Olivieri NF. Rapid healing of chronic leg ulcers during arginine butyrate therapy in patients with sickle cell disease and thalassemia. Blood 1994; 84:2378–2380.

Sher GD, Ginder GD, Little J, et al. Extended therapy with intravenous arginine butyrate in patients with beta-hemoglobinopathies. N Engl J Med 1995; 24:1606–1610.

Sherman M. Pathogenesis of disintegration of the hip in sickle cell anemia. South Med J 1959; 52:632–637.

Shields RW Jr, Harris JW, Clark M. Mononeuropathy I sickle cell anemia: anatomical and pathophysiological basis for its rarity. Muscle Nerve 1991; 14:370–374.

Shulman E, Natarajan M, McIntire LV. Pathophysiology and management of sickle cell pain crises. Lancet 1995; 346:1408–1411.

Sidman JD, Fry TL. Exacerbation of sickle cell disease by obstructive sleep apnea. Arch Otolaryngol Head Neck Surg 1988; 114:916–917.

Sidman JD, Brownlee RE, Smith WC, Fry TL. Orbital complications of sickle cell disease. Int J Pediatr Otorhinolaryngol 1990; 19:181–184.

364   REFERENCES

Siegel JF, Rich MA, Brock WA. Association of sickle cell disease, priapism, exchange transfusion and neurological events: ASPEN syndrome. J Urol 1993; 150:1480–1482.

Simmons BE, Santhanam V, Castaner A, et al. Sickle cell heart disease. Two-dimensional echo and Doppler ultrasonographic findings in the hearts of adult patients with sickle cell anemia. Arch Int Med 1988; 148:1526–1528.

Simni B. Sickle cell pain crisis. Lancet 1996; 347:261–262.

Simon EJ, Hiller JM. The opiate receptors. Annu Rev Pharmacol Toxicol 1978; 18:371–394.

Simon LS, Mills JA. Nonsteroidal antiinflammatory drugs [first of two parts]. N Engl J Med 1980; 302:1179–1185, 1237–1243.

Simons D, Travell J. Myofascial pain syndromes. In: Wall PD, Melzack R (Eds). Textbook of Pain. Edinburgh: Churchill Livingstone, 1989, pp 368–385.

Sinatra RS, Harrison DM. A comparison of oxymorphone and fentanyl as narcotic supplements in general anesthesia. J Clin Anesth 1989; 1:253–258.

Sinatra RS, Hyde NH, Harrison DM. Oxymorphone revisited. Semin Anesth 1988; 8(3):208–215.

Singh PN, Sharma P, Gupta PK, et al. Clinical evaluation of diazepam for relief of postoperative pain. Br J Anaesth 1981; 53:831–836.

Skjelbred P, Lokken P, Skoglund LA. Post-operative administration of acetaminophen to reduce swelling and other inflammatory events. Current Therapeutic Research 1984; 35:377–385.

Slovis CM, Talley JD, Pitts RB. Non relationship of climatologic factors and painful sickle cell anemia crisis. J Chron Dis 1986; 39:121–126.

Smith EW, Conley CL. Clinical features of the genetic variants of sickle cell disease. Bull Johns Hopkins Hospital 1954; 94:289–318.

Smith MT, Watt JA, Cramond T. Morphine-3-glucuronide: a potent antagonist of morphine analgesia. Life Sci 1990; 47:579–585.

Smith RJ. Federal government faces painful decisions on Darvon. Science 1971; 203:857–858.

Smith RJ, Berk SL. Necrotizing fasciitis and nonsteroidal anti-inflammatory drugs. South Med J 1991; 84:785–787.

Snyder SH. Opiate receptors in the brain. N Engl J Med 1977; 296:266–271.

Snyder SH. Drug and neurotransmitter receptors in the brain. Science 1984; 224:22–31.

Solanki DL, Kletter GG, Castro O. Acute splenic sequestration in adults with sickle cell disease. Am J Med 1986; 80:985–990.

Soll AH. Pathogenesis of peptic ulcer and implications for therapy. N Engl J Med 1990; 322:909–916.

Solovey A, Lin Y, Browne P, et al. Circulating activated endothelial cells in sickle cell anemia. N Engl J Med 1997; 337:1584–1590

Sowemimo SO, Meiselman HJ, Francis Jr RB. Increased circulating endothelial cells in sickle cell crisis. Am J Hematol 1989; 31:263–265.

Spector D, Zachary JB, Sterioff S, et al. Painful crises following renal transplantation. Am J Med 1978; 64:836–839.

Spence RJ. The use of a free flap in homozygous sickle cell disease. Plast Reconstr Surg 1985; 76:616–619.

Sprinkle RH, Cole T, Smith S, Buchanan GR. Acute chest syndrome in children with sickle cell disease. A retrospective analysis of 100 hospitalized cases. Am J Pediatr Hematol 1986; 8:105.

Stamatoyannopoulos G, Nienhuis AW. Hemoglobin switching. In: Stamatoyannopoulos G, Nienhuis AW, Majerus PW, Varmus H (Eds). The Molecular Basis of Blood Diseases, 2nd ed. Philadelphia: WB Saunders, 1993, pp 107–155

Stamatoyannopoulos G, Veith R, Al-Khatti A, Papayannopoulou T. Induction of fetal hemoglobin by cell-cycle-specific drugs and recombinant erythropoietin. Am J Pediatr Haematol Oncol 1990; 12:21–26.

Stamatoyannopoulos JA, Nienhuis AW. Therapeutic approaches to hemoglobin switching in treatment of hemoglobinopathies. Ann Rev Med 1992; 43:497–521.

Stambaugh JE, Lance C. Analgesic efficacy and pharmacokinetic evaluation of meperidine and hydroxyzine, alone and in combination. Cancer Invest 1983; 1:111–117.

Stanley TH, Hague B, Mock DL, et al. Oral transmucosal fentanyl citrate (lollipop) premedications in human volunteers. Anesth Analg 1989; 69:21–27.

Stanski DR, Greenblatt DJ, Lowenstein E. Kinetics of intravenous and intramuscular morphine. Clin Pharmacol Ther 1978; 24:52–59.

Steinberg MH. Hemoglobinopathies and thalassemias. In: Internal Medicine, 4th ed. St. Louis, MO: Mosby–Year Book, 1994, p 852.

Steinberg MH, Hebbel RP. Clinical diversity of sickle cell anemia: genetic and cellular modulation of disease severity. Am J Hematol 1984; 6:921–926.

Steinberg MH, Rosenstock W, Coleman MD, et al. Effects of thalassemia and microcytosis on the hematological and vaso-occlusive severity of sickle cell anemia. Blood 1984; 63:1353–1360.

Steinberg MH, Hsu H, Nagel RL, et al. Gender and haplotype effects upon hematological manifestations of adult sickle cell anemia. Am J Hematol 1995; 48:175–181.

Steiner RM, Ballas SK. Human immunodeficiency virus (HIV I) infection in sickle cell anemia: prevalence and outcome. In: Book of Abstracts, 21st Annual Meeting of the National Sickle Cell Disease Program, Mobile, AL, March 6–9, 1996, p 059.

Stephen JL, Merpit-Gonon, Richard O, Raynaud-Ravni C, Freycon F. Fulminant liver failure in a 12-year-old girl with sickle cell anaemia: favorable outcome after exchange transfusion. Eur J Pediatr 1995; 154:469–471.

Stevens MCG, Padwick M, Serjeant GR. Observations on the natural history of dactylitis in homozygous sickle cell disease. Clin Pediatr 1981a; 20(5):311–317.

Stevens MCG, Heyes RJ, Vaidya S, Serjeant GR. Fetal hemoglobin and clinical severity of homozygous sickle cell disease in early childhood. J Pediatr 1981b; 98:34–41.

Stiles M. The shining stranger: nurse-family spiritual relationship. Cancer Nurs 1990; 13:235–245.

Stimmel B. Pain, Analgesia and Addiction: The Pharmacologic Treatment of Pain. New York: Raven Press, 1983, pp 170–297.

Stovis CM, Talley JD, Pitts RB. Non relationship of climatologic factors and painful sickle cell anemia crisis. J Chron Dis 1986; 39:121–126.

Strauer BE. Contractile responses to morphine, piritramide, meperidine and fentanyl: a comparative study of effects on the isolated ventricular myocardium. Anesthesiology 1972; 37:304–310.

Stuart MJ, Stockman JA, Oski FA. Abnormalities of platelet aggregation in the vaso-occlusive crisis of sickle cell anemia. J Pediatr 1974; 85:629–632.

Styles LA, Vichinsky EP. Core decompression in avascular necrosis of the hip in sickle cell disease. Am J Hematol 1996; 52:103–107.

Styles LA, Schalkwijk CG, Aarsman AJ, et al. Phospholipase A_2 levels in acute chest syndrome of sickle cell disease. Blood 1996; 87:2573–2578.

Sunderland S. Blood supply of peripheral nerves, practical considerations. Arch Neurol Psychiatry 1945; 54:280–282.

Sunderland S (Ed). Nerves and Nerve Injuries. Edinburgh: Churchill Livingstone, 1978, pp 46–55.

Sunshine A, Olson NZ. Non-narcotic analgesics. In: Wall PD, Melzack R (Eds), Textbook of Pain, 2nd ed. New York: Churchill Livingstone 1989, pp 670–685.

Sunshine HR, Hofrichter J, Ferrone FA. Oxygen binding by sickle cell hemoglobin polymers. J Mol Biol 1981; 158:251–273.

Swerlick RA, Eckman JR, Kumar A, Jeitler M, Wick TM. $\alpha 4\beta 1$-Integrin expression on sickle reticulocytes: vascular cell adhesion molecule-1-dependent binding to endothelium. Blood 1993; 82:1891–1899.

Swift AV, Cohen MJ, Hynd GW, et al. Neuropsychologic impairment in children with sickle cell anemia. Pediatrics 1989; 84:1077–1085.

Sydenstricker VP. Discussion of paper: Sickle cell anemia from a pediatric point of view. Transactions of the Section on Diseases of Children of the American Medical Association 1924a, pp 77–88.

Sydenstricker VP. Further observations on sickle cell anemia. JAMA 1924b; 83:12–15.

Sydenstricker VP. Sickle cell anemia. South Med J 1924c; 17:177–181.

Sydenstricker VP. Sickle cell anemia. Med Clin North America 1929; 12:1451–1457.

Sydenstricker VP, Mulherin WA, Houseal RW. Sickle cell anemia: report of two cases in children, with necropsy in one case. Am J Dis Child 1923; 26:132–154.

Syroginannopoulos GA, McCraken GH Jr, Nelson JD. Osteoarticular infections in children with sickle cell disease. Pediatrics 1986; 78:1090–1096.

Szeto HH, Inturrisi CE, Houde R, et al. Accumulation of normeperidine, an active metabolite of meperidine, in patients with renal failure or cancer. Ann Intern Med 1977; 85:738–741.

Taiwo YO, Levin JD. Prostaglandins inhibit endogenous pain control mechanisms by blocking transmission at spinal noradrenergic synapses. J Neurosci 1988; 8:1346–1349.

Talacki CA, Ballas SK. Modified method of exchange transfusion in sickle cell disease. J Clin Apheresis 1990; 5:183–187.

Tanaka GY. Hypertensive reaction to naloxone. JAMA 1974; 228:25–26.

Tang R, Shimomura SK, Rotblatt M. Meperidine-induced seizures in sickle cell patients. Hosp Formul 1980:764–772.

Taub A. Opioid analgesics in the treatment of chronic intractable pain of non neoplastic origin. In: Kitahata LM, Collins D (Eds). Narcotic Analgesics in Anesthesiology. Baltimore: Williams & Wilkins, 1982, pp 199–208.

Tennant FS, Uelman GF. Prescribing narcotics to habitual and addicted narcotic users. West J Med 1980; 133:539–545.

Tennant FS, Uelman GF. Narcotic maintenance for chronic pain: medical and legal guidelines. Postgrad Med 1983; 73:81–94.

Terkonda R, Ebbinghaus S. Willoughby TL, et al. Protein C levels in sickle cell disease. Ann NY Acad Sci 1989; 565:430–431.

Teuscher T, Weil Von Der Ahe C, Baillod P, Holzer B. Double blind randomised clinical trial of pentoxiphyllin in vaso-occlusive sickle cell crisis. Trop Geogr Med 1989; 41:320–325.

Thomas AN, Pattison C, Serjeant GR. Causes of death in sickle cell disease in Jamaica. Br Med J 1982; 285:633–635.

Thomas JE, Koshy M, Patterson L, Dorn L, Thomas K. Management of pain in sickle cell disease using biofeedback therapy: a preliminary study. Biofeedback Self Regul 1984; 9:413–420.

Tien JH. Transdermal-controlled administration of oxycodone. J Pharm Sci 1991; 80:741–743.

Tobin DL, Holroyd KA, Reynolds RV, Wigal JK. The hierarchical factor structure of the Coping Strategies Inventory. Cognitive Therapy and Research 1989; 13:343–361.

Todd GB, Serjeant GR, Larson MR. Sensorineural hearing loss in Jamaicans with SS disease. Acta Otolaryngol 1973; 176:268–272.

Tonkin AL, Wing LMH. Interactions of non-steroidal anti-inflammatory drugs. Baillières Clin Rheumatol 1988; 2:455–483.

Topley JM, Rogers DW, Steven MCG, Serjeant GR. Acute splenic sequestration and hypersplenism in the first five years in homozygous sickle cell disease. Arch Dis Child 1981; 56:765–769.

Travell JG. Myofascial trigger points: clinical view. In: Bonica JJ, Albe-Fessard D (Eds). Advances in Pain Research and Therapy, Vol. 1. New York: Raven Press, 1976, pp 919–926.

Travell JG, Simons DG. Myofascial Pain and Dysfunction. In: Travell J (Ed). The Trigger Point Manual, Vol 1. Baltimore: Williams & Wilkins, 1983.

Travell JG, Simons DG. Myofascial Pain and Dysfunction. In: Travell J (Ed). The Trigger Point Manual, Vol 2. Baltimore: Williams & Wilkins, 1991.

Triadou P, Maier-Redelsperger M, Krishnamoorty R, et al. Fetal haemoglobin variations following hydroxyurea treatment in patients with cyanotic congenital heart disease. Nouv Rev Fr Hematol 1994; 36:367–372.

Turk DC. Rennert pain and the terminally ill cancer patient: a cognitive-social learning perspective. In: Sobel H (Ed). Behavior Therapy in Terminal Care. Cambridge: Ballinger, 1981, pp 95–123.

Turk D. Clinicians' attitudes about prolonged use of opioids and the issue of patient heterogeneity. J Pain Symptom Manage 1996; 11:218–230.

Turk DC, Meichenbaum D. A cognitive behavioral approach to pain management. In: Wall PD, Melzack R (Eds). Textbook of Pain, 3rd ed. Edinburgh: Churchill Livingstone, 1994, pp 1337–1348.

Twycross RG. Clinical experience with diamorphine in advanced malignant disease. Int J Clin Pharmacol 1974; 9:184–198.

Twycross RG. The use of narcotic analgesics in terminal illness. J Med Ethics 1975; 1:10–17.

Twycross RG, McQuay HJ. Opioids. In: Wall PD, Melzack R (Eds). Textbook of Pain, 2nd ed. Edinburgh: Churchill Livingstone, 1989, pp 686–701.

Twycross RG, Wald SJ. Long-term use of diamorphine in advanced cancer. In: Bonica JJ, Albe-Fessard D (Eds). Advances in Pain Research and Therapy. Vol. 1., New York: Raven Press, 1976, pp 653–661.

Umans JG, Inturrisi CE. Antinociceptive activity and toxicity of meperidine and normeperidine in mice. J Pharmacol Exp Ther 1982; 223:203–206.

Urquhart ML, Klapp K, White PF. Patient-controlled analgesia: a comparison of intravenous versus subcutaneous hydromorphone. Anesthesiology 1988; 69:428–432.

U.S. Department of Health and Human Services. Surgeon General's Workshop on Self-Help and Public Health. Rockville, MD: U.S. Department of Health and Human Services, 1987.

Valeriano-Marcet J, Kerr LD. Myonecrosis and myofibrosis as complications of sickle cell anemia. Ann Intern Med 1991; 115:99–101.

Van der Sar A. The sudden rise in platelets and reticulocytes in sickle cell crises. Trop Geogr Med 1970; 22:30–40.

Vandepitte J, Delaisse J. Sicklemie et Paludisme. Ann Soc Belge Med Trop 1957; 37:703–735.

Vane JR. Inhibition of prostaglandin synthesis as a mechanism of action for the aspirin-like drugs. Nature New Biol 1971; 234:231–238.

Vasudevan SV. Pain: A Four-Letter Word You Can Live With. Milwaukee, WI: SV Vasudevan, 1993.

Vaught JL, Rothman RB, Westfall TC. Mu and δ receptors: their role in analgesia and in the differential effects of opioid peptides on analgesia. Life Sci 1982; 30:1443–1455.

Ventafridda V, Ripamonti C, Bianchi M, Sbanotto A, DeConno F. A randomized study on oral administration of morphine and methadone in the treatment of cancer pain. J Pain Symptom Manage 1986; 1:203–207.

Ventafridda V, Bianchi M, Ripamonti C, et al. Studies on the effects of antidepressant drugs or the antinociceptive action of morphine on plasma morphine in rat and man. Pain 1990; 43:155–162.

Vermylen C, Cornu G. Bone marrow transplantation for sickle cell disease: the European experience. Am J Pediatr Hematol Oncol 1994; 16:18–21.

Vichinsky EP. Comprehensive care in sickle cell disease: its impact on morbidity and mortality. Semin Hematol 1991; 28:220–226.

Vichinsky EP, Lubin BH. Sickle cell anemia and related hemoglobinopathies. Pediatr Clin North Am 1980; 27(2):429–447.

Vichinsky E, Lubin B. Litigation and sickle cell disease. In: Book of Abstracts, 21st Meeting of the National Sickle Cell Disease Program, Mobile, AL, March 6–9, 1996, p 0113.

Vichinsky E, Styles L. Pulmonary complications. In: Sickle Cell Disease. Hematol Oncol Clin North Am 1996; 10:1275–1287.

Vichinsky EP, Johnson R, Lubin BH. Multidisciplinary approach to pain management in sickle cell disease. Am J Pediatr Hematol Oncol 1982; 4:328–333.

Vichinsky EP, Earles A, Johnson RA, et al. Alloimmunization in sickle cell anemia and transfusion of racially unmatched blood. N Engl J Med 1990; 322:1617–1621.

Vichinsky E, Williams R, Das M, et al. Pulmonary fat embolism: a distinct cause of severe acute chest syndrome in sickle cell anemia. Blood 1994; 83:3107–3112.

Victor AB, Imperiale LE. The pulmonary and small bone changes in infants with sickle cell anemia. NY State J Med 1957; 57:1403–1408.

Voskaridou E, Kalotychou V, Laukopoulos D. Clinical and laboratory effects of long-term administration of hydroxyurea to patients with sickle-cell/β-thalassemia. Br J Haematol 1995; 89:479–484.

Wade FA. Sickle cell crisis resembling obstructive (cholangiolar type) jaundice. Va Med Month 1960; 87:747–748.

Wainscoat JS, Bell JI, Thein SL, et al. Multiple origins of the sickle mutation: evidence from beta S globin gene cluster polymorphisms. Molecular Biology and Medicine 1983; 1:191–197.

Wajima T, Kraus AP. Leukocyte alkaline phosphatase in sickle cell anemia. N Engl J Med 1975; 293:918–919.

Walan A. Bader JP, Classen M, et al. Effect of omeprazole and ranitidine on ulcer healing and relapse rates in patients with benign gastric ulcer. N Engl J Med 1989; 320:69–75.

Walco GA, Dampier CD. Pain in children and adolescents with sickle cell disease. J Pediatr Psychol 1990; 5:643–658.

Waldman SD, Coombs DW. Selection of implantable narcotic delivery systems. Anesth Analg 1989; 68:377.

Waldrop RD, Mandry C. Health professionals' perceptions of opioid dependence among patients with pain. Am J Emerg Med 1995; 13:529–531.

Walker BK, Ballas SK, Burka ER. The diagnosis of pulmonary thromboembolism in sickle cell disease. Am J Hematol 1979; 7:219–232.

Walker BK, Brownstein PK, Burka ER, Ballas SK. Urinary retention in sickle cell syndromes. Urology 1980; 16:33–35.

Wall PD, Melzack R (Eds). Textbook of Pain, 2nd ed. New York: Churchill Livingstone, 1989.

Wall PD, Melzack R (Eds). Textbook of Pain, 3rd ed. New York: Churchill Livingstone, 1994.

Wallenstien SL. Analgesic studies of aspirin in cancer patients. Proceedings of the Aspirin Symposium. London: Aspirin Foundation, 1975, pp 5–10.

Walters MC, Patience M, Leisenring W, et al. Bone marrow transplantation for sickle cell disease. N Engl J Med 1996; 335:369–376.

Walters TR, Reddy BN. Sickle cell anemia and the NBT test. J Clin Pathol 1974; 27:783–785.

Wang WC, Geord SL, Wilimas JA. Transcutaneous electrical nerve stimulation treatment of sickle cell pain crises. Acta Haematol 1988; 80:99–102.

Ward SJ. Sickle cell pain crisis. Lancet 1996; 347:261.

Ware HE, Brooks AP, Toye R, Berney SI. Sickle cell disease and silent avascular necrosis of the hip. J Bone Joint Surg [Br] 1991; 73-B:947–949.

Warth JA, Rucknagel DL. Density ultracentrifugation of sickle cell during and after pain crisis: increased dense enchinocytes in crisis. Blood 1984; 64:507–515.

Washburn RE. Peculiar elongated and sickle-shaped red blood corpuscles in a case of severe anemia. Virginia Med Semi-Monthly 1911; 15:490–493.

Wasserman AL, Williams JA, Fairclough DL, Mulhern RK, Wang W. Subtle neuropsychological deficits in children with sickle cell disease. Am J Pediatr Hematol Oncol 1991; 13:14–20.

Wasserman CF, Phelps VR, Herzog AJ. Chronic hemolytic anemia in a white child due to thalassemia and sicklemia with a genealogic survey. Pediatrics 1952; 9:286.

Watson CPN, Evans RJ, Watt VR. Postherpetic neuralgia and topical capsaicin. Pain 1988; 33:333–340.

Watson CPN, Evans RJ, Watt VR. The post-mastectomy pain syndrome and the effect of topical capsaicin. Pain 1989; 38:177–186.

Watson RJ, Burko H, Megas H, Robinson M. The hand-foot syndrome in sickle cell disease in young children. Pediatrics 1963; 31:975–982.

Weatherall DJ. The thalassemias. In: Stamatoyannopoulos G, Nienhuis AW, Majerus PW, Varmus M (Eds). The Molecular Basis of Blood Diseases, 2nd ed. Philadelphia: WB Saunders, 1994, pp 157–205.

Weatherall DJ, Clegg JB. The Thalassemia Syndromes, 3rd ed. Oxford: Blackwell, 1981.

Weinberg AG, Currarino G. Sickle cell dactylitis: histopathologic observations. Am J Clin Pathol 1972; 58:518–523.

Weinstein SH, Gaylord JC. Determination of oxycodone in plasma and identification of a major metabolite. J Pharm Sci 1979; 68:527–528.

Weisman SJ, Schechter NL. Sickle cell anemia: pain management. In: Sinatra RS, Hord AH, Ginsberg B, Preble LM (Eds). Acute Pain: Mechanisms and Management. St. Louis: Mosby–Year Book, 1992, pp 508–516.

Weissman DE, Haddox JD. Opioid pseudoaddiction: an iatrogenic syndrome. Pain 1989; 36:363–366.

Weissman DE, Joranson DE, Hopwood MB. Wisconsin physicians' knowledge and attitudes about opioid regulations. Wis Med J 1991; December, 671–675.

Welch RB, Goldberg MF. Sickle-cell hemoglobin and its relation to fundus abnormality. Arch Ophthalmol 1966; 75:353–362.

Wethers DL, Ramirez GM, Koshy M, et al. The RGD study group. Blood 1994; 84:1775–1779.

Whelton A, Hamilton CW. Nonsteroidal anti-inflammatory drugs: effects on kidney function. J Clin Pharmacol 1991; 31:588–598.

White JM, Billimoria F, Muller MA, Davis LR, Stroud CE. Serum-α-hydroxybutyrate levels in sickle cell disease and sickle cell crisis. Lancet 1978; 1:532–533.

Whitten CP, Fischhoff J. Psychosocial effects of sickle cell disease. Arch Intern Med 1974; 133:681–689.

Wiesenfeld SL. Sickle cell trait in human biological and cultural evolution. Science 1967; 157:1134–1140.

Williams WJ, Beutler E, Erslev AJ, Rundles WR (Eds). Hematology, 2nd ed. New York: McGraw-Hill, 1977, p 506.

Williams WJ, Beutler E, Erslev AJ, Lichtman MA (Eds). Hematology, 3rd ed. New York: McGraw-Hill, 1983, p 595.

Williams WJ, Beutler E, Erslev AJ, Lichtman MA (Eds). Hematology, 4th ed. New York: McGraw-Hill, 1990, p 623.

Winnie AO, Pappas GD, DasGupta TK, et al. Subarachnoid adrenal medullary transplants for terminal cancer pain. Anesthesiology 1993; 79:644–653.

Winsor T, Burch GE. Rate of sedimentation of erythrocytes in sickle cell anemia. Arch Intern Med 1944; 73:41–52.

Wintrobe MM, Lee GR, Boggs DR, et al. Clinical Hematology, 8th ed. Philadelphia: Lea & Febiger, 1981, pp 851–852.

Wolfort FG, Krizek TJ. Skin ulceration in sickle cell anemia. Plast Reconstr Surg 1969; 43:71–77.

Wood PL, Richad JW, Thakur M. μ-Opiate isoreceptors: differentiation with κ agonists. Life Sci 1982; 31:2313–2317.

Wood WG, Pembrey ME, Serjeant GR, Perrine RP, Weatherall D. Hb F synthesis in sickle cell anemia: a comparison of Saudi Arab cases with those of African origin. Br J Haematol 1980; 45:431–445.

Woods GM, Parson PM, Strickland DK. Efficacy of nalbuphine as a parenteral analgesic for the treatment of painful episodes in children with sickle cell disease. J Assoc Acad Minor Phys 1990; 1:90–92.

Woods K, Karrison T, Koshy M, et al. Hospital utilization patterns and costs for adult sickle cell patients in Illinois. Public Health Reports 1997; 112:44–51.

Woolf CJ, Wiesenfeld-Hallin Z. The systematic administration of local anesthetic produces a selective depression of C-afferent evoked activity in the spinal cord. Pain 1985; 23:361–374.

World Health Organization. Cancer Pain Relief. Geneva, Switzerland: World Health Organization, 1986.

World Health Organization. Cancer pain relief and palliative care. World Health Organization Technical Report Series, 804. Geneva, Switzerland: World Health Organization, 1990, pp 1–75.

Wright CS, Gardner E. A study of the role of acute infections in precipitating crises in chronic hemolytic states. Ann Intern Med 1960; 52:530–537.

Wright SW, Norris RL, Mitchell TR. Ketorolac for sickle cell vaso-occlusive crisis pain in the emergency department: lack of a narcotic-sparing effect. Ann Emerg Med 1992; 21:925–928.

Wrightstone RN, Huisman JHJ. On the levels of hemoglobins F and A_2 in sickle-cell anemia and some related disorders. Am J Clin Pathol 1974; 61:375–381.

Wu KK. Cyclooxygenase 2 induction: Molecular mechanism and pathophysiologic roles. J Lab Clin Med 1996; 128:242–245.

Yaksh TL, Malmberg AB. Interaction of spinal modulatory receptor systems. In: Fields HL, Liebeskind JC (Eds). Pharmacological Approaches to the Treatment of Chronic Pain: New Concepts and Critical Issues. Progress in Pain Research and Management, Vol. 1. Seattle: IASP Press, 1994, pp 151–171.

Yang YM, Shah AK, Watson M, Mankad VN. Comparison of costs to the health sector of comprehensive and episodic health care for sickle cell disease patients. Public Health Reports 1995; 110:80–86.

Yang YM, Pace B, Kitchens D, et al. BFU-E colony growth in response to HU: Correlation between in vitro and in vivo fetal hemoglobin induction [abstract #1961]. Blood 1996; 88(Suppl. 1):493a.

Yaster M, Tobin JR, Billet C, Casella JF, Dover G. Epidural analgesia in the management of severe vaso-occlusive sickle cell crisis. Pediatrics 1994; 93:310–315.

Zeltzer L. Hypnosis in pain control. In: Hurtig AL, Viera CT (Eds). Sickle cell disease: psychological and psychosocial issues. Urbana: University of Illinois Press, 1986, pp 106–113.

Zeltzer L, Dash J, Holland JP. Hypnotically induced pain control in sickle cell anaemia. Pediatrics 1979; 64:533–536.

Zipursky A, Robieux IC, Brown EJ, et al. Oxygen therapy in sickle cell disease. Am J Pediatr Hematol Oncol 1992; 14:22–28.

Zola EM, McLeod DC. Comparative effect and analgesic efficacy of the agonist antagonist opioids. Drug Intelligence and Clinical Pharmacy 1983; 117:411–417.

Index